Oxford Medical Publications

Dementia
mind, meaning and the person

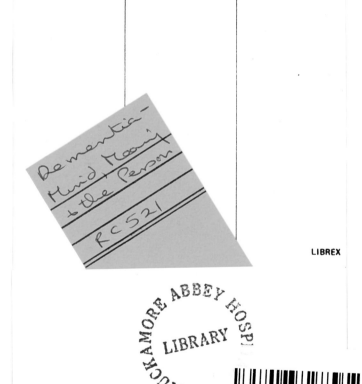

International Perspectives in Philosophy and Psychiatry

Series editors

Bill (K. W. M.) Fulford
Katherine Morris
John Z Sadler
Giovanni Stanghellini

Volumes in the series:

Mind, Meaning, and Mental Disorder
Bolton and Hill

Nature and Narrative: An Introduction to the New Philosophy of Psychiatry
Fulford, Morris, Sadler, and Stanghellini

The Philosophy of Psychiatry: A Companion
Radden

*Disembodied Spirits and Deanimated Bodies: The Psychopathology
of Common Sense*
Stanghellini

Values and Psychiatric Diagnosis
Sadler

Forthcoming volumes in the series:

The Oxford Textbook of Philosophy and Psychiatry
Fulford, Thornton, and Graham

The Philosophical Understanding of Schizophrenia
Chung, Fulford, and Graham (ed.)

Postpsychiatry
Bracken and Thomas

The Metaphor of Mental Illness
Pickering

Dementia
mind, meaning, and the person

Edited by

Julian C. Hughes
Consultant and Honorary Clinical Senior Lecturer
in Old Age Psychiatry
Northumbria Healthcare
NHS Trust and Institute for Ageing and Health
University of Newcastle UK

Stephen J. Louw
Consultant Physician in Medicine and
Geriatric Medicine
Freeman Hospital Newcastle upon Tyne
UK

Steven R. Sabat
Professor of Psychology
Georgetown University
Washington DC
USA

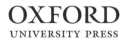

OXFORD
UNIVERSITY PRESS

01221224

OXFORD
UNIVERSITY PRESS

Great Clarendon Street, Oxford OX2 6DP

Oxford University Press is a department of the University of Oxford.
It furthers the University's objective of excellence in research, scholarship,
and education by publishing worldwide in

Oxford New York

Auckland Cape Town Dar es Salaam Hong Kong Karachi
Kuala Lumpur Madrid Melbourne Mexico City Nairobi
New Delhi Shanghai Taipei Toronto

With offices in

Argentina Austria Brazil Chile Czech Republic France Greece
Guatemala Hungary Italy Japan Poland Portugal Singapore
South Korea Switzerland Thailand Turkey Ukraine Vietnam

Oxford is a registered trade mark of Oxford University Press
in the UK and in certain other countries

Published in the United States
by Oxford University Press Inc., New York

British Library Cataloguing in Publication Data

Data available

Library of Congress Cataloging in Publication Data

Dementia : mind, meaning, and the person / edited by Julian Hughes,
Stephen Louw, Steven R. Sabat.
   p. ; cm.
   Includes bibliographical references and index.
   1. Dementia—Philosophy. 2. Identity (Psychology) 3. Self (Philosophy)
   [DNLM: 1. Dementia—psychology—Aged. 2. Personhood—Aged. 3. Professional-
Patient Relations—ethics. 4. Self Concept—Aged. WT 155 D376 2006]
I. Hughes, Julian. II. Louw, Stephen. III. Sabat, Steven R.
   RC521.D45564 2006
   616.8'3—dc22

                                                        2005019360

Typeset by Newgen Imaging Systems (P) Ltd., Chennai, India
Printed in Great Britain
on acid-free paper by
Biddles Ltd., King's Lynn

ISBN 0–19–856614–X (Hbk)   978–0–19–856614–4
ISBN 0–19–856615–8 (Pbk.) 978–0–19–856615–1

10 9 8 7 6 5 4 3 2 1

23 AUG 2006

For
Anne, Olli, Emma, Luke,
Stephanie and Anita,
And in memory of Gio, Irene, Jack, Rod, Sophia, Sam,
Terry, and Bob Grossman

Preface

Dementia is not the hottest topic in the philosophy of psychiatry. The excuses for this are several. In some countries, after all, it is dealt with by physicians (geriatricians or neurologists), not by psychiatrists. This is probably because it is readily thought of as a brain disease and not as a mental illness. In addition, the symptoms of a condition such as schizophrenia seem more likely to raise issues of interest to philosophers: thought insertion, delusions, hallucinations and the like. But the tendency to overlook the philosophical issues raised by dementia is a mistake.

For one thing, as the practitioners in this volume make plain, it is not *just* a brain disease. It affects the whole person. For this reason, as the philosophical discussions in this volume show, it is a condition that raises in a dramatic form issues about personhood. It should not be forgotten that people with dementia can also be troubled by hallucinations and sometimes by delusions, or at least confabulations. People with dementia can also become depressed, aggressive, apathetic, and seem to change personality and lose insight. Not everyone with dementia suffers in the same way and not all to the same degree. But it should be clear there is more than enough grist for the philosopher's mill. And our belief, in putting together this volume, is that philosophical contributions are valuable, because they can help to sharpen our thoughts about what we do as practitioners working in a variety of ways to help people with dementia.

For example, do people with dementia lose their minds? Do they lose their selfhood? What are the criteria employed in answering these questions and what supporting evidence is provided? Would our belief that such people have lost their minds and selfhood affect the ways in which we treat them? Does our treatment of them affect people with dementia and if so, how? If our behaviour does affect them in particular ways, what would that mean for them? Furthermore, as dementia becomes more common, society at large needs to think clearly about how it views and treats people with dementia.

The book stemmed from a conference with the same name that was held in Newcastle upon Tyne in late 2002. This is not simply a collection of the papers presented at that conference: not all of those involved with the conference appear in the book and not all of the authors attended the conference. The spirit of the conference, however, is maintained. The stated aim of the conference, which was a joint meeting of the Philosophy Special Interest Group and the Faculty for the Psychiatry of Old Age of the Royal College of Psychiatrists, was "to foster discussion of the philosophical issues and conceptual difficulties raised by dementia". The preamble continued: "The philosophical discussion will be informed by the realities of dementia and, we hope, will itself affect the way in which dementia and people with dementia are regarded. The interdisciplinary nature . . . is intended to encourage a broad understanding of dementia". These are the aspirations of the present volume too.

In drawing together such a volume we have faced an unavoidable difficulty. We hope it will be read by people from various disciplines and none. Inevitably, then, some people will know more about dementia, but will be unfamiliar with philosophical writings; others will be interested in philosophy, but know little about dementia. There may be the occasional "lay" reader who knows relatively little about either subject. There are two things to say. First, the authors have tried to write in a way that is as accessible as possible, whilst not detracting from the depth of their thoughts. Some chapters will be more challenging than others for particular readers, but—given our own different backgrounds as editors—we believe that the book will be read with profit by people with and without schooling in various disciplines. We hope so!

Secondly, we have written our own introductory chapter with the intention of sketching the field. We describe, albeit briefly, some basic features of dementia; we point towards sources of further information; we paint some of the philosophical and clinical background and set the chapters in context. You will have to judge to what extent we have been successful. The chapters that then follow move from philosophical to more practice-based discussions. Many of the chapters, however, contain insights from both philosophical reflection and from practical experience.

There are a number of people to whom we owe thanks. We have received ever patient and friendly help from the staff at Oxford University Press to whom we extend our sincere thanks: Richard Marley and (more recently) Martin Baum have acted as encouraging commissioning editors since the idea for the book arose; Carol Maxwell has been our main point of contact throughout the writing process and has dealt compassionately with our concerns and blunders; Diana Gallanaugh has provided meticulous and thoughtful copy-editing; whilst Helen Hill has directed the proceedings with great efficiency and care during the production phase. We must also thank our authors, who have put up with varying amounts of badgering, but who have remained remarkably friendly none the less. We shall remain extremely grateful to them for their considerable contributions. We should also thank the people with dementia, whose presence, generosity of spirit, honesty, and trust have informed and inspired many of the authors of the chapters that follow.

On a more personal note, we must thank Bill Fulford for encouraging us to work on this book in the first place. Little occurs in the world of philosophy of psychiatry without Bill's involvement. It has been a great support to have his enthusiastic backing throughout. Agnes Muse has provided a good deal of over and above secretarial help with the book. Joan Louw, Anne and Luke Hughes have provided last minute assistance with proof reading. We are enormously grateful to all those who have helped.

JCH
SJL
SRS

Acknowledgments

We are grateful for the kind permission given by Independent Newspapers Ltd. (Fig. 15.1), Oxford University Press (Fig. 15.2), the Alzheimer's Association, Korea (Fig. 15.3), the Confederación Espanola de Familiares de Enfermos de Alzheimer y Otras Demencias and Diego Alquerache (Fig. 15.4) and *Alzheimer's Disease International* (Fig. 15.5) to use the pictures that appear in Chapter 15.

Contents

List of contributors

F. BRIAN ALLEN is an Anglican priest and Chaplaincy Team Leader, Newcastle, North Tyneside and Northumberland Mental Health NHS Trust. He has been a Visiting Fellow at the Religious Studies Department of the University of Newcastle and managed the Christian Council on Ageing's Dementia Project which was based in Newcastle.

CARMELO AQUILINA qualified in Malta in 1986 and came to the United Kingdom in 1988 to train in psychiatry. He has trained in Liverpool and North London and worked as an old age psychiatrist in Sheffield and Eastbourne. Since 2000, he has worked in Croydon with the South London and Maudsley Trust. His research and clinical interests are self neglect in old age, health economic aspects of service delivery and end of life care.

MICHAEL BAVIDGE, before his retirement, worked at the Centre for Lifelong Learning at the University of Newcastle upon Tyne, where he taught philosophy and organised the Adult Education Programme. His published work includes *Mad or Bad?* and *Can We Understand Animal Minds?*, co-authored with Ian Ground, both published by Bristol Classical Press. Among his current interests are issues arising from medical practice, in particular pain management.

RON BERGHMANS is associate professor at the Department of Healthcare Ethics, University of Maastricht. His major publications and fields of interest concern ethical issues in mental health care, dementia care, death and dying, and research with human subjects. Together with Guy Widdershoven he is preparing a book on ethics and mental capacity (in Dutch).

HARRY CAYTON is National Director for Patients & the Public, Department of Health, London. From 1991–2003 he was chief executive of the Alzheimer's Society. His co-authored book for carers, *Dementia* (1997), has been published in seven languages. In 2004 he received the Alzheimer Europe Award.

LINDA CLARE is senior lecturer in psychology at the University of Wales, Bangor, and a clinical psychologist and neuropsychologist specialising in dementia research. Her research currently focuses on memory rehabilitation, awareness, and subjective experience.

PETER G. COLEMAN is professor of psychogerontology, a joint appointment between Psychology and Geriatric Medicine in the Faculty of Medicine, Health and Life Sciences at the University of Southampton. His primary research interests are in life-span developmental psychology and mental health issues of later life. He is the co-author (with Ann O'Hanlon) of *Ageing and Development: Theories and Research* (2004).

MURNA DOWNS holds a Chair in Dementia Studies and is Head of the Bradford Dementia Group, the Division of Dementia Studies at the University of Bradford. Her recent research interests include developing and testing the effectiveness of educational interventions for general practitioners, and quality of life in long term care. She serves on the Medical and Scientific Advisory Group for the Alzheimer's Society, the Executive Committee of the British Society of Gerontology and is a Social Care Advisor to Alzheimer Europe.

JOAN M. FORDYCE has worked as an occupational therapist, and as a psychoanalytic psychotherapist in private practice. She is a Member of the Victorian Association of Psychoanalytic Psychotherapists (retired) in Australia.

JULIAN C. HUGHES is a consultant in old age psychiatry at North Tyneside General Hospital and an Honorary Clinical Senior Lecturer at the Institute for Ageing and Health in the University of Newcastle. He studied philosophy before and after qualifying in medicine. His academic interests are in gerontological ethics and the philosophy of psychiatry. He currently chairs the Philosophy Special Interest Group of the Royal College of Psychiatrists.

A. HARRY LESSER is a senior lecturer in philosophy at Manchester University, author of a number of articles and editor or co-editor of two collections of papers in the field of bioethics, including *Ageing, Autonomy and Resources* (1999).

STEPHEN J. LOUW is a geriatrician and general physician based in Newcastle upon Tyne, UK. He is founder and chair of the Clinical Ethics Advisory Group within the Newcastle upon Tyne Hospitals NHS Trust and vice-chair of the UK Clinical Ethics Network. He was previously professor of geriatric medicine in the University of Cape Town. His publications reflect his interest in ethical reasoning, end-of-life decisions and the notion of personhood.

E. JONATHAN LOWE is professor of philosophy at the University of Durham, specializing in metaphysics, the philosophy of mind and action, and the history of early modern philosophy. His publications include *Subjects of Experience* (1996), *The Possibility of Metaphysics* (1998) and *A Survey of Metaphysics* (2002).

MICHAEL LUNTLEY is Professor of Philosophy at the University of Warwick. His research interests include: Wittgenstein; philosophy of thought; metaphysics of reasoning and judgement. Recent publications include, *Wittgenstein: Meaning and Judgement* (2003); 'The role of judgement' in *Philosophical Explorations* (2005). He was awarded an AHRB Innovation Award in 2003 to fund a pilot study of expert reasoning in classroom teachers

JENNY MACKENZIE is a senior lecturer in the Bradford Dementia Group, Division of Dementia Studies at the University of Bradford. She co-ordinates the MSc in Dementia Care and has recently completed research that examined the support needs of family carers of people with dementia from Eastern European and South Asian communities.

ERIC MATTHEWS is Emeritus Professor of Philosophy and Honorary Research Professor of Medical Ethics and Philosophy of Psychiatry in the University of Aberdeen. Previous publications include *The Philosophy of Merleau-Ponty* (2002). He is currently working on a book on the relevance of Merleau-Ponty's notion of the body-subject for psychiatry, forthcoming in this series.

JOHN McMILLAN is senior lecturer in medical ethics at the Hull York Medical School. He is a co-author, along with Grant Gillett, of *Consciousness and Intentionality* (2001). He is interested in the use of empirical methods to understand psychiatric ethics and he is currently working on a monograph that reevaluates the arguments of classic antipsychiatry.

CATHERINE OPPENHEIMER is a consultant old age psychiatrist in the Oxfordshire Mental Healthcare NHS Trust. She is co-editor with Professor Robin Jacoby of *Psychiatry in the Elderly*, Oxford University Press.

STEPHEN G. POST is professor of bioethics in the Case School of Medicine, Case Western Reserve University, and President of the Institute for Research on Unlimited Love—Altruism, Compassion, Service. His book *The Moral Challenge of Alzheimer's Disease: Ethical Issues from Diagnosis to Dying* (2000) has been a benchmark in the field of dementia and ethics.

JENNIFER RADDEN is professor and chair of the Philosophy Department at the University of Massachusetts, Boston Campus. She is author of *Madness and Reason* (1985), *Divided Minds and Successive Selves: Ethical Issues in Disorders of Identity and Personality* (1996), and editor of two collections, *The Nature of Melancholy: From Aristotle to Kristeva* (2000) and (in this series) *The Philosophy of Psychiatry: A Companion* (2004).

STEVEN R. SABAT is professor of psychology at Georgetown University. He earned his Ph.D. in neuropsychology at the City University of New York. The focus of his research has been the intact cognitive and social abilities of people with Alzheimer's disease (AD) in the moderate to severe stages, the subjective experience of the disease, and how communication between people with AD and their carers may be enhanced. He has explored these issues in depth in numerous scientific journal articles and in his book, *The Experience of Alzheimer's Disease: Life Through a Tangled Veil* (2001).

LISA SNYDER is the clinical social worker for the University of California, San Diego's Shiley-Marcos Alzheimer's Research Center, where she has counseled people with Alzheimer's and their families since 1987. She is author of the book *Speaking Our Minds—Personal Reflections from Individuals with Alzheimer's* (2000), and publisher of the international quarterly, *Perspectives— A Newsletter for Individuals with Alzheimer's or a Related Disorder*.

TIM THORNTON is professor of philosophy and mental health, University of Central Lancashire. He is co-author of the *Oxford Textbook of Philosophy and Psychiatry* (2005) and author of *Wittgenstein on Language and Thought* (1998) and *John McDowell* (2004) as well as a number of papers on philosophy and mental health.

GUY WIDDERSHOVEN is professor of healthcare ethics at the University of Maastricht. His main fields of interest are the ethics of chronic care, especially psychiatry, care for the elderly and care for people with an intellectual disability, and ethical aspects of end-of-life care.

1 Seeing whole

Julian C. Hughes, Stephen J. Louw,
and Steven R. Sabat

Introduction

Whole sight; or all the rest is desolation.   (Fowles 1978, p. 7)

There is a sense in which the story around dementia appears to raise no particular problems. We grow old and we decline. Part of this decline is mental. We become forgetful, which may be more or less of a problem. If the decline is too marked, or if it is too marked in a certain way, we shall need care and perhaps protection, perhaps from ourselves. If we suffer, we can be treated and the suffering comes to an end with death.

The sense in which the dementia story raises no particular problems is probably worth seeing. Dementia is an inevitable part of life now that we are an ageing society. We cannot avoid this fact about the world. Dementia signifies a deterioration in the person's brain and, hence, a loss of mental functioning. In a sense, then, dementia is like other physical illnesses; it causes specific disabilities that have characteristic consequences: failures in the person's ability to do certain things. These need to be compensated for by those around. The story about dementia is just the story of a chronic age-related disease, which in the end is terminal.

It would seem a travesty, however, to leave things like this. For a start, already there has crept into the account the idea that what makes dementia a disease is something to do with failure of action or 'ordinary doing', which is (intentionally) redolent of Fulford's work (Fulford 1989) on the nature of mental illness; and which should, therefore, alert us to the possibility that, *at the heart of the diagnosis of dementia lurks some sort of evaluative judgement.* And this should be something of a surprise; for dementia (out of all the 'mental' illnesses) is the most objective, most like a physical illness with definite pathology, objective tests, and rational treatments. Thus, just to take the three most common forms of dementia, *Alzheimer's disease* is typically a gradual, but progressive, loss of cognitive function, with 'forgetfulness' occurring early, but with the emergence of other deficits over the course of years, all of which can be correlated with the findings of particular pathological lesions in the brain (plaques and tangles); *vascular dementia* has a more sudden onset, where the problems in the person's mental powers reflect underlying damage relating to the blood vessels in the brain, either blockages or bleeds—that is, strokes or mini-strokes; and *dementia with Lewy bodies*, characterized more recently, usually presents with fluctuating cognitive deficits (which may be more to do initially with visuo-spatial skills than recall), well-formed visual hallucinations (often involving small animals or people), and the emergence of parkinsonism (for example, a blank expression and slowness of movements, tremor being milder and less common than in classical Parkinson's disease), with Lewy bodies (the lesions usually confined to structures towards the base of the brain and associated with Parkinson's disease) throughout the cortex.[1]

This all sounds rather definite, so in what sense is 'dementia' an evaluative notion? Well, although established criteria stipulate that a definite diagnosis can only be made post-mortem, so that the diagnosis of any of these conditions in life is only 'probable', there turn out to be no clear boundaries at the neuropathological level. Consider this, for instance, from experts in the field in one of the most influential textbooks on the subject:

> The pathology of [Alzheimer's disease] defies precise definition at present. This is because its individual components all occur to some extent in normal ageing. (Esiri and Nagy 2002, p. 107)

This is not to say, of course, that a definite diagnosis cannot be made. Clinically and pathologically some people have very clear-cut Alzheimer's disease. However, many have concomitant vascular pathology; and cortical Lewy bodies can be found in Alzheimer's disease too. Recognizing this lack of determinacy may be useful scientifically, because it may lead to a greater concentration on the ageing brain *as such*, rather than encouraging a focus on particular disease entities, which may or may not be natural kinds (of which more later). But what it certainly does is this: it lets the evaluative cat out of the factual bag. At the most objective end of 'mental' illness (that is, in the field of 'organic' dementias) it turns out there is no hard scientific boundary between disease and normality.[2] Lines can be drawn, but their exact location is a matter of evaluative judgement based on correlations between neuropathology and symptoms and signs. But which symptoms and signs? How much forgetfulness is pathological? What counts as normal ageing?

Of course, there is nothing new in this as far as mental illness is concerned. As Dickenson and Fulford (2000) point out, historically there has been a tug of war regarding the notion of mental disorder between those favouring a medical model and those favouring a moral model. Albeit there are important criticisms to be made of the tendency to favour the medical model—and a number of the authors in this book have made such criticisms extremely cogently here and elsewhere (cf. Chapter 15 by Downs and colleagues)—if things move too far in the direction of the moral model (leading to a refusal to acknowledge that any mental illness is caused by disease), bad consequences might ensue:

> Push the balance too far towards an exclusively medical model, and psychiatry slides from a properly medical role into coercive functions; . . . But push the balance too far towards an exclusively moral model . . . and we end up denying the resources of medicine to those who most desperately need them. (Dickenson and Fulford 2000, p. 55)

Similar dangers lurk in our judgements about what will and will not count as normal ageing and normal forgetfulness.

For the *cognoscente*, this will bring to mind concerns about the 'diagnosis' of mild cognitive impairment (MCI), which is thought of as a pre-dementia state—one in which not everyone will go on to develop the disease, but one for which drug treatment might one day be routinely recommended. This is the territory covered by Bavidge (Chapter 2) in his elegant discussion of the notion of 'the shape of our lives' and how this relates to the idea of human nature, which is an inescapable amalgam of facts and values and which in the end is inescapably shaped by our mortality.

In the face of diagnostic indeterminacy, it is worth bringing to bear philosophical thoughts about 'natural kinds', to which we have already alluded. Inasmuch as we can think of the dementias as disease entities, they could be accorded the description of natural kinds. These are 'a kind of event found in nature and hooked up to other events by laws of nature' (Hacking 1995, p. 59). Natural kinds are events in nature, but this means things or objects like books, animals, or instruments, or characteristics such as the colour gold. There is a sense in which the dementias are like this. They are (in a sense) disease entities: we can say without much doubt that so-and-so has dementia and that probably (by which we shall often mean that the chances are at least 90%) it is Alzheimer's disease. In addition, having this diagnosis will have causal consequences, in that certain types of deterioration can be predicted and certain forms of treatment will tend to help.

Yet our discussion of the neuropathology of the dementias, and the notion of MCI, and the indeterminacy with respect to normal ageing, all point to the conclusion that not every case of 'forgetfulness' or 'cognitive impairment' can be regarded as an example of a natural kind. These are neither always clear-cut entities in nature, nor in the clinic. Still, we may wish to say that they are kinds of some sort. Hacking usefully provides the notion of *interactive* kinds. Whereas natural kinds are *indifferent*—that is, to be a goldfish is simply *that* and you do not become more or less gold (or more or less fishy) by having been described in this way—an interactive kind is one that is affected by the description that it is given. Interactive kinds are such

> that, when known, by people or those around them, and put to work in institutions, change the ways in which individuals experience themselves— and may even lead people to evolve their feelings and behaviour in part because they are so classified. (Hacking 1999, p. 104)

Well, this is certainly the concern of many of the authors in this book who come from the background of practice. But their concern is not just about the margins, it is not just about the difficult cases in the clinic, it is about people who have barn door diagnoses, where the kind of dementia (pathologically and clinically) would seem otherwise to be appropriately described as a natural kind. The concern is that, because of the ways in which dementia is thought of, the diagnosis itself amplifies any disabilities that may result from the pathology.

From the philosophical side, the possibility is raised that many natural kinds in medical practice will be interactive, for, in human beings, the purely biological interacts (in some sense of that word) with the psychological, the social, the spiritual, and so on. In philosophical terms, what might be constitutive of something in the psychological realm is likely to have correlates in the physical or social realms. In brief, what is required philosophically is whole sight. And, of course, it is the lack of the 'holistic' approach in clinical work that often leaves patients and their carers frustrated. So, we can sketch a sort of circle in which real encounters with the problems surrounding dementia lead to the thought that there is an evaluative and interactive core to the type of thing that dementia is; which in turn leads to the requirement that people should be treated as wholes, with attention not only to their biology, but also to their psychology, their social and ethical concerns, and the cultural and spiritual aspects of their lives. We might add that the circle is hermeneutic: it has an interpretative basis. It brings in, therefore, not only causes but also meanings. And it is iterative, because the broader view of 'patients-as-persons' embedded in historical relationships and traditions should itself influence the ways in which science is conducted, the kinds of entities it seeks to delineate and the ways it sets about doing this.

Without entering these debates further, we should see the many other ways in which dementia is hugely problematic. From a clinical or practice-based view and from a philosophical point of view, every sentence of the supposedly unproblematic characterization we started with raises questions. To see this we need to see the whole picture. In the chapters that follow we shall see how philosophical analysis can help to paint the whole view. We shall also see how practice—the experience of interacting with people with dementia and their carers—can shed light on some of our philosophical concerns. This is the two-way traffic between philosophy and practice that has long been the aim and purpose of the philosophy of psychiatry (Fulford 1991).

Let us start by outlining how dementia can be hugely problematic. Then we shall take each of the notions—mind, meaning, and person—in turn and discuss the field that surrounds them. That is, we shall sketch the landscape to be covered in the rest of the book. Our recurring theme will be that the broad view, which philosophy encourages, should significantly enhance the two-way traffic between conceptual thought and practice. We hope to show that the philosophical view can be supplemented by the practice perspective, as well as that the clarification of concepts and arguments (typical of philosophical analysis) can be useful to clinical practice. But in providing an overview of what is to follow, we shall be suggesting a substantive conclusion too: people with dementia have to be understood in terms of relationships, not because this is all that is left to them, but because this is characteristic of all of our lives (even if *how* this is so can be disputed!). Seeing this is whole sight.

The burden of dementia

Dementia is a huge global problem. There are estimated to be 18 million people with the condition in the world, of whom 66% live in developing countries.[3] Furthermore, the prevalence of dementia is increasing as the population ages. The condition (that is, all forms of dementia) affects approximately 1% of those aged 60–64 years, but for those between 85–90 years the prevalence rate is over 20%.[4] Our purpose is not to review the epidemiology of dementia. After all, if there were only one person in the world with dementia, the condition would still raise the same conceptual puzzles. Nevertheless, the weight of the social burden that dementia poses for the developed and developing world, which includes its economic costs,[5] is part of the context within which the condition must be considered. These social and economic costs are a political reality that will shape the way we make decisions about the frail within our communities. Our conception of the person with dementia will (at least) influence the moral stance we take with respect to the treatment of people with dementia.

If dementia poses a socio-economic burden, it also poses a more immediate burden on informal (that is, non-professional) carers, who tend to be female spouses. They are prone to depression and high levels of stress (Cayton 2002). But many of the decisions they face are frankly ethical, so that they carry a 'moral burden' too (Baldwin *et al.* 2004). Again, therefore, how we think of people with dementia is not without practical and ethical significance. How people with dementia are positioned, how they are considered and referred to, can itself affect how they are as persons, how they behave, and how they inter-act (see Chapter 18, by Sabat). This can then be seen as a moral imperative. 'Our task as moral agents', says Post (in Chapter 14), 'is to remind persons with dementia of their continuing self-identity' (p. 229). Such 'moral respect' will surely reflect the ways in which we understand dementia: some ways of understanding—as Downs and colleagues ably demonstrate (Chapter 15)—will emphasize deficits and disease; others can reflect remaining capabilities and potential. There can be little doubt that our standing amongst other people is partly constructed by our interactions with them. Not only shall we be viewed and view from some distinct perspective, but also the possibility of mutual understanding will depend on the quality of our communications.

Detailed qualitative research, recorded by Snyder (Chapter 16), shows the potential for such mutual understanding even in the face of dementia. Hence, how we conceive of persons in general and persons with dementia in particular will set up a reflective pattern of behaviour or emotion, whereby our conceptions will tend to elicit certain responses. In turn, given that certain responses must be considered more dignified—in Cayton's terms, more adult (see Chapter 17)— the conceptions of the person that draw out such responses ought (morally) to be favoured.

Real encounters with people with dementia and their carers, as many of the authors in this book can testify, readily demonstrate the extent of the personal problem raised by this condition. In other words, it is not just a socio-economic problem and not just a moral problem for communities and for individuals, it is also a *critical* problem for a particular person. But this is not to suggest that the problem is necessarily wholly negative. We are using 'critical' to suggest Dworkin's idea of 'critical interests': those interests that give some shape to the person's life as a whole; those interests that give life meaning (Dworkin 1993, p. 201). According to Dworkin, critical interests link to the sense that our lives are intrinsically important, which in turn links with dignity:

> A person's right to be treated with dignity . . . is the right that others acknowledge his genuine critical interests: that they acknowledge that he is the kind of creature, and has the moral standing, such that it is intrinsically, objectively important how his life goes. (Dworkin 1993, p. 236)

So the *critical* problem is to do with negotiating a way through life, despite dementia, in order to preserve for as long as possible those aspects of our lives that are critical to us: we want Bavidge's 'alternative rather than impaired ways of experiencing life' (p. 49). Success or failure, as Oppenheimer (in Chapter 12) depicts so clearly from first-hand accounts and from her clinical experience, will depend on the biological ways in which the brain has been 'shattered' by the disease, on inner reserves certainly, on the quality of the care and communication of those around, and on the support and understanding of professionals, but also on aspects of the environment. The clinical challenge is to encourage the biological, psychological, social, and spiritual dimensions involved in a person's life to be optimally realized given the concrete circumstances. A philosophical issue concerns how these dimensions participate in, or constitute, personhood; and, more practically, what are the consequences of these dimensions being affected for the person with dementia?

Before considering personhood, we shall start with the simpler matters of the mind and meaning! The notion of dementia suggests being out of one's mind. The question we wish to pose ourselves is 'how are we minded?' And in connection with dementia, 'in what ways do our conceptions of the mind affect our view of people with dementia?' and 'are there good and bad ways to think about the mind in dementia?'

The mind as inside out

The background: a sketch of physicalism and dualism

One way to think of the mind is to equate it with the brain. This is materialism or physicalism.[6] In broad terms it suggests that mental states are just brain states. At its extreme, it becomes eliminativism, according to which all mental talk—that is, all use of language referring to mental states—will eventually be eliminated in favour of the more accurate talk of neurophysiological states (Churchland 1986). Perverse as this may seem to some, the suggestion is that instead of saying 'I remember the day when . . .', we shall instead say something like 'there has been the following flip-flop in my hippocampus . . .'. Of course, physicalism need not be so crude and it might even be asserted that we are all physicalists now! This would be true inasmuch as we all believe that the brain underpins (at least in some sense) our mental life. Thus, we read in a premier psychiatric journal,

> All mental processes, even the most complex psychological processes, derive from operations of the brain. The central tenet of this view is that what we commonly call mind is a range of functions carried out by the brain. (Kandel 1998)

Hence, when our brains are destroyed, so too are our minds. Less dramatically, but in a sense more decisively (because it could be argued that we have no way of knowing whether mental activity continues after brain death), when our brains are injured (as in dementia) our mental functioning is compromised. The link between the brain and the mind seems difficult to deny and can be regarded as a crucial plank in arguments about dignity, dementia and old age:

> Certainly, if brain degeneration can be held at bay, meaningful life will be prolonged, but in broad terms, reasonable cerebral function is the key to the quality of survival in the elderly. (Robertson 1982)

The bogy as far as physicalists are concerned is dualism. According to dualists, as epitomized by Descartes, the mind and the brain are separate sorts of stuff.[7] On the one hand, there are mental entities (thoughts, memories, and intentions) and on the other hand there is the stuff of the brain (neurons, neurotransmitters, and the neurovascular system). Whereas brain things can be measured and weighed, mental things have no such spatial existence. Of course, this raised for Descartes the problem of how the mind could act on or have influence in the world: how does mental stuff move physical beings as it seems so clearly to do? Descartes determined (on the basis of his neuro-anatomical knowledge) that the pineal gland was the seat of the soul, the place of interaction between the mind and the brain. Whilst this now seems a naïve suggestion, it should be recalled that the Nobel prize-winning neuro-physiologist, Sir John Eccles and the distinguished philosopher, Sir Karl Popper, developed a similarly 'interactionist' view of the mind and the brain as existing in separate but *interacting* worlds (Popper and Eccles 1977).

The dualism of Descartes led him into some contorted discussions, as in his letter to Father Mesland on 2 May 1644, where he made a distinction between 'memory of material things' and 'memory of intellectual things'. The former, apparently, depended on traces in the brain or cerebrum; whereas the latter depended on traces in the mind. He could not say much directly about these (latter) mental traces, but

> cerebral traces, on the other hand, render the brain liable to move the soul in the same way as before, and thus make it remember something; just as the folds in a piece of paper or a napkin make it more apt to be folded that way over again than if it never had been so folded. (Descartes 1644)

Perhaps Descartes should not have given way so much to the demands of physicalism. Perhaps he was right to press home the point about the radical difference between the mental and the physical. It was certainly Wittgenstein's view that 'a memory' and 'a trace' are two radically different things:

> An event leaves a trace in the memory: one sometimes imagines this as if it consisted in the event's having left a trace, an impression, a consequence, in the nervous system. As if one could say: even the nerves have a memory. But then when someone remembered an event, he would have to *infer* it from this impression, this trace. Whatever the event does leave behind in the organism, *it* isn't the memory.' (Wittgenstein 1980, §220)

Wittgenstein's suggestion is that the memory cannot be equated with some sort of physical representation in the brain. And he went on to suggest that the mechanics of the reproduction were neither here nor there when it came to considering what remembering actually amounted to:

> The organism compared with a dictaphone spool; the impression, the trace, is the alteration in the spool that the voice leaves behind. Can one say that the dictaphone (or the spool) is remembering what was spoken all over again, when it reproduces what it took? (Wittgenstein 1980 ibid)

This is not to say that Wittgenstein was himself a dualist, even if he wished to resist the pull of physicalism. But there have been modern defenders of dualism and it is worth noting their arguments. Lewis posed this passionate challenge to those who question dualism:

> . . . do they seriously deny that there is an ingredient in our behaviour, and in that of other creatures, which it is not plausible to reduce to purely physio-logical terms? Do we not feel pain, do we not perceive coloured entities, whatever their status, do we not hear sounds? And however full the explana-tion may be at the physical and physiological levels of all that occurs in this way, there is also, over and above all that, something vital for the proper understanding of such situations. This is where the dualist takes his stance. (Lewis 1982, p. 5)

There is something about our mental world that we do not wish to see reduced or eliminated. If, however, there are problems with various versions of both physicalism and dualism, is there an alternative? And, to revert to our original questions, what is the relevance of this discussion for dementia?

Dangerous concerns

It would be dangerous to make a quick move from a theory in the philosophy of mind to statements about how people with dementia should be treated without offering a raft of caveats. Part of the excitement of this book (we hope) is, however, that it does span the gap between philosophical theory and clinical practice. We are intrepid travellers here who must take risks because of the potential benefits, in terms of both theoretical and practical understanding, to be had from the journey. It seems reasonable, under the circumstances, for us to point out at the start that more work needs to be done to make the route clearer and it may be that we shall head down paths that turn out to be unnavigable. Others will have to follow and help to clarify the correct way.

So we shall, with a degree of temerity and being aware that the details of the relevant arguments would need to be worked out more fully, point to some concerns regarding the theories of the mind we have been considering. The concern over physicalism is precisely that it is too reductionist. If it reduces the mind (this is the concern and also an example of a big step that should be taken more cautiously) it also reduces the person. The concern is especially acute when the talk is of eliminating the mind. Even if this is incautious, it is not too reckless. After all, we do quite naturally make a link between minds and persons:

> For the only way we have of counting minds is by looking at the behaviour manifested by the persons whose minds they are . . . .   (Wilkes 1988, p. 166)

Moreover, we can point to those who link 'brain failure' to a lack of 'meaningful' existence as evidence that the path we are picking out is feasible, at least as a way of thinking that others have indulged. Thus we find the same Dr Robertson, whom we quoted above writing in 1982, writing a year later as follows:

> There is evidence . . . that many of the features of senility as seen in brain failure (mainly dementia and hemiplegic stroke) are medically unremarkable but are disturbing or offensive to those approaching old age and to the relatives of elderly patients . . . A common sequel is reference to a 'cabbage-like existence' and the wish that they in turn could somehow spare their offspring or spouses the unsavoury features of senility.   (Robertson 1983)

Robertson used his view of brain failure and the accompanying lack of dignity to argue in favour of advance directives to restrict treatment in cases of senility and the like. Now there may well be arguments in favour of using advance directives for such purposes. The concern we are expressing, however, is about how this stance, which is particularly aimed at 'senility', is encouraged by the linkage of brain failure to whether or not life is meaningful, dignified, disturbing, offensive, or unsavoury. The concern centres on the putative underlying assumption that 'brain failure' means 'person failure'; it gets there via a mixture of 'mind failure' and 'meaning failure'.

This type of concern is evident elsewhere, for instance, in the literature reviewed by Herskovits under the subheading 'Senility as monstrosity', where she writes

> . . . one can speculate that, now more than ever, people are afraid, sometimes terrified, of losing their minds as they grow old.   (Herskovits, 1995)

She also quotes Fontana and Smith (1989) saying that Alzheimer's disease robs 'the mind of the victim'. Herskovits talks about the 'Alzheimer's construct', which involves all of the social, cultural, and political discourse that surrounds the disease. But central to this discourse is the understanding of dementia as a 'progressive degeneration of the brain'. The negative discourse highlighted by Herskovits (and it has to be said that she is also able to find 'reparative' work that seeks to stress the ways in which the person or self can still be found in dementia) moves from the physical degeneration of the brain to images of a lost and monstrous self, albeit such images are found to be supported by broader social (for example, political and economic) pressures.

Robertson's article drew strong comment, including this sharp rebuke:

> Loss of dignity derives from the way we care for our sufferers from dementia, not from the illness itself. . . . More than at any other time of life the sufferer needs his personal identity preserved.   (Murphy 1984)

The thought that a person's identity can be preserved by others is one to which we shall return. It underpins much of what follows. It is a worry about the narrowness of the 'biomedical model', which involves symptoms and signs of dementia being attributed directly to neurological (that is, brain) impairment, which motivates the plea by Downs and colleagues (Chapter 15) for a more person-centred approach. In such an approach more would be made of the person's retained capacities, rather than simply their deficits. All of this is music to the ears of an ethicist such as Post, who has encouraged respect for older people, and for people with dementia in particular, over many years. Now he states that 'our task is to preserve identity' (p. 229). Similarly, Snyder (in Chapter 16) shows the value of people with dementia themselves coming together in a way that helps to preserve their individual identities and personalities. This was just what Murphy (1984) was after in her response to Robertson (1983). But it goes one step further, because in this case we find that it is not solely carers and others who are helping to support the personhood of people with dementia, it is the people with dementia themselves who form the groups and provide the reparative support.

Not only is there a concern that the focus on the brain may limit the view of dementia and stigmatize it, there is also a linked desire to show how much more can be done for, with, and by people with dementia if they are given a chance. Snyder's work (Chapter 16) shows how this might be so. Sabat (2001) also demonstrates that, even in marked dementia, people's retained abilities can be considerable, which must reflect underlying brain function even where others might wish to talk of 'brain failure'.

An example is found in the case of Dr B (discussed in more detail in Sabat (2001)), a retired academic and scientist who, according to standard tests such as the Global Deterioration Scale and the Mini Mental State Examination (MMSE), was in the moderate to severe stage of Alzheimer's disease. Despite his cognitive abilities being so compromised according to objective tests, his desire and ability to discern ways to maintain his feelings of self-worth remained intact. He was clearly interested in collaborating with one of the authors of this chapter (SRS) on what he called, 'The Project': an effort to help others understand the subjective experience of Alzheimer's disease. For it was to him, 'a sort of scientific thing' that would allow him to maintain a sense of self-worth. In referring to 'The Project', he commented that '. . . this is *real* stature to do' and 'others go with stature'. It was quite clear to him that, at the day centre he attended two to three times a week, he occupied no significant position within the larger group. As someone who held an advanced degree and whose lifelong inclinations and dispositions as an academic person were still very much alive in him, he sought to differentiate himself from the other participants, by not taking part in any of the activities and games that he described as being 'filler'—something 'that doesn't mean anything'. His desire to be seen as more than someone diagnosed with Alzheimer's disease who was merely a participant at a day centre is clear in the following conversational extract with SRS.

Dr B: Um, I, I, I'm groping as to how well can we do . . . I don't know if you get me right or wrong. I'm fishing for something.

SRS: Yes, I know.

Dr B: I'm finishing [fishing] for something because the phenomenon of, of, if I'm working with you, I can—look, I can work in here for 30 times and all that but in *this* group, I'm nothing. ['This group' refers to the day centre participants.]

SRS: Maybe—that is, we could be working together a lot.

Dr B: Yes.

SRS: But with the rest of the people in the day centre, you're nothing?

Dr B: I'm nothing.

SRS: What do you want to be?

Dr B: Well, I think in, in, very quickly, I think, I think it would be better, wait a minute. It takes on status . . . sometimes it's not a soft system between the two of us when I'm in the day tare [here he mispronounces 'care']. Maybe I'm crazy, but there's nothing that I can do about it.

SRS: Are you saying that you feel that you have no status with the rest of the day care people?

Dr B: Oh, absolutely. Absolutely! There, there, should be some hier, hierarty.

SRS: So you feel that you're a pretty bright guy, but that you're not really treated differently than people who aren't as bright?

Dr B: Ya, that's, that's forces me to do something like this. And I, I say that. Remember when you put the thing, when you gave me the letter? It was a very strong statement that I am something above, or something like that.

SRS: You feel that you're not treated with as much deference as you think you deserve. Is that accurate?

Dr B: Honestly, yes.

The fact that his cognitive decline, as measured by standard tests, was severe did not interfere with his ability to evaluate his social position at the day centre, to recognize that he was not being treated with the deference he believed he deserved as a person of academic accomplishment, and to seek means by which he could change that situation for the better. Clearly, then, the tests employed to assess his cognitive abilities did not tap his need, nor his ability, to maintain feelings of self-worth. Thus, the defects identified by such tests can detract from our ability to see a person's abilities.

The concern we have identified about physicalism is that it might encourage people to focus on brain deficits in dementia, to the detriment of other aspects of personhood. Similar to the dualists, we wish to encourage a broader view of what it might be to be a person and this starts with a broader view of what it is to be a minded person. So why do we not simply become dualists?

For one thing, dualism in any strict sense seems just too implausible. It might also encourage too 'gappy' a view of the person with dementia. Given the primacy of the mental for Descartes ('I am a thinking thing', he said), it could be that the physical is relatively ignored. But we know that a person's mental state will in large measure depend on their physical state. This is, indeed, the challenge for palliative care in dementia: the person may not be able to speak (the mental can seem inaccessible), but it may be that there are physical causes of psychological distress that require a physical and psychological approach (which may also incorporate social and spiritual aspects, and so on).[8] In the later stages of dementia especially, having a holistic view, which would not see soma and psyche as independent but as intertwined, would seem to be essential. Dualism would not preclude this approach, depending perhaps on the degree of interaction allowed between the mind and the brain, but *strict* dualism does tend to argue against the rational basis for integrated treatment. If what *I* am is my mind, then my body (including my brain) seems somewhat redundant, less worthy of care perhaps and (certainly in the absence of interaction) not the medium through which to treat mental distress in any obvious way. The gap between the mind and the brain in dualism does not help to support the need, suggested by Downs and colleagues in Chapter 15, for an integrated biopsychosocial approach. In which case, however, what are we to say about the mind that will square with, and be helpful towards, our understanding of dementia?

Narrative and subjectivity

Over against the dominating ideas of physicalism, which locate the mind and (inevitably) the person in the brain, we have anticipated the views of practitioners (recorded in later chapters) who wish to preserve the person's identity in dementia by the quality of care, by the nexus of relationships that surround people with dementia. In response to the charge that 'brain failure' means 'loss of mind', which in turn means 'loss of person', these authors are inclined to point to the environment (primarily the social environment) in which the individual's personhood is situated. What we would seem to require, therefore, is a theory of the mind that involves the environment. Luckily, there is one to hand! Before discussing 'externalism' of the mind, however, it is worth dwelling on the extent to which thinkers locate the mental outside the individual body. They point to the way in which our mental goings-on are located in, have to be understood within, a broader setting. Normally this setting is the story of our lives.

For example, here is a summary account of Gillett's 'narrative theory of the conscious mind':

> According to this view, we make discursive and narrative sense of ourselves as persons who live and move and have our being among others. The narrative is constructed out of the events that befall persons as detected by their information-gathering systems and rendered meaningful by their conceptual skills. The resulting story shapes holistic patterns of brain activity and thereby affects the neurophysiological stream that constitutes the proximal effect of one's doings in the world. In making sense of the world, we apply discursive skills and norms of judgment to what is going on in that stream to produce the narratives of our lives according to the framework we have made our own (on the basis of the kinds of things that normally go on around here). (Gillett 2004, pp. 29–30)

We do not propose to offer a thorough critique of this view (that must fall to other travellers who are better able to pick their way with more precision than we are able to do at present). But we shall make some observations.[9] First, this narrative view of the mind does not downplay the brain; in fact, it does the reverse. The brain is crucial to us as a means of, for example, 'information-gathering'. Second, however, the brain does not supply everything that we need to characterize the mental: we have to make discursive sense of ourselves as beings amongst others. This requires some skills, which will involve brain activity, but it also requires practical or social accomplishments, which are learnt in the world and typically involve discourse. This is not simply speech, but a complex set of rules that shape our conversations and reflect our deeply embedded nature as human language users. In turn, acquiring such social practices itself shapes the ways in which our brains work to manage our mental being in the world.

Third, this looks like a good account of mind from the point of view of those who have concerns about people with dementia. People with dementia will be experiencing problems doing things in the world at some stage. In part this will be because of cognitive (brain) problems. But being minded, having a mental life even in the context of dementia, also involves discursive skills in the world. Some of these, presumably, will be deeply ingrained, so that a degree of difficulty at the 'proximal' end of neurophysiology will not necessarily affect what happens at the 'distal' end, where we engage with the world. And this is what we see in dementia, where a person might perform poorly on a cognitive test, but still be able to function within the arena of discursive acts (Sabat 2001).

An example can be found in the case of Dr M, another retired academic who was diagnosed with probable Alzheimer's disease and whose MMSE score was poor enough for her cognitive decline to be termed 'severe' (Sabat 2001). That she was aware of the concept of reciprocity as a social norm in her culture was apparent many times. In the conversational extract that follows, she shows that awareness. Although she often expressed appreciation for the interactions she shared with SRS, she wanted the relationship to be mutual and not mostly of benefit to her.

> DR M: Now—then, I want to tell you something uh, that has some—I hope you're getting something out of this.
>
> SRS: Oh yes! Oh yes! No question about it.
>
> DR M: Because I, I feel, I don't want to, to use your time.
>
> SRS: You're worried that maybe my coming here might be wasting my time?
>
> DR M: Yes, exactly!
>
> SRS: Well, I'm assuring you that you're not.

Here, she has evaluated the situation in accordance with standards of fairness and is also expressing her desire to be of help. She does not want simply to be a 'receiver' of help but also a provider, a giver, of help to others rather than 'using' or 'wasting' another's time when there is no real benefit being gained. The concept of fairness, of mutuality, is not represented on standard neuropsychological tests of 'concept formation', but is clearly evidenced in the discursive act displayed by Dr M in the above extract. Indeed, neuropsychological tests administered 2 years before the above conversation occurred indicated that Dr M was deficient in concept formation 'consistent with a diagnosis of probable [Alzheimer's disease]'. To have concluded, on the basis of standard tests of concept formation, that Dr M was generally deficient in this area of cognitive ability was, therefore, a mistake.

As a potential corrective to this type of mistake, the narrative view in relation to dementia is one that can be found edging its way into the philosophical accounts in this book. McMillan (in Chapter 4) recalls his own work with Grant Gillett in which, following Kant, they suggested the expression the 'transcendental unity of narration' (Gillett and McMillan 2001, p. 162). The idea is that narrative, based on our 'webs of interlocution' (that is, our speech communities broadly conceived), can provide the unity that is a prerequisite (in this sense it is 'transcendental') for our sense of self. This idea, again, suggests the notion of our minds in some way reaching out into the community in order to provide the basis for an enduring sense of self. The idea of a narrative, that is, provides something public, something outside the head, even if connected to what might be occurring within, which can be shared and provide continuity beyond the necessity for the individual to be constantly self-conscious.

The idea of narrative is controversial. MacIntyre has been an influential advocate of the idea, suggesting that the unity of the self 'resides in the unity of a narrative which links birth to life to death . . .' (MacIntyre 1985, p. 205). MacIntyre went on to say, 'The narrative of any one life is part of an interlocking set of narratives' (MacIntyre 1985, p. 218). On the other hand, it may be that our narrative histories cannot be constructed in the single and continuous form suggested by narrative theorists; maybe narratives are more fictional and disjointed than we would like to imagine. Difficulties arise when the narrator can no longer tell the story, or participate in it as it is told by others. And it may even be that there are no others to tell the story. Nevertheless, the time-line of the story will persist as long as the person does, so there is at least a story to be told, even if the ending becomes less layered than it might have been earlier on. With such caveats in mind, Radden and Fordyce nonetheless suggest (in Chapter 5) that there is a likelihood that 'human activities share *some* of the formal properties of narrative . . .' (p. 77, emphasis added).

Talk of narrative certainly allows that an individual's story might be written both by the individual and also by other people. At the level of personality it is easy to see how this might be true: we are all influenced by those around us, who also determine to some degree how we present ourselves (see Sabat's Self 3, described in Chapter 9). At the level of mind it may not be so obvious, until we dwell on the extent to which our mindedness is also a matter of shared understandings (usually culturally shaped); here are Gillett and McMillan's 'webs of interlocution' in which we cannot help but participate. They are the prerequisite (the transcendental background) to our ability to present ourselves as selves of this (minded) sort in the world.

One of the factors at work here is the extent to which our minds can no longer be regarded as entirely 'inner'. As Aquilina and Hughes argue in Chapter 9, the boundaries between 'inner' and 'outer' are decidedly porous. It is not that there is no such thing as inner experience—the subjective world is not an illusion—it is just that the real world of the mental is not neat and tidy. In a messy way, it involves the outer world. But actually, this messiness is part of the fascination of the mind and of our place as minded people in the world:

> Our whole busy moral–aesthetic intellectual creativity abounds in private insoluble difficulties, mysterious half-understood mental configurations. A great part of our thinking is the retention, the cherishing, of such entities. 'Inner' can co-exist or fuse with 'outer' and not be *lost*. (What is inner, what is outer?) This is what *thinking* is like. (Murdoch 2003, p. 280)

The whole idea of the neatly circumscribed subjective, which derives from dualism, is challenged by Merleau-Ponty's conception of the 'body-subject'. As Matthews makes clear in Chapter 10, subjective thoughts and feelings are expressed in bodily form. Subjectivity has physical expression, but this does not deny (as a physicalist might) the reality of subjective experience. From the point of view of the person with dementia, a recognition of the importance of the body (not just because it is a body, but because it is a 'body-subject') becomes increasingly important. Some manifestations of the person's subjectivity will survive into severe dementia in a way, according to Matthews, that can identify the person. These elements of identity count against descriptions of people with dementia as being 'vegetables', akin to animals, or even like newborn children. Allowing this sort of talk adds to the likelihood that people with dementia will be infantilized and stigmatized, as Cayton persuasively argues in Chapter 17. The elements of identity that persist, even into severe dementia, are also demonstrated by the coherence and directedness that Radden and Fordyce point towards in Chapter 5 in what they refer to as 'coordination unity'. Again, this stresses the importance of the body as a medium that is not merely a physical object amongst others, but an object that conveys a certain sort of meaning, which derives from its connections to the person's life as a whole (perhaps this is the value of the conception of narrativity). In turn, the connection is to the person's proneness to subjectivity as signified by their body.

What we have seen, therefore, is that our minds and our subjectivity involve other people. The upshot for people with dementia is that, as persons, they have to be seen as interconnected, not as isolated, atomistic individuals. These ideas are underpinned by a broader conception of the mind, which we shall now sketch.

The externalism of mind

The idea behind externalism is that the mind requires the world of people and things; the mind is not and cannot be separate from it:

> Externalism . . . is a thesis about the relation between the mind and the world: it says that the world enters constitutively into the individuation of states of mind; mind and world are not, according to externalism, metaphysically independent categories, sliding smoothly past each other. (McGinn 1989, p. 9)

McCulloch uses a slogan to encapsulate what externalism amounts to: 'the mind just ain't in the head' (McCulloch 2003, p. 12). One of the implications of this idea, which we have already discussed, is that the objective cannot be excluded from the subjective. No doubt this requires considerable discussion, but externalism does seem to provide a way between the pitfalls of dualism and physicalism. The mind requires the world to give it content: 'Externalism . . . claims that mental (and linguistic) content depends upon, or is constituted by, states of the non-mental world' (Thornton 1998, p. 123). At the same time, subjectivity is as real as the world: mental content really does exist (mentally, as it were, but world-involving).

It is not that externalism is unproblematic,[10] but its major tenets are broadly accepted by many philosophers. The implications are wide and, in particular, relevant to theories of meaning, which partly inspire externalism and are partly influenced by it. We shall see how this is so in the next section. However, here we wish to return to our original quest. We can certainly say that philosophy broadens the view, but we also wish to push a substantive line and say that people with dementia have to be understood in terms of relationships, not because this is all that is left to them, but because this is characteristic of all of our lives.

As we conclude our discussion of the mind, let us just consider how we should interact with people with dementia if we were to take literally the pre-suppositions of physicalism. Then the person with dementia is simply another organism like us and, therefore, no doubt, there will be self-interested reasons for taking the other person seriously. But, at root, all of their concerns and interests are no more than manifestations of physical firings in their diseased brains and our concern for them turns out to be no more than similar neuronal activity. Meanwhile, the dualist must either believe that the person with severe dementia is mindless and, therefore, in some radical sense no longer a self or that the person's mind exists in some space or other, but the body can be regarded as an 'empty shell' (much as Mrs G seemed in Chapter 9). Albeit these are caricatures of complicated positions, it nevertheless remains true that physicalism and dualism do not map onto our experience of dealing with people whose mental powers have been affected by disease, nor do they give an adequate phenomenological account of what it is like to be a person (even without dementia) in the real world.

The key word in the descriptions of externalism is that this is a theory that says something about what *constitutes* the mind. This is not about what might *explain* mental phenomena. To give such an explanation we should indeed mention much about neurophysiology and the like. On the other hand, to say what *constitutes* a mental state, the state of being in love or of having certain intentions, requires something quite different. The requirement would be for descriptions of the state, but they would have to be meaningful. As we shall see, this entails that the concepts used in these descriptions should be shared publicly in order for meaning to be conveyed. Being minded, having mental content, conveying meaning, all require some sort of relationship (at least in principle) with other language users. Within such a discursive community, meanings can be conveyed, understandings can be achieved, intentions can be shared. And this then seems very relevant to people with dementia.

Whilst discussing phenomenology, McCulloch points out how reasonable it seems to ascribe certain mental states to someone on the basis of their outward behaviour:

> In this sense the phenomenological embraces some of the public aspects of thinking, speaking and understanding: sometimes, at least, when we are communicating with others, the shared contents are as much a part of the scene of which we are conscious as are the colours of nearby objects. (McCulloch 2003, p. 30)

He goes on to say that to understand another person's conscious life is 'interpretational' (McCulloch 2003). All of this squares with externalism. Our minds, on this view, reach out and embrace other minds, because we can share content. Part of what we do when we understand what someone else is saying can be thought of as grasping the same objects; we share the same world. Moreover, an implication is also that communication is not just verbal. As an approximation, we communicate by grasping (as it were) the shared object, whether this has been done verbally or by a more difficult type of interpretation.

McCulloch says:

> Rather than seeing the enterprise of interpretation as a way of fitting a plausible inner story to the given outward facts, one should see it as a way of gaining access to the phenomenology, the meaning-reality, of these outward facts themselves. Doings and sayings are the primary bearers of content. (McCulloch 2003, p. 105)

Once again, externalism's push outwards, whereby content becomes necessarily shared, or at least shareable, makes sense of the attitude towards people with dementia according to which, however muddled their language, it might still be possible to hear their meaning through genuine attempts to engage with them phenomenologically. We can still inhabit the world of the person with dementia, because it is the world we have always inhabited. Understanding meaning in this world is just to be minded as we are, with the potential for discursive interactions based on shared 'doings and sayings'.

It is an awareness of the importance of the particularities, the finer details of thoughts, motives, and actions, in their specific setting, that leads to the re-emergence of casuistry as an important form of moral reasoning, regarded by some as having greater validity than deductivism. Casuistry, as the term implies, starts with the particular *case*, whereas deductive methods of moral reasoning might start with principles and work back to the case (see Jonsen and Toulmin 1988; Murray 1994). It is, according to casuistry, through *immersion* in the nuances of the case and the *interpretation* of the issues in relation to moral theories that the right course of action may be discerned. Suffice it to say that this wholly justifiable system of reasoning requires, as a prerequisite, a comprehensive engagement with the details of the individual case (see also Louw and Hughes 2005). It follows, therefore, that if we wish to achieve a moral engagement with the person with dementia, we should strive to inhabit their world.

Talk of interpretation calls to mind the hermeneutic tradition, with its emphasis on empathic understanding. Externalism, as we have seen, tells us that mental phenomena are *constituted* by non-mental things of the world. Another account of the mind could tell us a *causal* story (indeed, the problem with physicalism is that it uses elements from a causal account to tell us what the mind *is*). Similarly, in describing the phenomena of dementia, we can either look for causal explanations, or we can seek a constitutive account and try to understand what it is actually like to have dementia. Empathic understanding is at the heart of hermeneutics and, as Widdershoven and Berghmans demonstrate in Chapter 11, it encourages us to take a different and broader view. Interpretation of behaviour can be useful as a way of seeing the views of the person with dementia, but as Widdershoven has stressed elsewhere, hermeneutics must address the whole context:

> The hermeneutic approach stresses that, in the definition of good care, the values of both parties—the person with dementia and the surrounding caregivers—are relevant. (Widdershoven and Widdershoven-Heerding 2003, p. 108)

So, we have seen how externalism of the mind pushes us into the world in a way that requires and allows understanding. Externalism sits very comfortably with the phenomenological goal of empathic understanding, where people, even with dementia, can occupy the same shared space of meaning. Hermeneutics encourages this sort of understanding and propels us forward to consider further the importance of context and relationships as a means of grasping the person's meanings:

> The hermeneuticians, then, repeatedly emphasize that, through understanding, we are given access to wholes and to relationships (Dilthey 1977). An experiential process becomes understandable only if we understand its relationships to other experiences of the person; a person's bodily gesture becomes understandable only if we understand its relationships to other expressions he or she makes; . . . Understanding, then, must contextualize or recontextualize any single item of experience by grasping its meaningful placement within and relatedness to other items that form the same context (Dilthey 1977). (Schwartz and Wiggins 2004, p. 355)

Grasping meaning involves a lot more than might be suggested by simple algorithmic accounts of language function. For instance, Mr R was in the moderate to severe stage of Alzheimer's disease (Sabat 2001). In SRS's initial encounter with him at an adult day centre, Mr R was speaking quite rapidly, clearly pronouncing virtually every word he uttered. Yet, the sum total of the words did not seem to make sense at all and there was not a single coherent sentence in almost 10 minutes of speaking. Accompanying his words was great emotional agitation, facial expressions dominated by frowns, and shaking of his head. He was clearly agitated and upset by something. Focusing on the extralinguistic forms of communication turned out to be vital as a way of engaging with Mr R. For when asked, 'Do you feel like crying?', he responded immediately with the first coherent sentence he spoke, 'You're damn right I do.' In this moment, Mr R realized that there was at least one other person at the day centre who understood his emotional state and could commiserate with him. Thus, it was possible to hear the meaning in Mr R's communicative act by listening not only to the words he spoke but, more importantly, to how he spoke them. And, in so doing, it was possible to communicate with him, attempt to comfort him, and win his trust as someone who could empathize with his situation.

In the case of Dr M (Sabat and Harré 1994), it was of great importance to have an understanding of her background and lifelong dispositions in order to appreciate deeply her present state of despair with regard to her word-finding problems. Dr M was, throughout her life, a literary person for whom it was of the utmost importance to use the *mot juste* rather than any ordinary word, for graceful eloquence was her way of speaking. The meaning of word-finding problems to her was quite different from that of other people with dementia who did not share her values about proper speech.

> SRS: You're not just any ordinary person who has some problems finding words. You're a person for whom words, words to you are kind of like a musical instrument.
>
> DR M: Um hum, um hum. That's exactly right.
>
> SRS: And so the kind of frustration you feel would be greater than for a person whose focus in life was not so literary. That could give you cause for a lot of grief.
>
> DR M: I think the issue is, that is, for me maybe especially this day for some reason or other, but for last, maybe 4 years, that I am not satisfied with myself because what I want isn't here. I've, uh, thinking of it and it makes me angry as well as, that is part of the . . . and I guess that is what is happening now. Don't you think?

Here again we see the importance of understanding the person with dementia in terms of their own lifelong values and dispositions, for only in so doing can we understand what the effects of dementia mean to *them* and without understanding the point of view of the person with dementia, empathic understanding is simply not possible. Yet, as these cases show, even in dementia (where initial communication might seem difficult), there can be a true meeting of minds through the creation of a shared public space.

Meaning: context and relationships

Having spent some time considering how we are minded, the groundwork has already been laid for an account of meaning that moves from internal designation to outward contextualization. The end-point, in a way that mirrors our discussion of the mental, will be a further emphasis on the importance of relationships. On the way we shall need to consider how relationships come into play: whether, in connection with meaning, they must actually come into play, or whether it is the potential or proneness for human encounters that gives us human meaning. Before all that, however, we should briefly acknowledge the enormity of the conceptual steps we are taking. From something as esoteric as the philosophical study of meaning we shall end up talking about the importance of the relationships in which, as human beings, we are embedded. This is the background insight to be drawn from our initial discussion, which follows, of a paper by Charles Taylor (whose work is also referred to by McMillan in Chapter 4 and Radden and Fordyce in Chapter 5). Taylor's insight is this: theories of meaning reflect and imply theories of the person. To understand the self correctly is to have a theory of meaning with the right amount of texture. The texture comes from the way in which meaning is embedded in practice, in the 'doings and sayings' referred to by McCulloch (2003). The 'right amount' of texture is the amount required to flesh out the theory of meaning such that it gives a realistic picture of real people in the real world. Our perception of people, including people with dementia, needs to be textured enough for them to be seen, not as parts, but as wholes.

From representation to public space

Taylor starts by describing a theory of meaning as *designation*:

> Words have meaning because they stand for things (or perhaps ideas, and thus only mediately for things). They 'signify' things . . . So you capture the phenomena of meaning if you see how words attach to their designata in this way. (Taylor 1985, p. 250)

This rather simple account of how words mean things has been supplemented by the Fregean idea that words only mean things in the context of a sentence. We have to know how the words work in order to understand them. It is not purely a matter of latching on to the connection between the designating word and the designated thing. The activity of speech becomes important. But what remains the same, despite the sophistication of Frege, is that theories of meaning are 'still founded on the notion of a representation' (Taylor 1985, p. 252). In other words, a theory of meaning must (on this view) focus on the ways in which speech acts depict reality. Taylor outlines how this account has been elaborated, but concludes that modern conceptions of language:

> take the primary linguistic phenomenon, the principal object of a theory of meaning, to be representation. What is it we have to understand in order to understand meaning? Primarily this, that with words we manage to frame representations.   (Taylor 1985, p. 253)

Taylor goes on to suggest an alternative approach to meaning, which has links with the philosophies of Heidegger and Wittgenstein (but for Taylor is derived from Herder, Humboldt, and Hamann). He outlines three aspects of this alternative approach, according to which language brings about explicit awareness of things, puts things into public space and thereby constitutes this space, and discloses the concerns that are essential to human beings (Taylor 1985, p. 263). We certainly could not hope to do justice in limited space to the elegance and subtlety of Taylor's analysis, but for our purposes we shall focus on the second aspect of the theory of meaning he is supporting, which relates to public space.

Language puts things out in the open. This means that whatever it is that emerges into public space becomes not just a matter for one of us, nor even a matter for each of us separately, but a matter for all of us together. The expression of something in a language creates rapport. In creating a public space, language creates 'a common vantage point from which we survey the world together' (Taylor 1985, p. 259).

Another alternative is to think of language as being a means of communication, where this is conceived in terms of one person giving *information* to another. But sometimes language is not used in this way at all, because there is perhaps no information to be passed on. Instead, the purpose of language is precisely 'to found public space, that is, to place certain matters before *us*' (Taylor 1985). Taylor later highlights the *expressive* dimension to language. Not only can language sometimes play this role without having any representative dimension to it, but the expressive role also helps to establish 'the kind of rapport which is peculiar to us linguistic animals' (Taylor 1985, p. 265). The problem with the view that the main function of language is to pass on information (or even representations) is that it ignores the ways in which, through language, we engage with one another. Hence,

> This is therefore another crucial feature about formulation in language. It creates the peculiarly human kind of rapport, of being together, that we are in conversation together. To express something, to formulate it, can be not only to get it in articulate focus, but also to place it in public space, and thus to bring us together *qua* participants in a common act of focussing.   (Taylor 1985, p. 260)

Putting aside (with reluctance!) Taylor's paper, we can see how this broader view of language and meaning is relevant to people with dementia. The idea of a public and the way in which language displays meaning in this sort of context brings grist to the mill of Widdershoven and Berghmans in Chapter 11. Here they set out how 'meaning-making' occurs through language, through communication. It is when the public space breaks down in dementia, because of the loss of the 'shared life-world', that meaning-making becomes difficult. The reaction, however, should not be to abandon the enterprise of trying to communicate, but to look for new interpretations (in line with hermeneutics) in order to re-create the shared public space insofar as this is possible; but it should not be assumed that this will be impossible, only that it might require effort. The effort is justified precisely because meaning-making *is* still possible, because—given some basic features of our shared humanity—we still inhabit the same world where public spaces have the potential to be created.

Communities and social construction

Our brief exegesis of Taylor's paper displays the move from seeing meaning as private designation (something that might happen inwardly) to seeing it as the dynamic creation of public space in which, of course, there must be participants (Taylor 1985, p. 280). One corollary of this line of thought is that an emphasis is laid upon the role of the participants in creating meaning. Unless people take part in the speech acts that create the public space of language there would be no language, no meaning. So meanings (in a similar way to 'the mental' in externalism) just ain't in the head either.

In a highly influential commentary on the later philosophy of Wittgenstein, where something like this line of thought can be found, Kripke (1982) developed what is known as 'the community view'. Roughly speaking, he said that the only foundation for meaning, the only basis for our confidence that the word 'green' will continue to mean what we all think it means, is community agreement. It is because we agree on the use of words and their meanings that there is meaning. This is not an empirical point, but a metaphysical one: there simply is no other conceptual basis to meaning. Individuals cannot interpret signs in language individually; signs (for example, words) have meaning as part of a communal practice. There is nothing other than this practice, for example, there is no heavenly (Platonic) form in which meanings are inscribed, to give foundation to the meaning that our words carry.

The community view, derived from Wittgenstein, is sometimes then used to support the notion of social constructionism. The link is made by Snyder in Chapter 16, where she is then able to show how communities of people with dementia can co-construct and define themselves through their interactions. Social constructionism also underscores the notion of selves developed in the work of Sabat (2001) (see also Chapter 9). The idea, crudely put, is that not only minds and meaning, but our selves too are constructed by our social encounters. We are who we are through our social interactions. It should be said that social constructionism is not a single theory, but is layered and is, in some ways, incontrovertible: some aspects of mental illness (including dementia, as Sabat (2001) has shown) have decidedly social roots (Church 2004). Nevertheless, in Chapter 8, Thornton launches a careful assault on some of the premises of social constructionism, which partly targets the discursive psychology of Rom Harré and Grant Gillett (Harré and Gillett 1994). Given the influence of Harré and Gillett, reflected variously in this book by McMillan (Chapter 4) and Sabat (Chapter 18), Thornton's arguments need to be taken seriously.

Constructionism (or constructivism) suggests that the meaning of a word, or the content of a psychological state (a memory for instance), is constituted by the continuing judgements that a speaker makes.[11] Thornton argues that these judgements require some backing, some further foundation, for them to do the job they are required to do. They were brought in by the constructivists precisely to provide a justification for our being able to use concepts in the ways that we do. Constructivism wishes to support the view that 'green' always means the colour green, but it does this by appealing to the on-going judgements of the community of language users and, argues Thornton, this just will not do. For, we can be sceptical about *these* judgements in the way that we can be sceptical about words having meanings in the old-fashioned sense of designations. We can be sceptical about how a word is bound to (designates) an object (viz. what is to stop the linkages slipping in ways that would make communication impossible?). Constructivism suggests that the community keep the links in place; but, in which case, what is to stop the judgements that make up the community view from slipping? In other words, once the sceptical challenge is mounted, it is difficult to stop it. To try to stop it with community agreement seems simply arbitrary.

The way to stop the sceptical regress is radical. It requires us to reject the idea that the key thing in understanding someone is to *interpret* their meaning (otherwise we might need an interpretation of the interpretation). Rather, meaning reflects *shared patterns of practice*. In understanding someone we share a public space, but we do not form the space by interpretation. It should be noted that, in this chapter, we have often stressed the importance of interpretation: it is central to much of hermeneutics and it was used in connection with the externalist account of mind. However, according to McCulloch, interpretation from the externalist perspective is a matter of entering the phenomenology, the real experience, of meaning:

> Rather than think of the semantic facts as "underlying", one should see them as public, since they are phenomenologically available when communication takes place. (McCulloch 2003, p. 105)

Hence, as we saw above, McCulloch goes on to say, 'Doings and sayings are the primary bearers of content' (McCulloch 2003). In other words, at least according to McCulloch, there is no need to appeal to the inner mental objects that then require interpretation, because the external world of practice (doings and sayings) is where the meanings just are in a way that does *not* require interpretation because they are contextualized. Hermeneutics need not make a mistake here either, because it too recognizes and requires the importance of the context.

If Thornton's criticism is convincing, does this undercut the approach to dementia commended by Downs, Sabat, and Snyder within this book and by others elsewhere? Helpfully, Thornton goes on to argue that social constructionism (1) is probably not required for some of the work that these authors wish it to do and (2) acts in any case as a useful heuristic. First, constructionism provides a strong reason for looking at the details of a person's speech. Second, it provides an incentive to strive to understand the person's meaning in order to respect their wishes. So constructivism may be a useful way to flag certain concerns about how we ought to engage and interact with others generally and with people with dementia in particular.

Approaching the other

A debate for philosophers is whether other people have to be involved in forming the patterns of practice that shape our meanings and underscore our language. Some, such as Kripke (1982), would argue that the community must actually be involved; whereas other philosophers (and Thornton, we guess, would be on their side) argue that there cannot be meaning without at least the *potential* for the appropriate patterns of practice, irrespective of whether or not the practices are instantiated (that is, irrespective of whether or not the patterns of practice actually exist or are lived out). There must at least be, on this view, the *potential* for such patterns in order even to conceptualize meaning. Either way, from our perspective, the point of this discussion is to force us to consider the other people—potential or actual—who must participate in the practices that underscore meaning.

Bringing in other people is fundamental when it comes to understanding people with dementia. It is certainly a concern for Oppenheimer, who makes a link between personal identity and 'mutual recognition between two people' (see p. 199). She talks of knowledge being 'preserved in the relationship' even when other cognitive skills have been lost. Elsewhere she has made clear how it is that relationships can play a role in determining whether a person flourishes or not:

> Old age psychiatrists daily see patients who experience some threat to their autonomy, and a minority of our patients, at some point in their lives, can scarcely be said to make autonomous decisions at all. Yet we see that these patients, for all their impaired autonomy, play an immensely significant part in the lives of the people who are connected to them. They are participants in relationships that can be joyful and rewarding; or troublesome, full of pain and guilt; relationships deeply rooted in the past, or fresh encounters between a new carer and the person needing care. It is the emotional context of these relationships (or their absence) that determine how much the person flourishes or withers, how much his potential for affection, enjoyment, humour, and the vivid communication of feeling, are stifled or expressed. (Oppenheimer 1999, p. 321)

In a similar way, Allen and Coleman (Chapter 13) point out the extent to which it is impossible to talk about ourselves without reference to others. They go on to use the Christian notion of the Trinity to show how, at the heart of the understanding of ourselves (as handed down by religious tradition), there is a recognition of the importance of relationship within *the person*. This stands against the more atomistic view of *the individual*, who seems—unlike the participant in Taylor's public space (Taylor 1985) and unlike the participants in relationship as described by Oppenheimer (1999)—disengaged, disconnected, and remote from others.

The notion of the profound interdependency of persons has long been established in African traditional thought. The Nobel Peace Prize winner and Archbishop Emeritus of Cape Town, Desmond Tutu, is credited with formulating a theology based on the African notion of *ubuntu*, which Tutu characterized thus: '. . . each individual's humanity is ideally expressed in relationship with others'; or, more straightforwardly, 'a person depends on other people to be a person' (Battle 1997, p. 39). Tutu's theology developed the idea that 'persons are ends in themselves only through the discovery of who they are in others' (Battle 1997, p. 43). On this view, persons will themselves be dehumanized when they dehumanize others. It follows that not only does the person with dementia retain aspects of their personhood in and through those around, but also that those caring for the person retain their humanity in remaining engaged with and exercising respect for the person who relies upon them for their care.

Allen and Coleman refer to the writings of the great Jewish thinker, Martin Buber (Buber 1937) and his emphasis on the person being thought of in terms of the 'I-Thou'. His work had a great influence on Tom Kitwood (Kitwood 1997) who, more than anyone, championed a new climate of care for people with dementia with the slogan 'person-centred care'. Kitwood's work is, not surprisingly, mentioned by many of the authors in this book.[12] Kitwood's notion of 'malignant social psychology', for instance, is deployed by Sabat in Chapter 18 to make a link with the idea of 'malignant positioning'. Both these ideas reflect a problem with others, a problem in the social environment, the effect of which is to undermine the individual's standing as a person. In line with Allen and Coleman's distinction, it is the isolated individual who loses *qua* person precisely because of the lack of connectedness with others.

Meanwhile, our tendency to move in the direction of relationships as a way to understand meaningful language, with the complementary tendency in the traditions of the spiritual realm to become aware of the other, does indeed find expression in the writings of Buber:

> And just as talk in a language may well first take the form of words in the brain of the man, and then sound in his throat, and yet both are merely refractions of the true event, for in actuality speech does not abide in man, but man takes his stand in speech and talks from there; so with every word and every spirit. Spirit is not in the *I*, but between *I* and *Thou*. It is not like the blood that circulates in you, but the air in which you breathe. (Buber 1937, p. 36)

Post (Chapter 14) also stresses the importance of a religious approach to people with dementia. He says our task as moral agents is to fill the gaps in the person's self-identity. We do this in the context of the public spaces which we share by engaging with the person. This need not be sharing at the level of rationality, but may involve affect and emotion. Our communications, by which we form public space and allow meaning, need not be only verbal, nor solely cognitive. Indeed, Post's great contribution to the ethical debates around dementia has been his persistent defence of a broader view of personhood. In particular, he has steadfastly attacked (what he has called) hypercognitive notions of personhood. Thus, we find him writing:

> When the capacity to seek meaning in the midst of decline gives way to more advanced dementia, as it will in the more severe stages of illness, then the experience of the person must be understood in relational and affective terms rather than in narrowly cognitive ones.   (Post 2000, p. 85)

In this section, therefore, in parallel to the moves made whilst discussing the mind, we have moved from meanings as inner representations to meaning as social construction to the notion of language as a pattern of practice that allows the formation of potential or actual shared public spaces. These spaces form the natural place for us to encounter others. Part of our humanity, indeed, is shown by our ability to make relationships through language, by which we convey information, and a lot more besides. The nature of relationship, which requires recognition of the other person, is a potent source of our spirituality, where this is understood to mean mutual engagement. The challenge in the case of people with dementia is to seek engagement where this might be difficult. The first step, however, is certainly to try to enter the world of people with dementia by understanding their doings and sayings.

Interestingly, the present Archbishop of Canterbury, writing in a psychiatric journal, stressed the importance of language in connection with the spiritual realm and the need to engage with people to care for them as persons (or as souls):

> Perhaps that is the real challenge of psychiatric care: to hold up a picture of what language actually is. Where communication is broken, dysfunctional, turned back on itself, persons are trapped: care for persons is care for their language, listening to the worlds they inhabit (to their souls) so as to engage with other worlds—neither reductively or collusively.   (Williams 2005)

The space of persons

Our discussion of mind and meaning has brought us, finally, to the idea of the person. So central, however, are the ideas of mind and meaning to our conception of persons that little more needs to be said, except that the issue of personal identity is the major topic for discussion by the philosophers in this book. Before concluding, therefore, we shall sketch the area of philosophical concern. In particular, we shall dwell on the notion of the transcendental unity of apperception, because it forms the basis to some of the discussion, but may not be familiar to non-philosophers. We shall also point to the broader view of the person that we see as emerging from our discussions.

Personal identity and psychological continuity

In Lesser's extremely clear account (Chapter 3), two senses of the term 'personal identity' are described and discussed. The same two senses are also picked up by McMillan (Chapter 4) and are reflected in Ricoeur's distinction between *idem* and *ipse* as described by Radden and Fordyce (Chapter 5). The first sense is the more philosophical sense of identity over time: being the same person both now and then. McMillan calls this the 'numerical' sense of identity and for Ricoeur it is *idem* or sameness. The second sense of personal identity, which Lesser ascribes to psychology and sociology, and which McMillan refers to as 'qualitative' identity, is referred to by Ricoeur as *ipseity*, implying 'self-hood'. This second sense involves understanding *who* the person is: it reflects the person's conception of thenselves, of the kind of person they are or ought to be.

Both Lesser and McMillan discuss the interplay between these two senses of personal identity. They both focus on the second (qualitative, *ipse*) sense. Lesser uses this to comment on the first sense of identity, whilst McMillan defends the view that this other (less traditionally philosophical perhaps) sense of qualitative identity should be given greater weight in philosophical discussions. Interestingly, Lesser and McMillan reach similar conclusions with a different emphasis. According to Lesser, understanding personal identity must involve understanding our 'boundedness', the way in which (as Bavidge suggests in Chapter 2) our lives have a shape, which includes a past and a future. Inevitably, then, our sense of our*selves* must include (at some level) an awareness of the inevitability of our decline, whether that be swift or prolonged, physical or mental (or both). Part of what we are, that is, involves the people we shall become. McMillan argues that qualitative identity—who the person is—can be maintained by others (to a degree), but he also acknowledges that there can be such a change in our ability to engage in 'value frameworks or webs of interlocution' (p. 70) that there may be moral grounds for allowing that the standing of one person with respect to another (for example, the wife to her husband with dementia) might radically change.

Radden and Fordyce, meanwhile, who (as we saw above) give grounds for appreciating the work that the idea of narrative can do, nevertheless suggest reasons for remaining sceptical that it can always do this work in severe dementia. On the one hand, then, they would tend to be not wholly impressed by the thought (inasmuch as it is based on narrativity *alone*) that others can keep the person's story going; but on the other hand, they see some benefit in the idea derived from Ricouer's work that 'characterization identity' (which equates to *ipseity*) can be collectively constructed or formed and (importantly) *sustained*.

Readers will have to judge the extent to which the contrasting accounts cohere or conflict. Interestingly, both McMillan and Radden and Fordyce make appeal to the work of Taylor, whom we discussed above. It is beyond our scope to discuss the place of narrativity in the thought of Taylor, or how the work of Taylor and Ricouer compare. And it needs to be recalled that the idea of characterization identity being collectively *constructed* or *formed* needs to be considered carefully if it is not to be open to the type of criticisms of constructivism, discussed above, levelled by Thornton.

What is clear, however, is that this discussion goes way beyond what can now seem like a more pedestrian discussion of whether sameness in the sense of *idem* identity is maintained by the body, the mind, the brain, or some mixture of these things. This is not to say that such discussions are facile—they are extremely sophisticated—but, unless notions of the mind and the person (and even the body) bring in the broader concerns already referred to, they seem to miss the crucial point of our being embedded in a multi-layered context of human interaction. We need to see, in particular, some inclusion of other people in our discussions of personhood.

All of this is quite inimical to the profoundly influential thoughts of the philosopher Parfit (1984), who has characterized personal identity in terms of psychological connectedness and continuity. Parfit's views, and their connection to the thought of Locke, are skilfully dissected by Matthews in Chapter 10. They are mentioned elsewhere in this book.[13] What we see, however, is a tendency, in part reflecting the influence of continental philosophy, to move beyond the confines of what might otherwise be narrowly regarded as 'psychological'. An externalist account of mind, for instance, gestures at the importance of the world outside the head in which real people participate, including people with dementia. Whilst philosophers, naturally enough, engage with Parfit's work, those who are at the practice end, as we have seen, look more naturally to the work of Kitwood in thinking about personhood. This is because the experience of practical engagement with people with dementia cannot but help to emphasize how it is that the person's identity (their *ipseity*) is more than simply the connections between their memories. People engage with each other, in everyday life and in care settings, in a bodily way and part of *what* they are, their quiddity, is their physical instantiation. But the point here is not simply that the body equates to the person; it is that our bodily interactions—our doings and sayings (amongst other things) *in the world*— make up our quiddity. The move, once again, is away from the inner world, which is also the world described by Post's notion of 'hypercognitivism', to the outer world of public space.

The transcendental unity of apperception

Philosophers have, however, raised deeper questions about what it is to be a self. Like the philosopher David Hume, when we look for ourselves, it may be that all we can find at any one time are bundles of perceptions and associated thoughts. This 'bundle theorist' view of the person is convincingly criticised in Lowe's analysis, in Chapter 6, of the philosophies of Locke, Hume, and Descartes. Lowe goes on to describe the Kantian notion of the transcendental unity of apperception. The notion of 'apperception' implies not just the mind's perceptions, but its perceptions of its own states. There always seems to be a single 'I' to regard the mental representations of the individual. But the 'I' is the possibility (and in this sense 'transcendental') of a unified view of the representations (thoughts or perceptions) that pass through the mind. Kant pointed to the idea that consciousness forms a unity—that self-consciousness has a single view—in that all conscious mental states appear to be the states of the same self.

Lowe reaches the tentative and agnostic conclusion that, although he has little doubt that he exists as an individual unified self, he has no firmer understanding of *what* he is, of his quiddity. It may be, as he says, that this was the point of Kant's transcendental self. One way of understanding Kant, therefore, is to say that we can locate a point of view, but one which is transcendental in the sense that it is a prerequisite to there being the sort of unity that we find to our perceptions and mental states. But we cannot go further and identify the item in the world that accounts for the unifying. The 'I', as it were, eludes us.

Well, but what is the relevance of this to dementia? Elsewhere in this book there are references to Iris Murdoch, the philosopher and author, whose dementia has been portrayed so vividly in books and in a film.[14] We have already made reference to her more philosophical work in this chapter. She also points to the elusive nature of the self that is self-aware. Our moment-to-moment existence in normal life passes by without us grasping it. She writes:

> One returns to the most obvious and mysterious notion of all, that this present moment is the whole of one's reality, and this at least is unavoidable. (The weirdness of being human.) Then one may again start reflecting upon the moment-to-moment reality of consciousness and how this is, after all, where we live. . . . What 'it was like' moment-to-moment we normally forget, it is as if we have to forget. This natural 'lostness' of the 'stream' may suggest its general nearly-non-existence and so its irrelevance. It may be thought of as only dispositionally extant, or at best an occasional indulgence of reflective people. On the other hand, surely it contains the whole chronicle of our existence, perhaps recorded by God.   (Murdoch 2003, p. 257)

What seems to be lost is, not only the stream that binds the moments together, but also the point of view of each moment. (And recall this is Murdoch reflecting on normal life, not on the life of the person with dementia who has lost Parfit's 'psychological continuity'. Thus she adds weight to Lowe's talk of the lack of difference between the afflicted and 'our own quotidian condition' (p. 102).) It is as if the transcendental *I* passes by too quickly to be recalled at any particular moment. It is at the extreme of our empirical reach and cannot be grasped, neither in health, nor in dementia.

Luntley also presents, in Chapter 7, an erudite and closely argued account of the thought of Locke and Kant. His conclusion is that the self, by which he means 'that which keeps track of things' (p. 105), can be conceived as being eroded by dementia. The self that he commends is decidedly the Kantian self. It is transcendental in that it is 'the ground for the possibility of keeping track of things' (ibid) and it is, thereby, not something that can be tracked itself. The person with dementia, therefore, on this view, does not lose track of themselves, but fails to keep track of outer things. The loss of this capacity amounts to the loss of the self. Luntley's view can be squared with an externalist account of the mind, because on his view the self—like the mind in externalism—is not an inner thing that can itself be tracked, but constitutively involves outer things, in that it is the ground for the possibility of keeping track of outer things.

One obviously challenging aspect of Luntley's account is that he goes on to suggest that the apparent ability to refer to the self, by saying things such as 'I am thirsty', does not constitute genuine self-reference if the person has lost the appropriate 'cognitive surround'. In other words, if the person's ability to keep track of things (in this case to keep track of bodily states, for example, being thirsty) is lost, then the self is lost and the statement 'I am thirsty' is meaningless. Although this is, at first blush, challenging, Luntley is careful to make the point that whether what he envisages is ever empirically true is another matter. His is a metaphysical point about the self. If his point is true, then it is at least possible that what he envisages might come to pass; whether or not it does is an empirical matter.

To this extent, if what he says about the self more broadly and the importance of the 'cognitive surround' is correct, Luntley's argument about the person with dementia saying 'I am thirsty' seems reasonable. As a matter of fact, however, it is difficult (empirically) to think of someone with dementia making an 'I' utterance that would be as meaningless as Luntley's argument requires. As the social constructionist talk of Self 1 suggests, first-person lexicals, mentioned by Aquilina and Hughes in Chapter 9, are important precisely because they appear to reflect the existence of the cognitive surround; that is, they appear to be meaningful. By the time the person with dementia gets to the stage where it is conceivable that there is no cognitive surround, language has usually gone, so there are no 'I' utterances. It is nevertheless true that 'I' utterances are sometimes wrong, showing that people with dementia can fail to track even their bodily states correctly. For instance, patients can sometimes say 'I haven't had my breakfast' when they have; and they might say 'I am hungry' despite continual, excessive eating. But in these sorts of cases the 'I' still seems to be doing some work: there is still tracking going on, even if the tracking mechanisms are awry.

Such cases only mean that the point at which the cognitive surround is gone needs to be pushed further back than Luntley's example suggests. The evidence provided by 'lucid intervals' and cases such as Mrs G's, as discussed by Aquilina and Hughes, ought to mean that the point where it is assumed that the self that tracks is lost needs to be put back quite a long way. Indeed, Mrs G's case, where it seemed clinically that she had 'gone' and could, therefore, be discounted from conversations, might be taken as a warning that the self that tracks could possibly be still tracking until very late in the disease. Sabat's work (Sabat 2001) also points in this direction. But these remain empirical points that do not dispute Luntley's more metaphysical assertions.

Luntley himself allows that his arguments do not need to be taken as a challenge to our moral attitudes towards people with dementia because, even if the self (on his conception) has been eroded, we would still need to pay attention to the individual's sentience, their ability to feel such things as pain and comfort. At this point, however, questions can be raised about the conception of the self being put forward. It is a highly cognitive view of the self: the self that keeps track, the self that involves a cognitive surround. This conception of the self would seem to be threatened by Post's attacks on 'hypercognitivism' (see Chapter 14) and by the appeal of those (represented in this book, *inter alia*, by Downs and colleagues, Snyder, Cayton, and Sabat, in Chapters 15–18) who emphasize the multi-layered nature of selfhood. Luntley's arguments work only if selfhood depends solely on the cognitive tracking ability he points to; but the question is why should the self be so restricted?

There are (at least) two arguments here. The argument from the other authors we have just mentioned in this book might amount to a stamp of the foot and an insistence that 'the self' simply should not be restricted in the way apparently suggested by Luntley. Is it not the case, they might reasonably ask, that selfhood—what it is that makes us the individual human creatures we are—involves capacities other than the capacity to keep track? Are we not also beings with motivations, with longings, with conation, with desires, with strivings, with humour, with emotions, with attachments, even with love? And do not these characteristics go beyond cognitive abilities and mere sentience? And may they not (empirically) persist in some form even into the very last stages of dementia in such a way as to undercut the cognitive denial of selfhood?

The second argument follows from this, but concerns the more metaphysical point about the self. Luntley might wish to argue that his conception of the self is the only one to provide the sort of unity over time that is an important part of our conception of what a self is. But this is because he has characterized the transcendental self as 'the ground for the possibility of keeping track of things', which is immediately to cast the self in a cognitive role. What if, as the previous (partly empirical) argument suggested, 'the self' were to be more broadly construed to include other things such as emotions, conations, drives, affections, and so on? Then perhaps the transcendental self would have to be characterized as 'the ground for the possibility of being a human person'. To be human is, after all, to be a human self. When we try to apprehend ourselves, then, what we find are various ways of being human in the world. In some ways, this may feel like an inner apprehension, but it involves an apprehension of the numerous ways in which we are human beings in the world. It is an apprehension of our place in the outer schema of things too.

The key (transcendental) point is, of course, that we never actually catch this point of view on the world, this ground of being human. It reflects, to use Iris Murdoch's expression, 'The weirdness of being human' (Murdoch 2003). The moment-to-moment nature of the self eludes us, even if we grasp at it in our thought and language. Perhaps aesthetic language takes us as close as we can go. This brings to mind Wittgenstein writing about philosophy and saying that it results in 'bumps that the understanding has got by running its head up against the limits of language' (Wittgenstein 1968, §119). The point is, our sense of ourselves as selves points us in the direction of something without which we would not be the individual human beings that we are; we never pin it down, however, partly because there is always some further way of characterizing ourselves; but mostly because (as the ground for the possibility of being the humans that we are) it is not a thing that is there to be designated or signified. It rather emerges through our 'doings and sayings' as human beings in the world. That is, we can never grasp its quiddity and the agnosticism of Lowe on this score (mentioned above), is perhaps the most appropriate reaction. Luntley's arguments help to bring out some of the possible implications and uses of Kant's notion of the unity of apperception; readers must judge whether the notion of the self seems empirically viable and whether the sense in which the self might disappear is one that challenges or squares with the experience of looking after people with dementia.

Personal space

The implication is that the metaphysical self may not convey all that there is to convey about the individual. Of course, the notion of the self or selves used by Sabat (2001) allows a broad interpretation, which certainly includes others. But it may be we are better off thinking of 'persons' rather than 'selves'. It is not that the philosophical notion of 'person' is uncontroversial (see Morton 1990), it is just that, whilst 'the self' can be construed in a metaphysical light (as something like 'the soul'), this is not the case with 'the person'. Persons are inevitably located in the world. Broad concerns inevitably come in, therefore, and cannot be abstracted away.

One of our themes in this chapter has been the move from within to without and we have already noted how this adds to the texture of the philosophical questions and answers. This move has partly been encouraged by an openness to continental thought. Thus we find Widdershoven and Berghmans (in Chapter 11) discussing Heidegger's notion of being-in-the-world. It is in this context that meaning-making occurs, which takes us back to our earlier discussion of meaning, contexts and relationships. Furthermore, Widdershoven and Berghmans demonstrate how our understanding of this philosophical notion can have an impact on how the fragmented sayings and actions of someone with dementia might be facilitated. The hermeneutic perspective brings in the idea of meaning-making as a joint venture and one that might be useful when clinicians are faced by ethical dilemmas. The approach epitomized by Widdershoven and Berghmans is a good example of how philosophy that engages with real cases can give a different view.

The way in which the 'metaphysical self' may not convey the entire picture, which is seen when we talk of persons, is most obvious when we turn to the discussion by Matthews (Chapter 10) of Merleau-Ponty's notion of the body-subject, mentioned previously. Matthews points out that a person cannot be thought of in terms of consciousness alone because of the way this ignores the body. The body also has an impact on the person's subjectivity. Moreover, Matthews goes on to argue that real respect for the person with dementia will involve care for the person's environment. For instance, it should encourage us to help people to stay in their homes for longer and it should support the view that institutional settings need to be as humane and homely as possible. The idea is that an individual's personhood can be maintained by attention to the surroundings: the public spaces they inhabit even when the ability to speak has passed.

This broadening in terms of how the notion of the person must be conceptualized is also conveyed (in Chapter 9) by the situated-embodied-agent view of the person (Hughes 2001). Implicit in this view is the idea that persons are embedded in an unspecifiable number of fields (social, ethical, legal, spiritual, and so on). The number of fields cannot be specified because the notion of personhood cannot be circumscribed. There is always a further way to describe a person, which means that persons can potentially always be situated in a new field. Thus, understanding a person is never complete. This way of thinking of persons provides a rich context in which to consider the numerous ethical issues that arise for people with dementia (Hughes 2002). Again, as in the discussion by Widdershoven and Berghmans in Chapter 11, the emphasis is on the person as a being-in-the-world where, for understanding to occur, there must be a grasp of the embedding context. And, as in the discussion by Matthews in Chapter 10, the person is regarded as a body as well as a subjective being, but as one who acts in the world, even if only by gesture and ingrained habits of behaviour.

The notion of the person, therefore, is a broad one. It has to be in order to accommodate the rich, multi-textured, and multi-layered ways in which an individual can be in the world. The person is in the world just as the mind is constitutively world involving. The person occupies public space: bodily, but also by the use of language, which—as in the case of meaning—involves, at least potentially, relationships with others. The person, in short, is situated and is partly constituted by this situatedness. That, too, applies to people with dementia and underpins the requirement that they should be treated with concern and with dignity.

Conclusion

We started this chapter by considering the idea, which is not immediately apparent because of the 'organic' nature of dementia, that the diagnosis of dementia was evaluative. Recognition of values brings into play a greater consideration of meanings. This becomes important when we consider the scale of the problems raised by dementia, both globally and individually. How we think of people with dementia will be crucially important in determining how we care for them.

We saw that our minds and our subjectivity seem to involve other people, although later we became more inclined to add the caveat that this involvement with others had to be at least potential if not actual. The notion of the externality of the mind pushed us further into the world and, in connection with meaning (and therefore meaning-making), we saw that it was in the public spaces formed by communication that this occurred. Again, despite the need to be cautious about the extent to which others *construct* meaning, there seems little doubt that our (at least potential) engagements with others are crucial to our standing as people who can convey meaning and use language. At the level of the person, the emphasis on the world is a corrective to the hypercognitivism that tends to reduce the notion of personhood to inner goings-on. Instead, we need to see the person as a situated human being, who engages with the world in a mental and bodily way in agent-like activities, showing (amongst other things) desires, choices, drives, emotions, needs, and attachments.

Our recurring theme has been the need to broaden the view, to move outwards to the world. We have seen how clinical practice takes us in this direction, by the emphasis from the practitioners on the importance of relationships. We have seen how philosophers also talk of public space (the space of meaning) and of the way in which the mind must (constitutively) engage with the world. Meaning-making takes place in the world between people, including people with dementia. So the emphasis is on seeing things whole. Perhaps this is best put by the philosopher Midgley:

> People sometimes say that the human brain is the most complex item in the universe. But the whole person of whom that brain is part is necessarily a much more complex item than the brain alone. And whole people can't be understood without knowing a good deal both about their inner lives and about the other people around them. Indeed, they can't be understood without a fair grasp of the whole society that they belong to, which is presumably more complex still. (Midgley 2001, p. 120)

Our substantive conclusion is that people with dementia have to be understood in terms of relationships, not because this is all that is left to them, but because this is characteristic of all of our lives. *How* this is so, as we shall see in the rest of the book, is a matter for fine debate. The philosophical disputes that may be unearthed will not be solved without further exploration.

But Midgley is surely right to draw our attention to the bigger picture, towards which we have been heading all along. Without this form of whole sight—the broader view of people with dementia that comes from the connection of practice and philosophy—our futures might indeed seem desolate.

Endnotes

1 This is a brief sketch of only some of the forms of dementia. For more details see a comprehensive standard text, for example, Burns *et al.* (2005).

2 Of course, there is nothing desperately new about this, nor is it a unique feature to psychological medicine. The 'normal' range of haemoglobin in the blood, for instance, is a matter of an evaluative judgement too, albeit there tends to be consensus concerning the number of standard deviations from the mean that will count as normal. Even so, by definition, there will be people whose blood haemoglobin falls outside the 'normal' range (for example, of two standard deviations from the mean for a particular laboratory) who are nevertheless fit and healthy. The upshot is that reference also has to be made to functional abilities before decisions are taken to act or not to act on any particular finding. This brings values more clearly into the picture. Things start to become more difficult once the values are disputed. All we are attempting to bring about here is an awareness of the extent to which there is room for value diversity in the field of cognitive impairment. The broader themes we are inevitably touching upon, for instance to do with definitions of disease, are fully discussed by Fulford (1989) and in several papers in Radden (2004).

3 See the Alzheimer's Disease International website: http://www.alz.co.uk/global/ (accessed on 14 March 2005).

4 See Jorm (2002).

5 See Wolstenholme and Gray (2002).

6 We can only sketch mind–brain theories briefly. For a more thorough philosophical treatment see Kenny (1989) and Lowe (2000).

7 Lowe discusses the thought of Descartes a little further in Chapter 6.

8 For further discussion of palliative care in dementia, see Post (2000, pp. 107–8 and 117–20); see also his mention of hospice care in Chapter 14 of this book, and Purtilo and ten Have (2004) and Hughes (2005).

9 We should quickly say that our observations do not necessarily reflect Grant Gillett's views exactly, although we suspect he would not object too strongly to what we have said.

10 See both McGinn (1989) and McCulloch (2003) for thorough discussions.

11 The closeness of this view to Taylor's talk of forming public spaces can be seen, although it would be wrong to ascribe constructivism to Taylor. Taylor was arguing that language formed public spaces, not that the judgements of individuals created meaning. Nonetheless, the roots of the various lines of thought can be seen to be enmeshed in ways that require delicate handling. What has to be understood, according to these ways of thinking, is the basis of meanings outside the head. In this chapter, we have been keen to support the idea that meanings are outside the head, because this provides (as Thronton suggests) a useful underpinning to the approach to people with dementia that we should wish to encourage.

12 By Aquilina and Hughes (Chapter 9), Allen and Coleman (Chapter 13), Post (Chapter 14), Downs and colleagues (Chapter 15), Snyder (Chapter 16), Cayton (Chapter 17) and by Sabat (Chapter 18). His social constructionist roots are more critically appraised by Thornton in Chapter 8.

13 Not only are they important to the discussions of McMillan (Chapter 4) and Radden and Fordyce (Chapter 5), but they also appear in Chapter 7 (Luntley) and Chapter 9 (Aquilina and Hughes) and they underpin some of Lesser's discussion in Chapter 3.

14 See Chapters 5 (Radden and Fordyce) and 9 (Aquilina and Hughes) for further references.

References

Baldwin, C., Hope, T., Hughes, J., Jacoby, R., Ziebland, S. (2004). Ethics and dementia: the experience of family carers. *Progress in Neurology and Psychiatry*, **8**: 24–8.

Battle, M. (1997). *Reconciliation—The Ubuntu Theology of Desmond Tutu*. Cleveland, Ohio: Pilgrim Press.

Buber, M. (1937). *I and Thou [Ich und Du]* (trans. R. G. Smith, 2004). London: Continuum.

Burns, A., O'Brien, J., Ames, D. (eds.) (2005). *Dementia* 3rd edition. London: Arnold Health Sciences.

Cayton, H. (2002). Carers' lives. In: *Psychiatry in the Elderly*, 3rd edn (ed. R. Jacoby and C. Oppenheimer), pp. 441–59. Oxford: Oxford University Press.

Church, J. (2004). Social constructionist models: making order out of disorder—on the social construction of madness. In: *The Philosophy of Psychiatry: A Companion* (ed. J. Radden), pp. 393–406. Oxford and New York: Oxford University Press.

Churchland, P. S. (1986). *Neurophilosophy: Toward a Unified Science of the Mind–Brain*. Cambridge, Massachusetts: Bradford Book, MIT Press.

Descartes, R. (1644). Letter to Father Mesland. In: *Descartes: Philosophical Writings* (ed. and trans. E. Anscombe and P.T. Geach, 1970), pp. 288–9. Sunbury-on-Thames: Nelson's University Paperbacks. (Originally, letter to Father Mesland, 2 May 1644, *Correspondence*, No. 347; Œuvres, A.-T., Vol. iv, p. 111.)

Dickenson, D., Fulford, K. W. M. (2000). *In Two Minds: A Casebook of Psychiatric Ethics*. Oxford: Oxford University Press.

Dilthey, W. (1977). *Descriptive Psychology and Historical Understanding* (trans. R. M. Zaner and K. L. Heiges). The Hague: Martinus Nijhoff.

Dworkin, R. (1993). *Life's Dominion: An Argument About Abortion and Euthanasia*. London: Harper Collins.

Esiri, M., Nagy, Z. (2002). Neuropathology. In: *Psychiatry in the Elderly*, 3rd edition. (Ed. R. Jacoby and C. Oppenheimer), pp. 102–124. Oxford: Oxford Unitersity Press.

Fontana, A., Smith, A. (1989). Alzheimer's disease victims: the 'unbecoming' of self and the normalisation of competence. *Sociological Perspectives*, **32**: 35–46.

Fowles, J. (1978). *Daniel Martin*. St Albans: Triad Panther Books. (First published 1977, London: Jonathan Cape.)

Fulford, K. W. M. (1989). *Moral Theory and Medical Practice*. Cambridge: Cambridge University Press.

Fulford, K. W. M. (1991). The potential of medicine as a resource for philosophy. *Theoretical Medicine*, **12**: 81–5.

Gillett, G. (2004). Cognition: brain pain: psychotic cognition, hallucinations, and delusions. In: *The Philosophy of Psychiatry: A Companion* (ed. J. Radden), pp. 21–35. Oxford and New York: Oxford University Press.

Gillett, G., McMillan, J. (2001). *Consciousness and Intentionality*. Amsterdam and Philadelphia: John Benjamin.

Hacking, I. (1995). *Rewriting the Soul: Multiple Personality and the Science of Memory*. Cambridge, Massachusetts: Harvard University Press.

Hacking, I. (1999). *The Social Construction of What?* Cambridge, Massachusetts: Harvard University Press.

Harré, R., Gillett, G. (1994). *The Discursive Mind*. Thousand Oaks, London and New Delhi: Sage.

Herskovits, E. (1995). Struggling over subjectivity: debates about the 'self' and Alzheimer's Disease. *Medical Anthropology Quarterly*, **9**: 146–64.

Hughes, J. C. (2001). Views of the person with dementia. *Journal of Medical Ethics*, **27**: 86–91.

Hughes, J. C. (2002). Ethics and the psychiatry of old age. In: *Psychiatry in the Elderly*, 3rd edn (ed. R. Jacoby and C. Oppenheimer), pp. 863–95. Oxford: Oxford University Press.

Hughes, J. (ed.) (2005). *Palliative Care in Severe Dementia*. London: Quay Books.

Jonsen, A. R., Toulmin, S. (1988). *The Abuse of Casuistry: A History of Moral Reasoning*. London and Berkeley: University of California Press.

Jorm, A. (2002). Epidemiology of the dementias of late life. In: *Psychiatry in the Elderly*, 3rd edn (ed. R. Jacoby and C. Oppenheimer), pp. 487–500. Oxford: Oxford University Press.

Kandel, E. R. (1998). A new intellectual framework for psychiatry. *American Journal of Psychiatry*, **155**: 457–69.

Kenny, A. (1989). *The Metaphysics of Mind*. Oxford: Clarendon Press.

Kitwood, T. (1997). *Dementia Reconsidered: The Person Comes First*. Buckingham: Open University Press.

Kripke, S. A. (1982). *Wittgenstein on Rules and Private Language: an Elementary Exposition*. Oxford: Blackwell.

Lewis, H. D. (1982). *The Elusive Self*. London: Macmillan.

Louw, S. J., Hughes, J. C. (2005). Moral reasoning—the unrealized place of casuistry in medical ethics. *International Psychogeriatrics*, **17**: 149–54.

Lowe, E. J. (2000). *An Introduction to the Philosophy of Mind*. Cambridge: Cambridge University Press.

MacIntyre, A. (1985). *After Virtue: A Study in Moral Theory*, 2nd edn. London: Duckworth.

McCulloch, G. (2003). *The Life of the Mind. An Essay on Phenomenological Externalism*. London and New York: Routledge.

McGinn, C. (1989). *Mental Content*. Oxford: Blackwell.

Midgley, M. (2001). *Science and Poetry*. London: Routledge.

Morton, A. (1990). Why there is no concept of a person. In: *The Person and the Human Mind: Issues in Ancient and Moral Philosophy* (ed. C. Gill), pp. 39–59. Oxford: Clarendon Press.

Murdoch, I. (2003). *Metaphysics as a Guide to Morals*. London: Vintage. (First published 1992, London: Chatto and Windus.)

Murphy, E. (1984). Ethical dilemmas of brain failure in the elderly (letter). *British Medical Journal*, **288**: 61–2.

Murray, T.H. (1994). Medical ethics, moral philosophy and moral tradition. In: *Medicine and Moral Reasoning* (ed. K. W. M. Fulford, G. Gillett, and J. M. Soskice), pp. 91–105. Cambridge: Cambridge University Press.

Oppenheimer, C. (1999). Ethics in old age psychiatry. In: *Psychiatric Ethics*, 3rd edn (ed. S. Bloch, P. Chodoff, and S. A. Green), pp. 317–43. Oxford and New York: Oxford University Press.

Parfit, D. (1984). *Reasons and Persons*. Oxford: Oxford University Press.

Popper, K. R., Eccles, J. C. (1977). *The Self and Its Brain*. Berlin, New York: Springer International.

Post, S. G. (2000). *The Moral Challenge of Alzheimer Disease: Ethical Issues from Diagnosis to Dying*, 2nd edn. Baltimore and London: Johns Hopkins University Press.

Purtilo, R. B., ten Have, H. A. M. J. (eds.) (2004). *Ethical Foundations of Palliative Care for Alzheimer's Disease*. Baltimore: Johns Hopkins University Press.

Radden, J. (ed.) (2004). *The Philosophy of Psychiatry: A Companion*. New York: Oxford University Press.

Robertson, G. S. (1982). Dealing with the brain-damaged old—dignity before sanctity (response). *Journal of Medical Ethics*, **8**: 173–79.

Robertson, G. S. (1983). Ethical dilemmas of brain failure in the elderly. *British Medical Journal*, **287**: 1775–77.

Sabat, S. R. (2001). *The Experience of Alzheimer's Disease: Life Through a Tangled Veil*. Oxford and Malden, Massachusetts: Blackwell.

Sabat, S. R., Harré, R. (1994). The Alzheimer's disease sufferer as a semiotic subject. *Philosophy, Psychiatry, & Psychology*, **1**: 145–60.

Schwartz, M. A., Wiggins, O. P. (2004). Phenomenological and hermeneutic models: understanding and interpretation in psychiatry. In: *The Philosophy of Psychiatry: A Companion* (ed. J. Radden), pp. 351–63. Oxford and New York: Oxford University Press.

Taylor, C. (1985). Theories of meaning. In: *Human Agency and Language. Philosophical Papers 1*, pp. 248–92. Cambridge: Cambridge University Press.

Thornton, T. (1998). *Wittgenstein on Language and Thought*. Edinburgh: Edinburgh University Press.

Widdershoven, G. A. M., Widdershoven-Heerding, I. (2003). Understanding dementia: a hermeneutic perspective. In: *Nature and Narrative: An Introduction to the New Philosophy of Psychiatry* (ed. K. W. M. Fulford, K. Morris, J. Z. Sadler, and G. Stanghellini), pp. 103–11. Oxford: Oxford University Press.

Wilkes, K. V. (1988). *Real People. Personal Identity without Thought Experiments*. Oxford: Clarendon Press.

Williams, R. (2005). The care of souls. *Advances in Psychiatric Treatment*, **11**: 4–5.

Wittgenstein, L. (1968). *Philosophical Investigations* (trans. G. E. M. Anscombe). Oxford: Blackwell.

Wittgenstein, L. (1980). *Remarks on the Philosophy of Psychology, Volume I* (ed. G. E. M. Anscombe and G. H. von Wright, trans. G. E. M. Anscombe). Oxford: Blackwell.

Wolstenholme, J., Gray, A. (2002). The economics of health care provision for elderly people with dementia. In: *Psychiatry in the Elderly*, 3rd edn (ed. R. Jacoby and C. Oppenheimer), pp. 177–97. Oxford: Oxford University Press.

2   Ageing and human nature

Michael Bavidge

Introduction

It is a truth universally acknowledged that 'all men are mortal' and yet the universality of ageing and death has not ensured that their significance has been universally agreed. Our dominant religious traditions have taught that we are not, at the deepest level, mortal, and that what matters most about us has nothing to do with mortality or even temporality. Now questions about the significance of ageing and death are coming from new secular and empirical sources. Increases in life expectancy have not just added a few more years to the average span of life. They are changing our experience of ageing and dying. The life sciences suggest that our deeply ingrained preconceptions about ageing and death may be wrong.

The signatories to the 'Position Statement on Human Ageing' thought it worth insisting that 'the prospect of humans living forever is as unlikely today as it has always been, and discussions of such an impossible scenario have no place in scientific discourse' (Smith and Olshansky 2002). This statement must have been directed at somebody, though appropriately the section in which it occurs, dealing with everlasting life, is the shortest in the paper. Immortality may never be on the scientific agenda, but new issues about the inevitability of ageing and death are arising because of scientific developments.

The idea of human nature is unavoidable because there is a need to distinguish what, if anything, is structural about our lives from what is individual and idiosyncratic. Are there relatively fixed parameters within which we act and create possibilities for ourselves? The most obvious boundaries to our activities are set by ageing and death itself. But if the realities of death and ageing are undergoing serious changes then the shape of our lives, as we experience them, must change also.

The shape of life

Personal lives have a shape. By 'shape' of life I mean life experienced as a whole, having a beginning, a middle, and an end and conceived as making some sort of sense. We talk about the 'Right to Life'. We do not just mean the right to go on breathing in and breathing out. People are the subjects of a life: they have the right, other things being equal, to live it *through*, to live it *out*, to shape it for themselves as best they can.

It is not an accident that biography and autobiography emerged as an important literary genre in Western societies with a liberal and Romantic ideology. Two things in particular are required from a biography: an account of the subject's childhood and disclosures about their personal relationships. We want to know how they came to be the people they are and we want to see them relating intimately to others because it is primarily in personal relationships and interactions that our personalities are disclosed.

Curiously in fictitious biographies that is enough. We feel we know David Copperfield very well because we know those sorts of things about him. But we do not know how his life ended. Well, that is just the way with characters in fiction. Their incomplete lives are left hanging in an imaginary world. Nevertheless, though we are told nothing about Copperfield's death, other people's deaths shape his life and intimations of mortality pervade his story.

Narrative and autobiography are important to our idea of ourselves and the loss of our ability to maintain them is central to dementia. What counts is not odd memories of the distant past, which demented people often have, but the ability to integrate past events into a meaningful, progressive pattern of experience, which the severely demented cannot manage. Without this pattern of experience our sense of ourselves disintegrates. Michael Luntley develops this thought when he writes, 'The failure to keep track of objects and events in the environment, if severe enough, can amount to a failure of self' (see p. 119 in Chapter 7).

We are complex creatures. We can distinguish between the end of our existence as animals, as human beings, and as persons. We have no guarantee that these different terminations will neatly coincide and harmonize with each other, even in an ideal world. One thing is clear: the shape of a human life, in the sense meant here, is not a purely biological matter. Human life can be thought of in both scientific and subjective terms. We want to take into account our factuality, objectively considered and to capture the shape of our experience and activity from the inside. The shape of our lives is, at least in part, a function of our imaginations and choices. But we do not act in a vacuum. There are biological structures within which we think and act and there are social structures which determine the options we take ourselves to have. And if our question is not to be a fantasy question it must take these determinants into account.

Human nature

What shape our lives have is part of the discussion about human nature. Unfortunately human nature has long been a suspect concept. There are many reasons for this: one is the difficulty of providing agreed content to the idea and another is that it offends against the requirement that we keep our facts and our values in separate drawers.

Neither of these objections deserves the respect they have been given. There will never be an unproblematic concept of human nature. Even though it is an unavoidable idea with an essential role in thinking about how we understand ourselves, it can only fulfil that role if it is contestable. Its content is one of the focal points for the development of ideas about how we ought to live and, more importantly, for practical 'experiments in living', as John Stuart Mill called them (Mill 1962, p. 211). Alex Mauron (Mauron 2001) in an article entitled 'Is the genome the secular equivalent of the soul?' cites as a reason for the equation of soul and genome that the genome determines 'both our individuality and our species identity' and 'contains a blue-print of human nature'. But the genome cannot fill the conceptual niche that human nature has occupied. As the Existentialists insist, human nature is not a blue-print that determines whether human beings are, for example, naturally aggressive, or monogamous, or religious. Nor can the concept of human nature settle once and for all demarcation disputes between nature and nurture.

Current disagreements about genetic determinism are connected with this issue. We want the concept of human nature both to be a quasi-scientific concept that outlines the determining elements of our species and a subjective concept that captures the shape of our experience and activity from the inside. The concept embodies the tension that Kant identified in his 'Third Antinomy'—the necessity and the impossibility of considering ourselves both to be totally part of the natural order and completely free and independent of it (Kant 1964).

The related, but more familiar objection is that human nature is a flawed concept because it is a horrible muddle of facts and values. The suspicion is that it is a hybrid concept, which confuses two domains of discourse both of which are perfectly legitimate if kept separate, but when fused produce bad science and moral special pleading. There has been a push, evident since the Enlightenment, towards morally neutral science on the one hand and pure morality uncluttered by factual considerations on the other. Neither of these reciprocal objectives is realistic, particularly not in medical science. If there were no such concepts as health, disease, and nature—all of which have factual and evaluative functions—we would have to invent them. Being carers, we cannot avoid taking up a point of view on behaviour at which moral and factual considerations intersect. The value-free world could only appear in a report from a place no one has ever occupied.

Our question then becomes, given current and future developments in the understanding and control of ageing, what changes can we expect in our ideas about human nature? To what extent are we likely to have to change our ideas about what sort of animals we are and what sort of future we can expect for ourselves and what a worthwhile human life should be like?

Professor John Harris anticipates profound social, economic, and political consequences of increased longevity and of better health in old age. He has speculated that the prospect of overcrowding and competition between old and young for jobs could create a situation in which society decides a fair age for its members' survival and withdraws medical care beyond that age (Harris 2000). Alternatively, he suggests, it might be that people would be offered the chance of a longer life in return for agreeing not to have children. These scenarios sound alarming enough but they are predicated on the basis of perfectly possible advances in medical science. More dramatic speculations are possible if we allow our imaginations greater scope.

Stories of immortality

In *Gulliver's Travels*, Swift offers us satirical fantasies that are related to Professor Harris's utilitarian thoughts about the consequences of longevity (Swift 1976). He describes the plight of the Struldbruggs. They are a group of people in the land of Luggnagg who have the misfortune to be born immortal. When Gulliver first hears about these creatures he imagines all the wonderful advantages they must have: what prosperity they could achieve in an endless life of industry and effort; what advantages eternal lifelong education would bring: 'I should be a living treasury of knowledge and wisdom, and certainly become the oracle of the nation' (Swift 1976). But to Gulliver's amazement, the Struldbruggs are in a pitiable condition. Swift's account of their decrepitude is cruel and misanthropic:

> ... they had not only all the follies of other old men, but many more that arose from the dreadful prospect of never dying. They were not only opinionative, peevish, covetous, morose, vain, talkative, but uncapable of friendship, and dead to all natural affection, which never descended below their grandchildren. Envy and impotent desires are their prevailing passions. (Swift 1976, p 171)

Swift presents this sad picture as a portrait of beings that are both immortal and live out their 'perpetual life under all the disadvantages that old age brings along with it'. But he underestimates the conceptual strain that the idea of immortality would produce. We would have to imagine a form of life completely outside the present natural order. He does not go that deep. His Strudlbruggs are odd-balls born randomly into a normal mortal population.

In fact, Swift's pessimistic picture consists of the miseries that would probably attend a life much the same as our own, which, though not eternal, was significantly extended and which, though not blissful, was qualitatively improved. The Struldbruggs' problems have nothing to do with immortality. Nor do they arise just because the ills of vast old age go on for longer. They arise because their life would lose its shape and therefore the meaningfulness that life has for the mortal inhabitants of Luggnagg.

Another literary example is the short story 'Miranda's tale' by Tom Kirkwood (Kirkwood, 2001). This yarn is set two or three hundred years in the future when 'fraitch technology', which repairs cell damage, has been developed. People do not age or die. But if they have the full quota of children that the State allocates to them, they forfeit the right to further fraitches, so they become the 'Timed Ones' and they die after a few decades.

Professor Kirkwood has interesting things to say about the psychological problems people would face in this new world:

> In the early centuries after fraitch technology was developed, the emotional burden of a long life was poorly understood and the suicide rate grew alarmingly high. Psycho-fraitching of the mind quickly became as important as the regeneration of the cells and tissues of the body. (Kirkwood 2001, p. 100)

If life without end is a meaningless life then psycho-fraitching can only be a technique for obscuring that fact. Professor Kirkwood speculates that people may be psychologically impelled to conform to the old fallacious idea that there is a natural pattern to life that ends in ageing and death.

Trivializing temporality

These are exercises in imagining the consequences if ageing and even death were abolished or very different. There are long-established philosophical lines of thought that are not meant in any way to be fantasies but do raise questions about the significance of ageing and mortality. They claim to analyse and explain aspects of our real and present lives. Utilitarianism, for example, prides itself on being an economical theory that can explain morality in terms of maximizing welfare across a population. A commonly perceived weakness of the theory is that it treats people simply as receptacles of benefits. Moral concepts that attach to people on non-utilitarian grounds are rejected. Bentham, for example, thought that rights were nonsense and natural rights were nonsense on stilts (Bentham 1962, p. 501). There are no rights because no one is entitled to put limits on what the utilitarian administrator can do in allocating benefits in order to maximize general welfare. For similar reasons Utilitarians would probably resist the idea that the shape of human life has any moral relevance. Prioritizing exercises in public health provision that are based purely on utilitarian calculations have widely been thought to discriminate against older people. Benefiting the young gives a greater return than the same treatment allocated to the old. But these attitudes seem to discount essential aspects of our moral lives. What is morally valuable is not there being lots of enjoyable experiences or episodes, but that people achieve personal satisfaction through living a *meaningful* life. And we cannot live a meaningful life without conceiving how our lives should end.

Another example of a line of philosophical thought that plays down the idea that lives have a shape that is morally relevant can be found in Thomas Nagel's article, 'Death', in *Mortal Questions* (Nagel 1979). He argues that death terminates the enjoyment of satisfactions to which there is no intrinsic end, for example, the pleasures of conversation with friends or the enjoyment of nature and of art. It would always be good to have more of these things:

> Observed from without, human beings obviously have a natural lifespan and cannot live much longer than a hundred years. A man's sense of his own experience, on the other hand, does not embody this idea of a natural limit. His existence defines for him an essentially open-ended possible future containing the usual mixture of goods and evils he has found so tolerable in the past. (Nagel 1979, pp. 9–10)

The clash between the inevitability of death and the essential open-endedness of personal experience means 'a bad end is in store for us all'.

Nagel's argument suggests a sort of dualism: insofar as we are organisms, our lives have a natural termination in death; but as persons, with our own subjective experience, there is no built-in ending. From a moral point of view, we may as well be immortal.

This tendency to trivialize the temporality of our experience produces suspect idealizations of life. For example, in the context of a disagreement with Dame Mary Warnock, Professor Harris writes that,

> the question of whether or not an individual is a person just is the question of whether it is morally important; and in particular of whether it shows what-ever moral importance normal adult human beings have. (Harris 1992, p. 30)

That line of thought risks leading us to dangerous conclusions about how we should behave towards those at the beginning and end of life who do not come close enough to the normal adult ideal—and to run that risk by ignoring the fact that human beings are really temporal in all aspects of their existence.

Two patterns

Shakespeare describes the 'Seven Ages of Man' in a famous portrait of a human life in *As You Like It*, in which he tracks a human being, or at least a male human being from infancy, through childhood and romantic adolescence, to warrior and responsible citizen, to old age concluding:

> Last scene of all, That ends this strange eventful history, Is second childish-ness and mere oblivion, Sans teeth, sans eyes, sans taste, sans everything. (Shakespeare 1951, Act 2, Scene 7, 163–66)

This picture has at least the satisfaction of presenting life as a symmetrical movement, from infancy to old age, a return to the place from which we came. It may be a dispiriting picture but it does provide us with a pattern and a conclusion to which we can aim at least to submit ourselves. It echoes the ancient advice we get from Lucretius that we should not fear death because post-mortem non-existence is no more alarming than non-existence prior to conception. He wrote: 'one who no longer is cannot . . . differ in any way from one who has never been born' (Lucretius 1951, p. 122). We are not horrified by the fact that we did not exist when Julius Caesar marched about; nor should we be discomforted by the thought that shortly we shall return to non-existence.

The trouble with these symmetrical pictures of human life is that they do not take temporality seriously enough. Time counts. There is a big difference between non-existence, timelessly considered and the non-existence that follows life and death. The first may induce a momentary metaphysical vertigo; the second fear and anxiety. Similarly losing one's competence and personality after a long life is a very different prospect from the incompetence that characterizes the infant.[1] The symmetry that Shakespeare and Lucretius suggest is merely rhetorical.

The 'Seven Ages of Man' was a familiar theme in medieval writing before Shakespeare got his hands on it (Burrow 1986). But it does not sit comfortably with an entirely different view of human life, the Christian linear view in which we are in progress towards a perfect life post-mortem. In Christian anthropology, human beings are not naturally (in one sense of 'naturally') mortal. The difficulty of reconciling the notions of eternal life and the Resurrection with the apparently obvious biological pattern of birth, growth, and decay tested the ingenuity of theologians. Aquinas speculates that our bodies will be resurrected in their prime:

> Man will rise again without any defect of human nature, because as God founded human nature without a defect, even so will He restore it without defect. Now human nature has a twofold defect. First, because it has not yet attained to its ultimate perfection. Secondly, because it has already gone back from its ultimate perfection. The first defect is found in children, the second in the aged: and consequently in each of these human nature will be brought by the resurrection to the state of its ultimate perfection which is in the youthful age, at which the movement of growth terminates, and from which the movement of decrease begins. (Aquinas 1920)

Aquinas is committed to a theological view that attributes an inferior status to both childhood and old age. The former is a preparation for, the latter a decline from adult competence, which in the next life will be stabilised (if not frozen) in eternal aspic. Our terrestrial life has to be seen as secondary, if not illusory, against the background of the supernatural drama in which the life of the spirit goes from strength to strength.

Both the circular and the Christian linear views, though for different reasons, underestimate the impact that time has on the shape of our lives. The topography of the human mind manifests temporality at all levels. Sensations last for measurable periods. Perceptions are perceptions of a changing scene in space and time. We rely on memory to maintain coherent patterns of thought and action and to establish our sense of ourselves. Our most rational thoughts are discursive, that is, when we work things out, we go round the houses and it takes time.

When people try to take the idea of immortality seriously they have to seek out some aspect of human life that seems, in some way or other, to escape the constraints of time. Arguments for the immortality of the soul often take the form of inferring from the fact that some truths are timeless to the conclusion that the contemplation of them could be atemporal. But it is surely cheating to argue from the abstract nature of certain types of thoughts to the timelessness of certain types of thinking.

Ageism

Granted that temporality is embedded in all aspects of human experience, there is still a question about the unavoidability of ageing. It may be inevitable that being around for a long time will cause the wear and tear that constitutes ageing. It looks as if there will always be a price to pay for the innumerable hits that just living makes on our organisms. But old age is not itself a pathological condition.

We are very conscious of old people's forgetfulness, shortened attention span, decreased capacity to solve problems, and so on. We are equally aware of the cognitive and executive weaknesses of childhood but we are not as inclined to regard them as symptoms of pathology. Mild cognitive impairment (MCI) is a worrying category. Criteria for MCI include deficiencies in attention, memory, visio-spatial abilities, language use, and reasoning skills. The controversial issue is whether it is possible to establish MCI as a condition that falls short of dementia but which is distinguishable from the cognitive changes associated with normal ageing. At what stage should we regard the set of characteristics covered by MCI to be pathological? There is a danger that these characteristics of old age become a syndrome because they can be relatively easily measured. We could amuse ourselves by inventing conditions of youth that match MCI but which no one is tempted to regard as symptoms of disease, for example, mild information deficit and severe preoccupation with oneself.

These ageist prejudices arise partly because the ageing process makes us liable to the diseases of old age, but also because we too readily assume that the differences in attitudes and competencies that characterize old age are *deteriorations*.

Sabat and Harré, in their paper 'The Alzheimer's disease sufferer as a semiotic subject', make similar points even in relation to people who are suffering from moderate to severe dementia. They summarize their research by saying,

> The discourse of Alzheimer's disease sufferers, studied in depth, is found to reveal the afflicted as being semiotic subjects, that is, persons, for whom meaning is the driving force behind their behaviour. (Sabat and Harré 1994, p. 146)

They conclude that accepting this enables 'better treatment of the sufferers and clearer communication between the afflicted and others' (Sabat and Harré 1994, p. 159).

None of this suggests that dementia is other than a serious condition that can be desperately distressing for sufferers and their loved ones. It does not mean that Alzeihemer's disease and the other conditions that cause dementia are not thoroughly undesirable and ought to be managed as well as possible and eliminated, if possible. Nevertheless the findings of Sabat and Harré provide a cautionary tale against our tendency to dismiss the experience of the elderly.

The thought that human consciousness emerges, develops, and ages should remind us not to pathologize old age. We have a pretty high opinion of ourselves. We are, as far as we know, the only rational, self-conscious, freely choosing beings on earth—possibly anywhere. What we pride ourselves on is not a single phenomenon or a narrowly defined set of capacities. There are many ways of being a rational animal; many stages that we go through. During a human life there is a multiplicity of ways of experiencing the world. If we try to list them we tend to produce dichotomies: young/old, healthy/ill, male/female, rational/emotional, lucid/demented. There is a danger that we interpret these as alternatives: one of which is good, the other bad. But there are mixed costs and benefits attending all stages of life. It is only when these become dysfunctional that we should start treating them as pathological symptoms. We should think of old age as offering alternative rather than impaired ways of experiencing life.

The elderly have been around the block, seen it all before, and developed habitual ways of responding. Their interests and behaviour are motivated by different ambitions, concerns, and anxieties from those of the young. There is a freshness and enthusiasm we enjoy in children who are facing situations for the first time. But there are also distinctive and valuable qualities in the experience and the attitudes of the elderly who have been in similar situations many times before.

An important part of shaping our lives is locating ourselves in the generations. We are somebody's children and grandchildren. We come to see ourselves as the grown-ups, the parents, eventually the elderly. We would be seriously discomforted without this perspective on ourselves and our relations to others. As we have seen, Aquinas speculates that on the Last Day our bodies will be resurrected in their prime. Are we to be in Heaven with our parents and grandparents all the same age? I suspect that the continuation of human life and society that resurrection is meant to guarantee could be undermined by this prospect.

It is interesting in thinking about the generations, that there is a direct biological link between sex and death (Kirkwood 2001). Sexual reproduction involves the separation of two principal lines of cells, the germ-line and the soma. The soma buys specialization and enormous diversity at the price of losing its reproductive function. Consequently there is little evolutionary value in preserving the soma in good nick and we are our soma. At this point, biology seems to support the traditional view that our mission is to be born, to mature, to reproduce, and to die. It is interesting that Utopias populated by Immortals have always to break the link between reproduction and caring, between children and parents.

However positive our attitude to old age becomes and whatever improvements may be introduced into the experience of ageing, it seems uphill work not to see a down side to it. People sometimes say that it is not death they mind, but dying. This is not a foolish thought but still people would not take such a negative view of the process of dying if it did not end in being dead. Similarly there are many positive aspects to ageing and we can imagine these being significantly deepened as the diseases of old age are controlled or eliminated. Nevertheless, as long as death awaits us, ageing will be seen as a process we would at the end of the day prefer not to engage with.

Experience and death

The temporality and finitude of human life is the central theme of Heidegger's thought. The title of his book, *Being and Time*, advertises the point (Heidegger 1980). One of his favourite formulae for characterizing human life is 'being-unto-death'. He does not mean just that all men are mortal. He means that progress through time towards death is an internal, constitutive feature of human experience. Death is not just the final end of our lives as organisms; it modulates our experience. It is our recognition of the inevitability of our own deaths that gives us the sense of our own individuality and the inalienable value of a person's life.

Heidegger writes in *On the Way to Language*,

> Mortals are they who can experience death as death. Animals cannot do so. But animals cannot speak either. The essential relation between death and language flashes up before us, but remains still unthought. (Heidegger 1972, pp. 107–8)

Joshua Schuster gives this interpretation of Heidegger's meaning: 'There is no death without mineness. . . . Only a being with mineness can die (much later Heidegger will remark that animals do not die, they only perish)' (Schuster 1997). Only creatures who are self-consciously aware of their own individuality can die; but equally only creatures who are aware of their own deaths develop the notion of themselves as individuals in the strong personal sense.

Our lives are characterized by project and possibility.

> A man's life includes much that does not take place within the boundaries of his body and his mind, and what happens to him can include much that does not take place within the boundaries of his life. (Nagel 1979, p. 6)

The end of a person is not like the end of anything else in the natural world, because the life of a person is a life of self-conscious possibilities.

The force of Heidegger's thought comes home when we realize that even if genetic engineering and prophylactic interventions mean that we could live indefinitely, we would still be mortal. Accidents will happen. We would still be subject to violent assault. Genetics cannot rid us of al Qa'ida or the IRA. And it certainly cannot stop the next meteorite from colliding with the earth.

Closer to home, genetics cannot change the fact that suicide will always be a possibility. And not just one possibility among all the others. It is, in a unique sense, my possibility. Mortality will always be there, because we can always bring our lives to an end. The question for the new Immortals would not be 'Why do we have to die?' but 'Why does death remain a possibility for us?' Wittgenstein unhelpfully reminds us, 'death is not an event in life: we do not live to experience death' (Wittgenstein 1922). We can, however, envisage the possibility of the end of all possibilities—and not only envisage it but choose it. We do not experience death, but we do experience life in which death is a permanent possibility. What bites in relation to human nature is not the inevitability of death but its irremovable possibility. We would remain mortal even if by some technological miracle we could survive indefinitely.

Medical advances have already altered our self-image and we can expect the evolution to continue. Increased life-span, a healthier old age, and the elimination of dementia will change people's views of themselves, their expectations, the structure of their lives as they experience them. But they will not touch our natures as being-unto-death, as finite, as contingent. The possibility of fatal accident or suicide is not just some external hazard that we will never be able to guarantee avoiding. It is an internal possibility that will always structure the experience of our lives.

It is a version, suitable for a scientific age, of an old story. We will be in a new paradise created and maintained by biological technologies, an enchanted garden of endless delights, but there is one fruit we must not eat. The fact is that personal death will always be there as threat or option and it will be *the* special threat or option—the only possibility that brings all the other possibilities to an end, the only one that ends a life.

Conclusion

There are at present inescapable drawbacks about old age. If you want to avoid a whole series of serious diseases, do not be old. But we are discovering that many of the deteriorations associated with old age are not the essential attendants of advanced years, but are features of diseases that we can reasonably expect to manage more effectively in future.

The success of gerontology in enabling us to experience old age and the ageing perspectives on the world in as disease-free state as possible, as lucidly as possible, should encourage us to look more positively—and not just out of compassion—on old age, even old age that shows signs of wear and tear.

Gerontology will not offer us or threaten us with an escape from ageing and death, but it does offer the possibility of experiencing ageing and death more comfortably and lucidly. It can give us more control in undergoing these processes. It will give us new choices, including the various options around euthanasia, which we may prefer we did not have.

Human life is unique. Its end is not like the end of anything else in the natural world. The claim that our ageing and our deaths are unique phenomena raises the suspicion that we are victims of a Ptolemaic illusion: the processes of ageing and dying seem different from any other sort of end process because *that's how it looks from here*. But perhaps on this occasion we are right to think we are special. We are self-conscious to a high degree and we are consciously ageing and heading towards death—and that makes us unique. It is the 'Third Antinomy' again. From an objective point of view human ageing and death is in principle no different from ageing and death throughout the animal world. But from a personal, experiential point of view, the end of a person is like no other ending.

Endnote

1 For further discussion of this point see Harry Cayton's comments in Chapter 17.

References

Aquinas, T. (1920). *Summa Theologica: Supplementum Tertiae Partis*, 81: 1. (From *The Summa Theologica of St Thomas Aquinas*, 2nd edn (trans. Fathers of the English Dominican Province).) (Available at http://www.newadvent.org/summa/508100.htm (copyright Kevin Knight, 2003) (accessed on 29 March 2005).)

Bentham, J. (1962). Anarchical fallacies. In: *The Works of Jeremy Bentham, Volume 2* (ed. J. Bowring). Boston, Massachusetts: Elibron Classics.

Burrow, J. A. (1986). *The Ages of Man*. Oxford: Clarendon.

Harris, J. (1992). *Wonderwoman and Superman*. Oxford: Oxford University Press.

Harris, J. (2000). Intimations of immortality. *Science*, **288**: 59.

Heidegger, M. (1972). *On the Way to Language*. New York: Harper and Row.

Heidegger, M. (1980). *Being and Time*. Oxford: Blackwell.

Kant, I. (1964). *Critique of Pure Reason*. London: Macmillan.

Kirkwood, T. (2001). *The End of Age*. London: Profile Books.

Lucretius (Titus Lucretius Carus) (1951). *On the Nature of the Universe*. New York: Penguin.

Mauron, A. (2001). Is the genome the secular equivalent of the soul? *Science*, **291**: 831–2.

Mill, J. S. (1962). On liberty. In: *Utilitarianism* (ed. M. Warnock), pp. 126–250. Glasgow: Collins, Fount Paperbacks. (First published 1859.)

Nagel, T. (1979). *Mortal Questions*. Cambridge: Cambridge University Press.

Sabat, S. R., Harré, R. (1994). The Alzheimer's disease sufferer as a semiotic subject. *Philosophy, Psychiatry, & Psychology*, **1**: 145–60.

Schuster, J. (1997). Death reckoning in the thinking of Heidegger, Foucault, and Derrida. *Other Voices*, **1**: 1 (March). (Electronic journal published by the University of Pennsylvania, available at http://www.othervoices.org/jnschust/death.html (accessed on 29 March, 2005).)

Shakespeare, W. (1951). *As You Like It*. In: *William Shakespeare: The Complete Works* (ed. P. Alexander), pp. 254–83. London and Glasgow: Collins.

Smith, J. R., Olshansky, S. J. (2002). Editorial: position statement on human aging. *Journals of Gerontology, Series A, Biological Sciences and Medical Sciences*, **57**: B291.

Swift, J. (1976). *Gulliver's Travels and Other Writings*. Oxford: Oxford University Press.

Wittgenstein, L. (1922). *Tractatus Logico-Philosophicus* (trans. C. K. Ogden). London: Routledge and Keegan Paul.

3 Dementia and personal identity

A. Harry Lesser

Introduction: the two senses of 'personal identity'

In psychiatry and philosophy the term 'personal identity' has in effect two distinct senses; and, to complicate matters further, both of them have a technical and a non-technical use. In one sense the term refers to being the same individual person over time, being, for example identical with the person who committed a crime or to whom an obligation is owed. Philosophy has been mainly concerned with identity in this sense and with the question of what makes a person the same person over time—whether it is simply the physical continuity of a particular body and brain or whether there is some persisting soul or self, that is, some persisting mental entity. Moreover, those philosophers who have thought there must be such a persisting self have had very different theories about its relation to the physical body and whether it can survive bodily death. We should also note that in the last century there have been many philosophers who have located personal identity in the person itself, as a being which is both mental and physical, and have denied that it is possible to split up or analyse a person into mind and body. Indeed, some philosophers, like some psychiatrists, have thought that this is a moral issue as well as a metaphysical one and that the false conception of humans as simply bodies, or minds, or even minds and bodies interacting, rather than as persons, is positively harmful in its effects on how we see people and therefore how we treat them.

But all these theories have been attempts to answer the question of what makes a person the same person and have been concerned with personal identity in this sense. More accurately, one may say that they have been concerned with two related issues, a metaphysical question of what makes a person the same person over time and an epistemological question of what criteria we use, or ought to use, to decide this. The answers given, whatever they may be, then influence the answer to a further question: whether personal identity always persists at least from birth to death, or whether, so to speak, a life history should sometimes be regarded as involving more than one person. It is this further question, as it relates to people with serious dementia, that is the subject of this chapter. But to see this we must consider the other main sense of 'personal identity'.

Personal identity as conception of oneself and as persistence

This other sense of 'personal identity' refers roughly to a person's conception of themselves and the kind of person that they are and/or should be: this is the sense used by psychology and sociology and in this sense of identity the same person may have different identities at different times during their life, as a result, for example, of a change of job, marriage or divorce, or a religious or political conversion. Dementia, if it is more than mild, clearly affects a person's identity in this second sense, possibly (at its worst) removing it altogether. This chapter will consider the implications this has for what we should say about their identity in the first sense; and then whether this in turn should affect our attitude to the threat to identity posed by dementia.

However, at this point it might well be asked 'Does it matter?' Is not this first sense of 'identity' sufficiently abstract and metaphysical to be ignored? The answer to this is that, as with many abstract issues, one's view of it turns out to have important practical consequences. One of these is mentioned above: the way we treat each other may be affected in a number of ways, according to whether we believe that what is essential is the mind, the body, the mind and body in interaction, or the personhood. Equally important is the question to be considered here, about persisting identity. This question is important in many contexts. For example, it matters a great deal whether the person being punished really is the person who committed the crime, whether the person in possession of the house really is the person who bought it, and so on. Now, this applies not just to formal relationships, concerned with justice, but also to emotional relationships— love, friendship, family relations—where a crucial element is often the memory of a shared past and hence where the appearance of dementia, and the loss of this memory, confronts us with the question 'Is this the same person?'

In trying to answer this question, one may take one of two approaches—to use the jargon, one may be descriptive or revisionary. One may try to make explicit the conceptual scheme we actually use, or one may argue that we ought to abandon this scheme in favour of a better one—one that is, for example, simpler, or more accurate or more useful. Although I think that revisionary metaphysics, like revisionary science, can be perfectly legitimate, my approach here will be descriptive. Within this approach one can, as indicated above, tackle two questions: first, what personal identity actually consists in and second, by what criteria we decide whether someone is or is not the same person, in the philosophical sense. The first issue, involving not only the question raised above—as to whether the self is something mental, physical, or both—but also the more basic question concerning whether there really is something, mental or physical, persisting throughout a person's existence, or simply a very complex chain of causation involving physical and mental processes in which nothing actually persists, is fascinating but very difficult. Fortunately, the relevant question here is the second one.

Moreover, the relevance to dementia becomes very quickly apparent. It seems clear that, whatever the metaphysical truth of the matter may be, the main criterion we use, and have to use, to decide whether person X (for example, the suspect) is the same as person Y (the criminal) is bodily continuity: evidence that a person who is physically the same as X or a person physically continuous with X ('a younger X') committed the crime is evidence that X did. We operate by recognizing people physically, or by recognizing their physical connection with an earlier person: and we could not do anything else. But there is another important criterion of identity, which is memory: for oneself, it is one's memories that settle the question 'Was I the person who did so-and-so?' As long as a person's memories fit with what other people saw them doing or experiencing, there is no discrepancy and thus no problem. But once they come apart, a problem arises. Sometimes the problem is easily solved: perhaps there is a reason why the person has no memory of this part of their past. For instance, perhaps they were too young, or drunk, or other people thought they saw them but did not (for example, they had an identical twin). But sometimes, in the absence of a plausible explanation, the discrepancy persists.

I suggest that this is the problem with dementia and personal identity. By normal criteria, which are physical, a person with even serious dementia is still the same person; but there are gaps in their memory, especially short-term memory. They do things they then do not remember doing and fail to recognize people they have been intimate with for years. They may also have personality changes, as a result of memory loss and these changes may well be of a distressing type, involving, for example, an inappropriate loss of self-control, or even violence. The question is 'Should we say this is the same or a different person relative to the pre-dementia person?'

One thing we could say, if the psychological discontinuity with the 'previous person' is sufficiently severely disrupted, is that what we have is a new person. That is, the gaps in memory and changes in personality are sufficiently serious for it to be appropriate to consider the previous person as having ceased to exist, so that we should not consider the pre-dementing and post-dementing person as one and the same. People do indeed sometimes talk as if this were the case: 'He's not there any more' is sometimes said. But it seems fairly clear that, whatever they say, this is not something they literally believe. Indeed, one might suggest that if this were what people really did believe they should be less distressed by the dementia of a relative: it should be easier to accept that a loved person has gone away and been replaced than that they are still here but unable to recognize their family or continue the relationship with them.

So we cannot say that the person with dementia really is a new person without doing violence to what people in general actually believe—and believe on good grounds, given our normal criteria for personal identity—even though in some ways this might reduce the distress of the family. Can we go, as it were, to the other extreme and say that this is in principle, and with regard to its effect on personal identity, no different from any other significant psychological change? People throughout their lives change their tastes, their skills, their moral qualities, the things they can remember or tend to forget, and so on, sometimes for the better and sometimes for the worse. Indeed, when these changes are radical we have a whole vocabulary and way of talking about ourselves as well as about other people that suggests that there is now a new person. This may be seen positively—'She's a new person'—or negatively— 'He's not himself any more'. But in neither case is it to be taken literally. Once again, we may note that these things might not be said with the same distress, or the same pleasure, if they were meant literally and they could not be said about oneself at all. This point is in a way summed up by the jokes about the man who came back from holiday saying, 'I'm another man: I'm myself again' and the one who took a long swig of schnapps and said 'I'm another man. I'll give the other man a drink'. Similarly, psychological changes caused by dementia, it might be said, become sometimes, as time goes on, particularly extensive and particularly distressing; but in no way do they affect a person's identity in the philosophical sense, though they do, of course, alter their psychological identity.

But once again, to take this line would not do justice to how the situation is actually perceived and how people feel. Indeed, things might be less distressing for the person and their family if the dementia could be seen just as a change, like many others. But it seems to be different, even from changes in psychological identity, in both degree and kind. This is because dementia, if it becomes severe enough, seems to produce—or to threaten the production of— a loss of identity, rather than a change: the fear is that there will be not a new person, but life without personality at all; not that there is a different person from the person one has loved or been friends with, but that this person has turned into a non-person. The assumption behind this, whether or not it is consciously expressed, seems to be that to be a person one must have a certain mental unity, an awareness of oneself as a persisting being and not just a physical continuity. This awareness is compatible with great changes in emotions, tastes, abilities, and so on and even with gaps in memory; but if it seems to have been lost or to have become only intermittent, then the fear arises that, though one is in the presence of the same physical being as before, one is no longer with the same person, or perhaps with any person. The question then is whether this fear and this reaction, however natural and intelligible, are in fact rational and appropriate. To consider this, we need to return to consider identity in the philosophical sense and whether this shows anything about psychological identity.

Identity incorporates growth and decline

In considering what in this strict sense makes a person the same person, we need to distinguish between what we actually observe and experience—experience in our own case, observe and, perhaps more importantly, relate to in the case of others—and what may or may not lie beyond this. There are perfectly legitimate questions as to whether we existed in any form before this life, whether we will survive death in any way, and whether we have any persisting self, physical or mental. But what we experience empirically is that we are born, we undergo constant change mentally and physically, and we die. That is to say, our identity has to be the identity of an impermanent and changing being, relating in all kinds of ways to other beings, especially other persons and remaining the same through these changes because of the special links to its own past and future. So I suggest that both philosophical and psychological personal identity have to include 'boundedness' (like it or not, we are all subject in the end to birth, development, decline, and death), connections to both the past and the future, and being involved in all kinds of relationships with other people. Bavidge (Chapter 2, p. 41) refers to this boundedness as the 'shape of our lives'.

If it is correct that boundedness is an essential feature of identity, two consequences may be discerned. The first is that, though serious dementia damages the awareness of identity, it does not destroy identity itself, in either the philosophical or the psychological sense. This is because it is part of our identity, like it or not, that we will certainly die and probably decline. Even though how much decline (for example, whether mentally as well as physically) varies hugely from person to person, that we are liable to decline is an essential part of what we are—just as is the fact that we have developed in all sorts of ways since birth. This is not to deny that it is a misfortune and a very distressing one, not only to the person themselves, but also, sometimes even more, to their friends and family. Nor is it to deny that decline is different from change in general. It is to claim that experience demonstrates that to be a person is to be liable not simply to change but also to gain and lose strength and ability, both mental and physical: a person is not only the sort of being that has memories and a sense of self, but also, like it or not, the sort of being that can lose memories and can lose the sense of self. This is sad and painful; but we ought not to make matters still worse when this happens to someone (mercifully, it does not happen to us all, although we are all liable to it and all vulnerable) by adopting the false idea that the identity of that person has been destroyed. We may say, metaphorically, that this has happened, as a way of indicating how sad it is that a person has largely lost awareness of their identity. But it is a metaphor: the decline is part of being a person, not part of ceasing to be one. Ceasing to be a person does not occur before death—and perhaps not even then, in the opinion of many.

This is reinforced by a second consideration. Part of our identity is our connection with our past and our future. For identity by definition is not momentary: questions of identity are not about whether a thing is at any moment identical with itself, which it obviously is, but whether it is identical with something earlier. In particular, the identity of a constantly changing being—and we really are changing physically and mentally from moment to moment, even if the changes are very small—cannot lie in how it is at any particular moment, but must essentially involve the relationships between what is happening at that moment and what has happened and will happen. Two things are involved: the relation to the future and the relation to the past. For example, our relationships with children, especially (but not only) our own, are coloured by our awareness that they are growing and developing, that is, by our awareness of the relation of present to future. We ask them what they want to be when they grow up; we make them do things that we hope will aid their development; we try to stop them doing things which may damage their development. Those parents who try, consciously or unconsciously, to 'stop the clock' or to make it go too fast, are rightly considered dangerous people.

Now this relationship to the future still exists even when there is little future left and the process is one of decline rather than growth. It is true that, though we have to die, we do not have to decline in the way in which we have to grow; and it is also true that if we could stop the clock in old age this would not be damaging in the way it would be if children could be prevented from growing older. But it remains true that the total arresting of change is impossible. Indeed it may well be that if one tried to work out the implications of such an idea one would find that it is not simply an idea of something that does not in fact happen, but of something which is actually unintelligible or senseless. Also, if we were not changing beings, we would not decline, but we also would not develop. So we have to accept not only that being liable to decline is part of being a person, but also that we could only avoid being liable to decline if we were unchanging beings who could cease at some point to have a future. This notion, though, (1) is unintelligible and (2) if it were possible, could only become reality at the price of losing our ability to develop, so that much more would be lost than gained. In other words, being liable to decline cannot be separated from being able to develop; and we could not have the one without the other. Both, moreover, are necessary consequences of being creatures that change; and this is so much part of us that we cannot even in imagination really make sense of the alternative. Hence we come to the same conclusion as that in relation to boundedness: being liable to decline is not merely part of being a person but something which must, like it or not, necessarily be part of a person and without which all that is good would also be lost. Finally, we should note that even when decline is what is mainly in evidence, there are often at least moments of development and advance, even in old age and even when dementia is progressing.

To this it might be replied that in practice, even if it is true, it is cold comfort. It may be true that being liable to decline as well as grow is a necessary part of being what we are and without it our lives would inevitably be much poorer. But being mortal is a necessary part of what we are and being immortal and still physical might inevitably be the horrific state of ever-increasing senility portrayed in Swift's *Gulliver's Travels*. Nevertheless, people die at different ages and the fact that mortality is universal is little comfort when people die before their time. Similarly, the fact that we are inevitably the kind of beings that are liable to dementia is of little comfort when faced with a relative or partner who is actually in that state. This is true, but what it shows is that the dementia gives no reason for ending the relationship or ceasing to love the person: it was a possibility, and a possibility that could not be eliminated, from the very beginning. It is not just, to repeat the point, that we are liable to decline and that for some the decline takes this very distressing form: it is also that a relationship is necessarily a relationship with someone who is, over time, both able to develop and liable to decline.

The other aspect of identity is its relation to the past. Our relation to others is coloured by what has happened and this persists even beyond the grave: many of us feel we have a relation to the dead, for example, to our deceased parents; and this is independent of whether or not we believe in survival. Because this is so, then even when a person has lost awareness of some, or much, of their past, this does not alter the value of what happened in the past or destroy their relationships with people who shared some of that past with them. The feeling exists that the present dementia somehow invalidates the healthy life of the past, but in fact it leaves it untouched; and the feeling should be rejected as being neither rational nor helpful.

To this it might be objected that, though the past cannot be altered, our attitude to it can and should be changed by later events. An obvious example would be moral changes: if a person repents of what they have done and reforms their behaviour, their previous life ought no longer to be held against them. But this applies to what a person does voluntarily: that they themselves are no longer able to remember what they shared with others, or to share those activities, does not make what happened any less valuable. On the contrary, those events have a forward effect and help to make the relationship, despite everything, still meaningful.

Conclusion

So, if we consider philosophically the question whether a person with even serious dementia retains their identity, the answer is that they do. They always were, like the rest of us, liable to such things as dementia: unfortunately, in them the liability was actualized, but this does not make them someone different. The effects of dementia do damage the awareness of one's identity and can be particularly serious and troubling. But they give us no philosophical ground for saying that the identity has been destroyed, or that the relationship with them has been destroyed or should be ended, or that the past has been in any way invalidated. In this way philosophy provides us with some consolation. The consolation is limited and cannot do a lot by itself. But it saves us from one or two errors that can destroy or damage hope and make a bad situation worse. With this modest role we should be content!

4 Identity, self, and dementia

John McMillan

Introduction

This chapter begins by distinguishing philosophical notions of personal identity from folk views of identity. Philosophers are primarily interested in identity as a 'numerical' or how it is that we know that a person is the same person over time. Folk notions of identity focus more upon 'qualitative' identity or the features that a person has. Both notions are relevant to self and dementia but folk theories are especially so. I will suggest that what people often worry about is character change and that this can be fruitfully interpreted by Charles Taylor's suggestion that there is an important connection between agency and an individual's frameworks of the good.

In 1994 the Royal Institute of Philosophy published a collection of papers from a lecture series that was promoted by the Philosophy Special Interest Group of the Royal College of Psychiatrists. *Philosophy, Psychology and Psychiatry* contains a paper on personal identity and psychiatric illness written by Tony Hope (Hope 1994). It is a paper that deserves greater attention than it has had thus far, because of the important questions that it raises about personal identity and personality change as a result of dementia.

Hope considers the case history of Mr D. This chapter will revisit the case of Mr D and make a number of related points about qualitative identity or what we might also call a person's sense of self.

Parfit on qualitative and numerical identity

It is important when thinking about personal identity and persons to draw a distinction between qualitative and numerical identity.

The evening before an important lecture I could sneak into the lecture theatre and paint the lectern yellow. The lectern that will be found in the lecture theatre the next day will look different and we would be justified in saying that the lectern is not the same. Qualitatively, a feature or property of the lectern will be different, so we are justified in saying that the qualitative identity of the lectern has changed.

Although this act would be a fairly strange and juvenile thing for me to do I might, instead, opt for an action that is even odder. I could sneak into the lecture theatre with a lectern that is exactly the same as the lectern already there and replace it with my own. If I was successful in avoiding detection then tomorrow it might be that no one apart from me knows that the lectern is not the same lectern. This is an example where the numerical identity of the lectern has changed.

One way of thinking about this is that this distinction furnishes us with two different ways of calling something 'the same'. Sameness can consist in having the same properties or it can mean that a thing is identifiable as the same thing even though many of its properties may have changed.

This distinction can be applied to the identity of persons too. Qualitatively I am a different person from the person that lived in New Zealand 6 years ago, yet there is little reason to doubt that numerically I am the same John McMillan who lived in New Zealand 6 years ago. When philosophers discuss personal identity they are usually, but not always, interested in numerical rather than qualitative identity. When most people are concerned about identity and the effect of a different outlook on life, a new job, a new relationship, or dementia they are concerned with qualitative identity. There is a complicated relationship between numerical and qualitative notions of identity that becomes important when thinking about personality change brought about by dementia. One plausible view of what numerical personal identity consists in is that it is a set of mental features of the person. John Locke (Locke 1990) thought that personal identity consists in memory over time. So it is the fact that I remember past actions and events that are the defining mark of me being the same person over time.

There is a famous objection to Locke's conception of personal identity— one that was noticed soon after he published *An Essay Concerning Human Understanding*. The problem is that our memory is all too fallible. Locke seems to imply that if I committed a crime in the past and if I cannot remember it, then I cannot be held responsible for that crime, because I am not the person that committed the crime.

Most philosophers opt for a theory of personal identity that is Lockean to the extent that it relies upon psychological components as the properties that make a person the same person over time. Parfit thinks that what he calls psychological connectedness and psychological continuity are both important for personal identity. '*Psychological connectedness* is the holding of particular direct psychological connections', while 'Psychological continuity is the holding of overlapping chains of *strong* connectedness' (Parfit 1984, p. 206).

As we are all too aware, it is very common for people to change qualitatively through dementia. Given that dementia has a profound effect upon an individual's mental life, it is entirely possible they may change so much that it raises serious doubts about whether there exists the degree of psychological continuity and connectedness necessary for numerical personal identity. Tony

Hope (1994) explores this question in his chapter in *Philosophy, Psychology and Psychiatry*. While I have a view about numerical identity, in this chapter I am going to make some suggestions about how we can frame some aspects of qualitative change in dementia.

A summary of Tony Hope's case

Mr D taught classics at a boy's preparatory school. He loved music and played the piano. He married at 25 years of age and had two daughters. He retired at age 63 because his workload was beginning to become too much for him. Soon after retirement he was diagnosed with Alzheimer's disease. At first he enjoyed retirement, but life gradually became more difficult. After about a year he became less affectionate to his wife. Things deteriorated to the point where, for the first time in their married lives, they slept in separate beds. As time went on he started to do less and less. His indifference to his wife started to become active hostility and this hostility became directed to his daughters as well. About 4 years after retirement he wandered out of the house when his wife was out shopping. The police brought him back after complaints that he was 'molesting little girls'. Apparently he had said some things to a group of schoolgirls in a shop and the shopkeeper was concerned and called the police. His physical aggression has never extended beyond pushing his wife away. He can feed himself and is fully continent. There are times when he appears to know who she is, but for much of the time he does not appear to know her.

His wife's attitude towards him has changed radically over the years. At first she did not see the changes as being the result of an illness—she thought that he had ceased to love her. The second stage was when she accepted he was ill and that he needed her help. But over the last year her attitude has changed again . . . She says that he must go into a home permanently. 'I don't see why I should have him in the house at all. It's like living with a stranger. He's not the man I married—that man has been dead for at least 2 years.' (Hope 1994, p. 133)

There are a number of ways that we might take Mrs D's statement. At face value she appears to be making a point about numerical identity in that she literally does not believe that the demented man called Mr D is the Mr D she married. She might also be taken to be saying that Mr D is so different qualitatively that the ground upon which their relationship and mutual commitment was built has been eroded.

Hope proceeds at this point to consider whether we ought to consider the demented Mr D after dementia as being a literally different person from the pre-dementia Mr D. This is a very important question, because the answer that we give will have a number of important implications in terms of how we regard Mr D's interests. If he is numerically a different person, then he would have no right to Mr D's property and other interests. Also, Mrs D and her daughters would have no moral obligations to Mr D as spouse or father over and above those that they would have to any other person with Alzheimer's disease.

I shall now turn to some considerations regarding a related dimension of the issues raised by the case of Mr D, namely the way that he has changed qualitatively or what we might also call changes in his agency or self.

Frameworks of the good and webs of interlocution

In *Sources of the Self*, Charles Taylor (1989) attempts to establish that 'selves' are necessarily tied to frameworks of value and that any investigation of human selfhood cannot escape discussion of its associated frameworks. He argues for a deep connection between selfhood and conceptions of the good. Taylor believes that frameworks that allow a consciousness of value are the result of culturally produced ways of life and that living within such frameworks constitutes the self. He says:

> ... the claim is that living within such strongly qualified horizons [or frameworks for value] is constitutive of human agency, that stepping outside these limits would be tantamount to stepping outside what we would recognise as integral, that is, undamaged human personhood.   (Taylor 1989, p. 27)

If we apply this line of thought to Mr D, it is already obvious that Alzheimer's disease has damaged his personhood. His personhood, or the things that made him the person that he was, have been radically altered by his illness. What is unclear at this stage is *how* Alzheimer's disease has caused him to step outside these frameworks, or for that matter whether this is a useful way to think about the way he has changed.

Narrative and self-conception

One of the more interesting ideas in *Sources of the Self* is the idea that knowing, forming, and articulating a sense of self is a discursive or narrative process.[1] Taylor says:

> My self-definition is understood as an answer to the question 'who am I?' And this question finds its original sense in the interchange of speakers. I define who I am by defining where I speak from, in the family tree, in social space, in the geography of social statuses and functions, in my intimate relations to the ones I love, and also crucially in the space of moral and spiritual orientation within which my most important defining relations are lived out. (Taylor 1989, p. 35)

This claim is very close to the thesis that Grant Gillett and I developed in *Consciousness and Intentionality*, namely that our identity or sense of self is defined with reference to the 'webs of interlocution' within which we live

(Gillett and McMillan 2001, p. 162). Webs of interlocution are the networks of interpersonal relations that we are immersed in, which play an important part in our formulation of a sense of self.

An interesting literary example of this is Roskolnikov, Dostoyevsky's character from *Crime and Punishment* (Dostoyevsky 1991). In his relative isolation as a penniless law student in a big city, he forms a conception of who he is and wants to be. But the fact that he knows who he is, in that sense, does not mean that he has arrived at a robust and sustainable belief in the good. In order to achieve the latter he later has to be drawn into webs of interlocution, in part by the horror of his act and in part by his real engagement with others, which provided 'defining relationships' within which his life could move forward. It seems that, by acquaintance and intentional participation, knowledge of our social relations is necessary in order to have a sense of identity. Even then our consciousness of having an identity and a self worth caring about is not totally given by any framework, but is given in addition by what goes on between people who in part constitute that framework.

Conveying a sense of who you are to another person will often involve telling them a story about your 'webs of interlocution'. Psychotherapy, for instance, demands that such reflection upon oneself takes place. It attempts to facilitate the construction of personal narratives that provide sustainable identity explanations to which one can commit oneself and which will support one at points of threat or disorientation.

This 'narrative approach' to personal identity is consistent with Kant's ideas on the matter. Kant (1929) thought that to explain agency we needed to distinguish between the empirical self and an a priori principle of apperceptive unity that is necessary to all our perceptions and reasoning. Roughly speaking, the empirical self is just like the narrative self formed in accordance with webs of interlocution: it is a potential object of thought and therefore you can think of it as existing in the past or present. The principle of apperceptive unity (the Transcendental Unity of Apperception) records the possibility that, as well as this product of conceptualization and experience there is a subjective aspect of self that can take its own mental life as an intentional object and so become self-conscious. An author engaged in writing the events of his life can, as it were, step outside the stream of narrative and see how he is getting on.

One way of taking these thoughts (about our sense of self or qualitative personal identity) is as an extension of this interpretation and amplification of the Kantian theory. We have suggested that we might call this a Transcendental Unity of Narration (Gillett and McMillan 2001, p. 162). Kant, at some points, did not stress the importance of a speech community's influence upon general (or discursive) concepts. Narratives formed on the basis of our webs of interlocution can fill in the gaps that might be read into the Kantian theory. Such theories imply that to discover (or make sense of) who the empirical self is, we must think how this self fits into spheres of interaction, how its actions are consistent, and why it performed certain actions (Harré and Gillett 1994).

Although Taylor is quite right about the narrative nature of creating a sense of identity, we should not think that agency is simply constituted by the value frameworks or webs of interlocution in which we live. Paying attention to the other half of Kant's theory of the self will help to avoid this pitfall. There must exist some faculty with which to reflect upon the meaningfulness of the empirical self, which can, as it were, distance itself as subjectivity from the narrative of lived conscious experience and hold it up to the light of reflection. This does not mean that you have to accept what Kant says about the matter. Yet some story must be told about how it is possible, without some such faculty of self-distancing, to consider one's life meaningful and able to be reformed according to one's current assessments of value. When we speak of agency we mean not just our empirical selves, but also the faculty by which we make meaningful choices and through them influence the unfolding nature of the empirical self. We must, however, guard against the mistake of reifying an extensionless point of willing that drives the self this way and that without significant constraint from within the lived narrative. This would be, in a sense, a denial of the progressive formation of self and consciousness by lived experience with others.

Taylor thinks there is a fatal flaw in the conceptions of personal identity espoused by Locke (1990) and Hume (1956) and carried through into the writings of Derek Parfit (1984), where we lose sight of the unifying, morally committed narrator altogether. Taylor says,

> . . . what has been left out is precisely the mattering. The self is defined in neutral terms, outside of any essential framework of questions. In fact, of course, Locke recognises that we are not indifferent to ourselves; but he has no inkling of the self as a being which essentially is constituted by a certain mode of self-concern—in contrast to the concern we cannot but have about the quality of our experiences as pleasurable or painful.

> This is what I want to call the 'punctual' or 'neutral' self—'punctual' because the self is defined in abstraction from any constitutive concerns and hence from any identity in the sense in which I have been using the term . . . Its only constitutive property is self awareness.   (Taylor 1989, p. 49)

Taylor might be making a mistake here, because Locke, Hume, and Parfit should be read as being primarily interested in numerical identity. Where Taylor is right is that we do want an account of identity that does justice to the sense of coherence and meaningfulness that our notion of agency implies. Without considering the narrative nature of our construction of the empirical self it is hard to arrive at such a conception.

Mr D and the qualitative self

I have suggested that our webs of interlocution are the foundation upon which our sense of self or qualitative identity is formed and that a typical instance of self-articulation involves developing a first-person narrative about our webs of interlocution. At first this does not look like a promising way to think about the changes in Mr D. Given the extent to which his dementia has altered his ability to think, reflect, and act upon what is important to him, he is not going to produce an account of his change in identity. However, when thinking about numerical identity the aim is to come up with an account of how it is that we can identify an individual as the same individual over time. These are conditions that can be applied in a third-person way. I think that we can make a similar move for Mr D. Given his past dedication to family and marriage, his wife's views about his change are crucially important. She has been married to him for most of their lives and knows, possibly almost as well as the pre-dementia Mr D would have known, what his webs of interlocution or frameworks of value were. So she is in a good position to give a narrative account of his agency and how dementia has damaged it.

Of course, it might reasonably be pointed out that Mrs D's narrative will be shaped and coloured by her recent experiences and her perspective as the spouse of Mr D. Furthermore, she does not have direct access to Mr D's mental life and it may be that he kept things from her. However, third-person perspectives can be relevant for self-conception. If I have a picture of myself as a charming and kind person, this is open to refutation by evidence to the contrary from those who know me well. I might come to revise my self-conception in the light of such evidence, but it is also possible that I might remain in ignorance and a third party might have a more accurate view on the kind of person I am. In such a case my first-person perspective of my self-conception would contain a falsehood.

There is an alternative way to take Mrs D's comment that 'It's like living with a stranger. He's not the man I married—that man has been dead for at least two years.' We know that there have been profound changes in Mr D. He has gone from being an active person to one who is very inactive. His not knowing who she is when they have shared most of their lives together must be deeply hurtful to her. The interpersonal nature of a long-term relationship is such that it would have been a very significant component of Mrs D's sense of who she is. When this is coupled with his antisocial behaviour towards her and other women—all behaviours radically at odds with who Mr D was—this disruption of their webs of interlocution could lead someone to say that the person that was Mr D is now dead, in the sense that he is a completely different kind of person. If all of the most significant components of what it was that made him the kind of person he was have changed, then Mr D may be said to have become like another person.

While this does not have the same radical implications that a change in numerical identity might have, it could have a number of moral implications. The kind of person that Alzheimer's disease has produced is so different from the man that Mrs D knew for all those years, it might mean she no longer feels she has the obligations to him that she once had. These obligations were built upon mutual concern and respect, as well as the projects that they undertook as a married couple. Since Alzheimer's disease has stopped Mr D's engagement in these value frameworks or webs of interlocution, it has undermined the basis for their mutual obligation.

While questions about the numerical identity of those with dementia are important, I think that we also need to be mindful of accounts that illuminate the qualitative features of personhood. In this discussion I have attempted to show that the changes brought on by dementia go beyond the narrow questions about whether a person is, in a numerical sense, the same person.

Endnote

1 This idea is also developed by Rom Harré and Grand Gillet in *The Discursive Mind* (Harré and Gillett 1994).

References

Dostoyevsky, F. (1991). *Crime and Punishment*. London: Penguin.

Gillett, G., McMillan, J. (2001). *Consciousness and Intentionality*. Amsterdam and Philadelphia: John Benjamin.

Harré, R., Gillett, G. (1994). *The Discursive Mind*. London: Sage.

Hope, T. (1994). Personal identity and psychiatric illness. In: *Philosophy, Psychology and Psychiatry* (ed. A. Phillips Griffiths). pp. 131–43. Cambridge: Cambridge University Press.

Hume, D. (1956). [1738] *A Treatise of Human Nature, Book One*. London: J. M. Dent.

Kant, I. (1929). [1787] *Critique of Pure Reason* (trans. N. Kemp Smith). Hampshire: Macmillan Press.

Locke, J. (1990). [1689] *An Essay Concerning Human Understanding*. Oxford: Oxford University Press.

Parfit, D. (1984). *Reasons and Persons*. Oxford: Clarendon Press.

Taylor, C. (1989). *Sources of the Self: The Making of Modern Identity*. Cambridge: Cambridge University Press.

5 Into the darkness: losing identity with dementia[1,2]

Jennifer Radden and Joan M. Fordyce

Introduction

That some sort of personal identity is lost when dementias ravage the brain seems indisputable. But what kind of identity is lost and what unchanged aspect of the person other than the endurance of the body, might—at least for a time—be retained? One short answer lies in philosophical traditions deriving from Locke's discussion, wherein personal identity depends on the very memory whose failure is a harbinger of dementia: from the onset of the disease, on such an account, identity disappears. Personal and self-identity are complex, multi-stranded concepts, however, which show up in many different discourses. This is particularly evident in English-language writing on the identity of persons, which has undergone a sea change in the last 15 or 20 years. Such writing now reveals greater acknowledgement of Continental European traditions and reflects emotional valences absent from previous discussions. Our guiding presumption here is that there are several ways of talking about identity—so when some forms of identity are eroded through dementia, other forms may yet be ascribed. These more enduring aspects of identity, it is our hope, can illuminate certain ethical quandaries over how to feel about and respond to those suffering from the conditions that cause dementia.

In Part 1, we introduce some variations on traditional discussions of identity and personal identity from Leibniz and Locke, respectively. These variations include Paul Ricoeur's contrast between *ipse* and *idem* identity and aspects of one loose but influential sense of identity informing present day identity politics. In Part 2, we explore the implications of these alternative conceptions of identity in relation to dementia and to some of the ethically troubling questions it raises.

Part 1: oneself as another

Ipse and *idem* identity

Paul Ricoeur begins his volume *Soi-meme comme un Autre* (*Oneself as Another*) with an explication of his title and a fundamental distinction: that between identity understood in terms of the Latin *ipse* and *idem* (Ricoeur 1990, 1992). *Idem* identity he takes as the equivalent of 'sameness', *ipse* identity, or *ipseity* as 'selfhood'. *Idem* or sameness identity is in some respects closer to philosophical conceptions of personal identity in the English-speaking tradition from Locke. Of this *idem* identity, Ricoeur says that it concerns the question 'What am I?' and 'unfolds an entire hierarchy of significations . . .'; of these, 'permanence in time constitutes the highest order, to which will be opposed that which differs, in the sense of [being] changing or variable' (Ricoeur 1992, p. 2). *Ipse* or selfhood, identity in contrast, concerns the question of 'Who am I?'. *Ipse* identity involves 'the dialectic of *self* and *other than self*' (Ricoeur 1992).[3]

Now we begin to understand Ricoeur's title: the selfhood of oneself implies otherness to such an intimate degree, as he puts it, that 'one cannot be thought of without the other, that . . . one passes into the other, as we might say in Hegelian terms'. The meaning here is not merely a matter of comparison, he stresses. It is rather an 'implication': not oneself as similar to, but oneself 'inasmuch as being' another (Ricoeur 1992, p. 3).[4]

For those who have struggled to understand dementia within the constraints of the philosophical traditions deriving from Locke's discussion, welcome new possibilities and fresh questions emerge with each aspect of Ricoeur's distinction. Unlike identity judgements, judgements about the sameness of two or more items sometimes admit of degree. By replacing the absolute judgement of identity with the relative judgement of 'sameness', we can perhaps better accommodate the elusive remaining elements of the earlier person left by dementia. To support and bolster that lingering sameness, we may be able to attribute aspects of selfhood, or *ipse*, identity to the person with dementia. When all thought processes and memory appear to have been eroded, there might yet be sense to speaking of the person with dementia as remaining themselves 'inasmuch as being' another. And such an expanded notion of personal identity will perhaps help us with some ethically puzzling questions about the person with dementia: what is owed them—in treatment, in attitudes, in rights? To what are they entitled, not merely out of respect for their humanity generally understood, or in honour of the person they once were, but *because they are still that person*?

Along with Ricoeur's notions of *ipse* and *idem* identity, but looser and more political, conceptions nourished by some of the same influences as Ricoeur's will prove fruitful as we explore these possibilities. Familiar from Anglo-American political and feminist philosophy and from what is sometimes known as identity politics, such conceptions of identity are associated with what has come to be called the politics of recognition. These discussions will encourage us to consider unexplored and under-emphasized continuities on the basis of which we may speak of the person with dementia as the same as their old self. And acknowledging the role of others in identity construction will invite a theme we develop in this chapter: that other people might sustain someone's identity as her own capacity to do so is eroded.

Identity in the politics of recognition

Several distinguishable strands contribute to the identity of identities politics and questions of political recognition. Apparently growing out of a Hegelian, communitarian, and relational sense of self, this way of speaking portrays identities as constituted by their culture and affiliations. This 'identity' plays a central part in a range of discourses today—from the public, political, and legal, to the personal, private, and literary.

Two further features are now widely accepted as constitutive parts of the identity of persons. Such identity deserves public or political 'recognition' and is attributable as much (or more) to collectives as to their individual members.[5] This kind of identity is associated with ethnic, racial, class, and gender politics. But arguably, it will also help us see how to respond in the face of the depleted identity of those with dementia.

Characterization identity

New terms and contrasts have been introduced to separate the more political, and more recent, types of identity discourse. Marya Schechtman speaks of identity as concerning *characterization* (Schechtman 1996). (The identity associated with earlier theorizing in the Lockean tradition she designates *reidentification* identity, in contrast.) For Schechtman characterization identity is 'the set of characteristics each person has that make her the person she is', so that 'a person's identity is defined in terms of her characteristics, actions and experiences' (Schechtman 1996, p. 74). A person's identity comes in the form of a self-narrative in the work of many who employ these categories, including Schechtman. The actions and experiences making up that narrative comprise the personal story of which the subject stands as 'author'.[6]

The notion of characterization identity captures other presuppositions found in less formal discussions of identity as well, particularly those associated with the politics of recognition. We shall adopt the term 'characterization identity' and focus attention on a handful of these presuppositions and emphases—the active role of the subject in identity construction; the idea of collective authorship; certain emotional valences; and the notion of narrativity. These several foci are laid out below, along with the ways in which Ricoeur's *ipse* or *selfhood* identity both echoes and also diverges from this notion of characterization identity.

Active, collective authorship of the self-narrative

Characterization identity emphasizes and presupposes activity and active involvement on the part of the subject (and others). First, identity is achieved through creative construction by the 'author(s)' of the self-'narrative'. This is portrayed as a complex, active engagement involving selection, imaginative appropriation, emphasis, interpretation, framing, and forgetting. Moreover, it is a continuing, if not continuous, activity: once achieved, the person's identity must be maintained through the same active process, as life unfolds and new experiences affect the self. Identity, it is often emphasized, entails the *on-going* integration of possible perspectives and versions of who an individual is into a coherent and meaningful life story (Taylor 1989; Benhabib 1992, 2002; Alcott 2000). The active aspect of (narrative) identity construction is a central element in Ricoeur's account also: self-understanding is for him an *interpretation* of the self, which

> finds in the narrative . . . a privileged form of mediation [involving] . . . the *interweaving* of the historiographic style of biographies with the novelistic style of imaginary autobiographies. (Ricoeur 1992, p. 114, our emphasis)

Also presupposing an active subject is the effort of identification by which one embraces the affiliative constituents representing one's identity (one's nationality—Australian-ness, gender—femaleness and femininity, professional role, and so on) and identifies with one's affiliates (others so identified, such as Australians, women, and so on). This emphasis on the active process of 'identifying with' also comports with Ricoeur's account. To a large extent, he says,

> . . . the identity of a person or a community is made up of these *identifications* with values, norms, ideals, models, and heroes *in* which the person or the community recognizes itself. . . . The identification with heroic figures clearly displays this otherness assumed as one's own . . . . (Ricoeur 1992, p. 121, our emphasis)

So in constructing oneself, and in identifying with others, one is an active participant in the formation of one's own characterization identity.

Nor are the narratives of characterization identity solely 'authored' works. These identities are constituted, it is widely agreed, by a complex interaction between first-, second-, and third-person perspectives (Nelson 2001; Baier 1985, 1991; Taylor 1989, 1995; Code 1991; Alcott 2000). The very self-awareness required to possess an identity depends upon and grows out of the contribution, and particularly the recognition, of other persons, as well as deriving from otherness as such (Glas 2003, in press). From Hegel to Foucault, as one recent analysis observes, 'the Other . . . is accorded the power to recognize, to name, even to constitute one's identity' (Alcott 2000, p. 332). Emphasis on the part played by others in the construction of an identity is nicely secured by Hilda Lindemann Nelson's definition of identity as a relationship between more than one person. Identity, she notes, means 'the *interaction* of a person's self conception with how others conceive her' (Nelson 2001, p. 6, our emphasis).

These conceptions of the part played by others in identity construction run contrary to much in North American culture, where individualistic and narcissistic presuppositions and, we might say, (socially inscribed) delusions, lead to a systematic under-statement of our dependency on other people in most of our endeavours (Baier 1985, 1991). They also challenge the individualistic self found in the traditional Anglo-American political philosophy deriving from Hobbes and Locke. In such work, as more recent corrections from feminist theorists and communitarians have made clear, identity is misleadingly portrayed as a self-creation unaided by other people (Sandel 1982; Shanley and Pateman 1991; Meyers 1997).

Reflecting the Hegelian traditions from which these less individualistic ideas arose, the other authors of a person's characterization identity are sometimes referred to as the Other (as in the quotation from Alcott above). Yet 'the Other' is ambiguous in theorizing today, often referring to other people, sometimes to those persons and qualities defined in contrast to a given norm or norms, and sometimes, simply, to otherness or difference. Recognizing this ambiguity, Ricoeur speaks of the *polysemic* character of otherness, which implies that, as he puts it, the Other 'is not reduced to the otherness of another person' but has additional meaning as well (Ricoeur 1992, p. 317). To avoid confusion we henceforth refer to the second and third persons participating in the construction of identity as 'others' or 'other persons'.

In restricting our interpretation of 'oneself as another' to the collective authorship of characterization identities by other people we diverge from Ricoeur, who weaves into his account of *ipse* identity two of the meanings of Other (other people and otherness or difference). The Other, as he puts it, 'stands opposite the Same, in the sense of oneself (*soi-meme*)' (Ricoeur 1992, p. 318). Otherness understood as the intrinsic duality that binds and separates the self from 'other than self' is for Ricoeur a constitutive characteristic of *ipse* identity.

That being said, however, the present exploration is less theoretical than practical and our focus is on other persons rather than otherness as such. Without denying their importance to a complete account of *ipseity*, we set aside here those other dualities between mind and body, subject and experience, and self and conscience through which Ricoeur completes his account of ipseity.[7]

The part of others in self-constitution introduces limitations. My identity can be, and indeed must be, selective. It is, after all, a partly aspirational construct. The possible versions selected in the construction of a coherent and meaningful self-narrative are not entirely idiosyncratic, nor unlimited, though. They are rather, as Benhabib puts it, 'part of a cultural web' of narratives, any one of which will be '*available* to the individual' (Benhabib 1992, p. 56). Though the resulting story will be, in Ricoeur's words, '. . . an unstable mixture of fabulation and actual experience', the ingredient of fabulation will be a *constrained* fabulation (Ricoeur 1992, p. 162).

In contrast to this emphasis on the active, social process required for characterization identity, the notion of personal identity in traditions deriving from Locke leaves the subject, in a sense, inert. Identity is not actively constructed through any intentional or particular efforts by the subject or by others and questions about the collective or sole authorship of identities do not arise—or remain without salience—in discussions of such identity.

Recognition

Modern day characterization identity is associated with certain fundamental emotional valences, or attitudes. The impulse for recognition as an identity is one of these. That impulse is the engine fuelling identity politics and the movement of groups demanding minority rights, for example. I identify as a member of—and identify with—some group; at the same time I demand recognition for that group's identity along with my own (Fraser, 1997). This is portrayed as an important moral and political right, moreover, not merely a widespread psychological inclination. In Taylor's words 'The withholding of recognition can be a form of oppression' (Taylor 1995, p. 232). We return to the moral significance of this point later in this chapter.

Focus here is on the impulse toward recognition understood as a psychological attribute. We do not mean to deny the underlying theoretical bases of such a conception derived from Hegelian writing. However, our limited goal here is to explicate the notion of characterization identity as it has emerged in recent, English-speaking political philosophy, rather than to uncover the whole, theoretical superstructure to which the psychological attribute can be traced.

In some political and psychoanalytic accounts the impulse for recognition as an identity is an almost irresistibly strong tendency. Thus, for instance, Judith Butler portrays us as prepared to pay the price of the misrepresentation (interpellation) of our identity for achieving its recognition. (As Butler graphically explains it, '. . . a subject is hailed, the subject turns around, and the subject then accepts the terms by which he or she is hailed' (Butler 1997, p. 106); and she speaks of 'a certain readiness to be compelled by the authoritative interpellation'(Butler 1997, p. 111).) However weakly or strongly it is understood, most theorizing implies that, today at least, this impulse for recognition is a universal one.[8]

In contrast to this emphasis on identity recognition, classical accounts of personal identity in the Lockean tradition ignore this aspect of identity recognition or at most represent a subject indifferent as to its identity.

Narrativity

Like Riceour's *ipse* identity, characterization identity is closely tied to notions of a self-narrative. But the substance of that narrative, and particularly its degree of coherence and unity, are issues generating extensive controversy.

Some thinkers not only insist that human existence is fundamentally temporal but also imply that it is experienced as a single, continuous narrative. Others reject the notions of both a unified self or author and of a coherent and unified self-narrative, insisting that individual experience is too fractured, uncertain, and contingent to permit full narrative structure. Those writing about narrativity range themselves between these two extremes, as James Phillips has shown in a recent discussion (Phillips 2003). Phillips aligns himself with Ricoeur (and Alasdair MacIntyre (MacIntyre 1984)) in accepting narrative identity as closer to a task or project accomplished by the individual than to a 'simple unified story . . . laid down in advance'. Yet narrative identity has a fictive, imaginary dimension in that '. . . it is the challenge of each individual to take the raw, given features of his or her life and to mold them into a meaningful and intelligible narrative structure'(Phillips 2003, p. 315).

Because of these differing understandings of narrativity, we refrain from linking any one account of narrativity with characterization identity as it has been outlined thus far. Whichever version of narrative identity is adopted, however, there will likely be acknowledgement that human activities share some of the formal properties of narrative—particularly that of deriving intelligibility from historical sequences with beginnings, middles, and endings.

Part 2: some ethical implications

The person with dementia eventually may lose all self-awareness and with it any sense of their own identity.[9] Arguably, however, the loss of an awareness of self-identity is distinct from loss of identity as such. Here we set aside more rigid, memory-based conceptions of personal identity, from the Lockean tradition, in favour of looser ones of sameness or 'survival'. The exploration which follows will involve two parts. We consider first the sense, other than the immediate bodily one, in which the person remains the same, survives, or remains a unity, when severe dementia compromises memory. Our second inquiry is into whether—and, if so, how—the efforts of others may be sufficient to sustain a person's characterization identity, at least for a time, as the dementia worsens. The guiding assumption is that the account of characterization identity sketched here, bolstered by appeal to Ricoeur's *ipse* identity with which it has much in common, offers us the means of approaching some of the practical, ethical problems we encounter when confronting advanced dementia.

Dementia, sameness, and singularity

Identity conveys not only sameness but oneness, a point perhaps insufficiently stressed in Ricoeur's account of *idem* identity with its emphasis on sameness through time. Such sameness is compatible with an enduring plurality, so to

Ricoeur's emphasis on sameness must be added separate acknowledgement of singularity. In non-empirical theories of the self such as the Kantian one, the transcendental self or subject ensures oneness as well as sameness: there, the self remains unchanged through time as well as being a unified and coherent whole. But in psychological theories of self, each aspect of identity—sameness or survival, on the one hand, and singularity, on the other—must be addressed on its own.

Our exploration, thus, actually involves two questions. First, even in advanced dementia when memory becomes defective, there might remain some enduring attributes—other than spatio-temporal continuity and the unchanging persistence of bodily properties—sufficient to entitle us to say that the person has, to some degree, and for a little more time, survived. What enduring attributes might they be? Second, and separately, might there remain a coherence, singularity, or oneness to the person even when stricken this way?

Before considering the quest for some unchanging, non-bodily attributes sufficient for personal survival, it is necessary to introduce the language of survival, which serves the same purpose as Ricoeur's 'sameness' in this discussion and functions as 'sameness' would. This language (of survival) is associated with Derek Parfit (Parfit 1984), whose rejection of the metaphysical presuppositions of a transcendental subject of experiences opens the possibility that the continuity and connectedness between earlier and later stages of the purely empirical, psychological self admit of degree; Parfit emphasizes that such 'survival' will not be a discovery, but a decision. On a suitably adjusted survival threshold, the sameness or survival of a handful of attributes, or even a single attribute, may entitle us to pronounce some degree of survival between the earlier person we knew and the much-changed person with dementia we now encounter. We may elect to say that person X survives or is the same person with their affliction, even if they retain only their characteristic good manners and apologetic smile.[10]

Other than by adopting a suitably adjusted survival threshold along the lines proposed by Parfit, can we make the case for sameness with any plausibility? Certainly a person is more than their cognitive capabilities. Agnieszka Jaworska begins her important discussion of persons suffering Alzheimer's disease and the capacity to value with a quote from Luria: '[A] man does not consist of memory alone. He has feeling, will, sensibilities, moral being . . .' (Jaworska 1997). This passage is emblematic for Jaworska: having a normative conception of oneself, and what she calls a 'practical identity', she insists, '. . . need not involve pondering the narrative of one's whole life' (Jaworska 1997, p. 119). It can involve being a 'valuer'. This trait of being a valuer, fortunately, long remains intact in the person with Alzheimer's, who apparently values, savours, and appreciates experiences with some intensity and with the appearance of a rationale (Jaworska 1997, p. 120).

Anecdotal evidence is rich with examples of the persistence of personal traits even after extensive memory loss: the enjoyment of music, food, and simple repetitive games and activities, the feel of another's hand stroking the face. Such simple pleasures persist and are stable and they outlast more seemingly sophisticated and more cognitive traits.

Jaworska provides some neurobiological support for her claim. At the early stages of Alzheimer's disease, she notes, the neuronal damage affects primarily the hippocampus, whose functions include the acquisition and processing of long-term explicit memory for facts and events and transforming fresh short-term into lasting long-term memories. Moreover, other regions of the brain are primarily responsible for interactions of reasoning and decision-making processes—especially those concerned with personal and social matters—with feelings and emotions. And damage to these regions is most likely to compromise a person's ability to value (Jaworska 1997, p. 122).

In drawing attention to the way the ability to value is relatively unaffected in Alzheimer's sufferers and to the stability of their value preferences, Jaworska's purpose was to unseat a conception of autonomy that places too much emphasis on the states and capabilities reliant on certain aspects of memory. But regardless of its role in autonomy, at least the well-sustained capacity to value, as Jaworska understands it, apparently constitutes a set of traits that remain relatively unchanged through time. As a *valuer* if not as a *rememberer* of the narrative of her life, the person survives the effects of Alzheimer's.

Further into the darkness, we know, even the valuer will be lost. Eventually, little but spatio-temporal continuity and enduring physical properties will remain to warrant a judgement of sameness-based identity here. Yet this leads us to the second question asked above—whether there might remain a singularity or oneness to the person even when, except for bodily unity, all else seems to have disappeared.

Embodiment conceals several different forms of unity (Radden 2003). Rather than scattered across space and time, my body is a single entity, pursuing its own, unique spatio-temporal path. In addition though, embodiment provides an everyday, minimal identity or agency which ensures, for example, that when I move, I do so as a coordinated and unified whole. And this unity, we suggest, will be slow to disappear.

The predictable sequence of disabilities that, at least as Shenk portrays it, seems exactly to reverse the order of a young child's developmental milestones, ends with the loss of the infant's first four achievements. Initially, the dementia patient can no longer walk unaided; then they can no longer sit up without assistance; next, they cannot smile; and finally, they cannot hold up their head (Shenk 2002, pp. 122–23).

This poignant progression is strikingly sad, but it is also telling in a way relevant to our discussion. Long after more complex, memory-dependent capabilities have been lost and perhaps, too, after the 'valuer' has disappeared, the patient continues to move as a coordinated, unitary whole. They walk; later when they cannot walk, they sit unaided, and smile. Even the last to go, the simple ability to hold up their head, reflects evidence of a certain coherence and directedness that bespeaks executive function.

Its very ubiquity makes this particular kind of (what might be called) 'coordination unity' easy to overlook. After infancy, human beings are deprived of it only in the rarest of instances (Gazzaniga 1979). One such instance is the neurological disorder known as 'anarchic hand syndrome', where separate limbs move as if from separate volition; another is post-operative commissurotomy patients who occasionally exhibit behavioural incoherences suggesting not uncoordinated, but *separately* coordinated, hand movements.

Coordination unity is far from full agency: at most it suggests what Jaworska calls the 'margins' of agency. Nonetheless, through that long decline until the patient can no longer lift their head, some faint hint remains of the unified, executive core we associate with full agency.

Collective authorship and the right to recognition

Theoretical accounts of the part played by others in the construction of characterization identities raise certain questions and tensions. Forming one's own identity seems to be part of the widely accepted, apparently *individually, as well as* collectively exercised, political right to self-determination. Yet it is also acknowledged that our identity construction is for, and must be answerable to, the judgements of others and that without the recognition of others and the assistance they provide in identity construction, such characterization identity would be impossible. In addition, people around us place limits on identity construction and maintenance: as we saw earlier, the self-narrative is constrained by a range of options conforming to consensual realities.

In the case of dementia this tension around the role of others in characterization identity construction becomes more pronounced. The delicate, usually wordless, collective effort that results in the construction and maintenance of normal characterization identities will not long be unaffected by the social disruptions resultant from such disorder. The customary tacit negotiation between first-, second- and third-person perspectives will likely be severely compromised by the disabilities, dysfunctions, and deficits associated with conditions like Alzheimer's disease; it will also be affected by the responses those deficits engender in others.

On analogy with the notion of collectively wrought characterization identity construction, we want to explore collective characterization identity maintenance or sustenance. Ricoeur's emphasis has been on the way the *formation* of a person's *ipse* identity depends on and is matched by the ipsiety of those around them. But his account readily allows us to extend the 'bipolar' or reciprocal phenomenon to cover the *sustaining* of the dementia sufferer's *ipse* identity though the attention of others.

The model of collective identity sustenance requires others to do more and to do it differently. (This will be familiar, of course, to anyone whose loved one suffered dementia.) Increasingly, others must remember, reinforce, and reinscribe the identity of the person with dementia. In Ricoeur's terms, this involves others holding and preserving the dementia sufferer's *ipse* identity as, and to the extent that, their own grasp on it weakens.

The construction and sustaining of the person's characterization identity have been, until the deficits of dementia make themselves known, collective efforts conducted largely tacitly. Increasingly, as these deficits erode aspects of the person's memory and self-awareness, the task will come to include the provision of explicit identity recognition—a response that says, in some form, 'this is who you are and what you are like'. This increasing task of explicit identity recognition is matched by the multitude of ways those around them increasingly maintain the persons's identity *without* recourse to words of any kind. In seeking to bring comfort to the 'valuer' after the 'rememberer' has disappeared, other people provide favourite experiences, honour long-preferred ways of doing things, recognize and cater to idiosyncratic habits, and so on. (One elderly woman for whom personal appearance had always been especially important, was faithfully taken for hairdressing and manicuring and attired elegantly long after she had lost the power to request such attention or to see to or even—apparently—to appreciate these niceties herself. Another was provided the simple pleasures of ice cream and the feeling of beach sand between her toes.)

Until now, also, to the extent that others were called on to sustain the identities of those around them, this task will have been largely mutual. Other people will have helped sustain, just as they helped constitute, my identity at the same time as I helped maintain (and constitute) theirs. Now, however, the task of holding and preserving the identity of the person suffering dementia will come to be placed more squarely on the shoulders of others (often, these are the shoulders of second persons, intimates, and the customary societal carers, women).

The most noticeable initial problem with this model is perhaps the discomfort and sense of falsity it sometimes brings upon those others left with the burden of sustaining the identity of a loved one through these processes of holding, reinforcing, and reinscribing. Although perhaps a distorted reaction, the response is often angry and disappointed. The loved identity seems to have gone—replaced by an alien changeling, it sometimes seems, or by no one. '*This is what you were and were like*' we want to say to the dementia sufferer, '*but no more!*'

The sadness, frustration, shock, disorientation, anger, and even antipathy in those others whose task this has become will often make it a painful and challenging one. (Ricoeur's treatment of the body as both part of, and alien from, oneself, may explain some of the negative feelings evoked in other people by the dementia sufferer: their repugnance is to this demonstration of the body as alien and other, as Phillips has pointed out.[11])

The heart-breaking aspect of this task of sustaining characterization identity cannot be ignored. Nonetheless, it is an enterprise apparently required by the very notion of characterization identity as that identity has been defined and explained here.

The demands on those caring for the person with dementia, which derive from the notion of characterization identity, are several and fall into what looks to be a group of separable imperatives. First, such identity, we saw, is an evolving, not a static condition: as life experiences affect the person, their characterization identity, and thus their self-narrative, adjust to accommodate those changes. So the elegiac finality of 'this is who you were, and were like' is, arguably, an inappropriate and even a morally insufficient response. New experiences and realities can and perhaps should be woven into the narratives other people now increasingly construct.[12]

This proposal has significant practical consequences. When a family decides to spare a person with dementia from painful news (the fact that a grown child had divorced his spouse, or become ill, for example), this suggests they may be failing to honour the on-going nature of this characterization identity. Though it will provoke suffering (albeit a short-lived state), perhaps the patient should be told. Even interpretations of the disease's symptoms and course may perhaps be required of those undertaking this difficult sustenance task.

The second imperative is theoretical as well as practical. To turn away from the task of sustaining the characterization identity of the person with dementia suggests a failure to acknowledge the extent that the construction of the identity before the illness was a product of others as well as of the person themselves. Consistency suggests that what was begun by others should be continued by them. And this point would not so readily be lost from sight were the distorting ideology of individualism, which casts each person the master of their fate and captain of their soul, to be replaced with more realistic, collectivist assumptions—as it surely should be. This is a task that, due to their part as co-constructors of others' characterization identities, carers and loved ones may owe the person with dementia.

Next, if we accept the modern political conception of characterization identity we understand that the urge for recognition has significant moral as well as theoretical and psychological status. To return to Taylor's words, quoted earlier, the withholding of recognition may be a form of oppression. In failing to sustain the characterization identity of the person with dementia, we may be failing to honour what is believed a universal political or liberty right to recognition. It is true that the patient with advanced dementia may have lost the desire for an identity. But that may not exempt us from the obligation to sustain such an identity for them. In other cases, notably that of infants, human rights are not curtailed because of the rights bearers' inability to understand or demand what is owed them. So it is difficult to see why they should be in the case regarding the right of the person with dementia to (identity) recognition.[13]

Each one of the preceding points constitutes a moral and theoretical rejoinder in the face of the repugnance intimate others sometimes feel when shouldering the burden of sustaining characterization identity. A final, more positive consideration is that the effect of sustaining characterization identity seems likely to enhance and support the autonomy of the person with dementia; it will help them set and meet goals and to make meaningful practical decisions within their capabilities.

Preferences and proclivities, values and ideals, form a central and as we have seen a relatively stable and enduring, part of any characterization identity. And such traits are the building blocks of meaningful practical decisions, because such decisions regularly require a choice between competing courses of action based on preferences. In fact, as Jaworska has emphasized, autonomy requires a valuer. So the steps we can take to support autonomy on the one hand, and on the other hand to sustain identity in the way described—and pre-scribed—here, will often go hand in hand. Sustaining characterization identity will serve to enhance autonomy and supporting autonomy will prove one important way of sustaining characterization identity. Such entwining is evident in the following account of the way two adult sisters helped their father (J) decide, when he left the family house for alternative accommodation, to replace a piece of furniture—his worn couch. (Rather than a rare case of a decision made possible and partly constituted by others, we stress the everydayness of this account: others frequently help in such ways, of course.)

> The 30-year-old couch was a reminder of happy family times; it bore repairs J had completed himself; it was of a quality difficult to replace today; even the damaged upholstery, scratched by his dog, reminded this old man of companionably sharing the couch with the dog for recent afternoon naps. Yet there were equally compelling, competing considerations. The couch was beyond mending; it was disagreeably shabby; indeed it was so worn and unattractive that its very presence would serve as a discouragement to the visitors and guests whose company J hoped to enjoy in his new accommodations. Remembering and evaluating this complex and incommensurable set of facts, preferences, and memories to reach a decision over the couch proved, at first, a daunting challenge because of J's advancing dementia. He wavered and hesitated, forgot, remembered, and began over, entirely unable to keep in view all the factors and their respective weights. Once they recognized the complexities that placed this task beyond J's capabilities his daughters were able to find a way to assist. In one long, concentrated discussion, they supported J through the decision process by keeping in their minds all the strands and significances he seemed beyond retaining, and proffering them when they were called for. Thus prompting and reminding J as he proceeded, they helped him work towards a resolution of this dilemma. Afterwards, J's daughters served as witnesses to the decision and to the reasoning by which it had been reached; they were able to remind him that, how, and when, the determination to replace the couch had come about.

This was a collective effort that supported and assisted J while allowing him to participate in what was, in a certain qualified way, 'his' decision. But—and this was the point of the example—it also served to reinforce and reinscribe important aspects of J's characterization identity: his role as provider, fixer, and appreciator of good furniture; his fondness for and appreciation of the dog; his hopes for the pleasures of a new home and the social opportunities it would provide. In rehearsing each of the considerations affecting J's decision, his daughters served to sustain, reinforce, reinscribe, and so to *recognize* his characterization identity. Supporting his autonomy proved a way to sustain his identity as well.

Commenting on the contested interpretations of the self as 'author' of the self-narrative in his discussion, Phillips makes reference to the erosion or loss of a narrating subject with the advance of dementia. The tragic absence of narrative identity in dementia, as he puts it, 'requires a looser, minimized . . . notion of the narrative self' (Phillips 2003, p. 326). About the same diminution of the narrator and narrative wrought by advanced dementia, Gerrit Glas has observed that there remains a deep intuition that 'even when all narrativizing has gone' there is a residual personhood that 'should not be violated'(Glas 2003, p. 349). This dimension of personhood, Glas insists, 'transcends the sphere of self-determination and sees personhood from a second person perspective, that is, the perspective of who I am in the eyes of others'(Glas 2003).

The example of J's couch will again prove useful as we try to understand these observations. First, theories of narrativity are grounded in the normal case, yet, as these authors acknowledge, pathology such as J's forces us to speak of narrativity as a matter of degree. Second, theories of self-narrative such as Ricoeur's comprise two features, that of the narrating subject, or author, on the one hand, and temporality, on the other. These are inextricably linked in such theorizing, particularly for Ricoeur.[14] But such theorizing is again based on the normal case. In the psychopathology of dementia illustrated by the above example, each element is weakened and reduced ('minimized'). Moreover, the reduced, minimized notion of narrativity revealed by that example also allows us to disaggregate the factors of authorship and temporality.

Once a weakened narrativity is acknowledged to have occurred in cases of dementia such as J's, we suggest, the entwining of narrative and narrator might also be questioned. Thus, the account of J and the couch illustrates a fairly simplified temporal sequence and a minimized narrator, although not perhaps in equal measure. Arguably, this 'story' retains the sequence and temporal pattern of a narrative regardless of whether it can be said to reflect an author in the sense associated with most accounts of the narrative subject. The narrative of J's decision to discard the old couch certainly possesses some of the quality of temporality. Most obviously, J deliberated at t_1, decided at t_2, and agreed at t_3 to allow the couch's removal. But the question of authorship may be considered separately. As the central focus of this narrative, J remains, in one sense, its subject. Yet the extensive on-going assistance required for his story to unfold (the way J's personhood or *who he is*, as Glas puts it, requires the eyes of his daughters) seems to limit the extent to which he may be cast as either 'author' or 'co-author' of any first-person narrative. This then may be an instance where the aspects of temporality and authorship, respectively, do not keep pace as they decline. If this is so, the unravelling of narrativity that occurs with dementia, we suggest, serves to throw light on the concept of narrativity as it can be derived from the work of theorists such as Ricoeur.

Conclusion

The advance of dementia is a source of real and pressing ethical puzzles: how one should feel about, and what attitudes and responses one should adopt toward, its sufferer; how ought we to understand them, what is due them, morally speaking, and why?

We undertook the preceding exploration in the hopes of clarifying and perhaps resolving some of those puzzles. Eventually, as the disease progresses, almost all hint of the person we knew will likely be *eclipsed*, leaving only the body—maybe itself barely recognizable—to taunt us with its empty endurance. But breaking from Lockean concepts and instead acknowledging the self 'as another' in Ricoeur's words, has revealed ways to salvage for a little longer a little more, not only of the sameness of the dementia sufferer but also, perhaps, aspects of their *ipseity* or selfhood. In addition, it has uncovered a way of honouring the identity of that person that is not so dependent on mere sameness. We have found moral reason to respond to that person as we would the person they once were. Not merely physically, but in important other ways they remain, for a while, that person.

An embrace of these new conceptions of identity, we have argued, seems also to invite a new set of prescriptions. Our duty to sustain the characterization identity of the person with dementia as long as is possible, we saw, may be demanded by that patient's right to identity recognition.

The tentative language employed here reflects the provisional nature of our conclusions. If there is a coherent sense of characterization identity, we have argued, which borrows from Ricoeur's *ipseity* and is able to disaggregate conceptions of narrativity, then that conception of a person's identity may allow us to derive practical steps and moral duties as we encounter dementia in those we know and care for.

Endnotes

1 In what her husband John Bayley regarded as a startling moment of understanding as she succumbed to dementia, Iris Murdoch described herself as sailing into the darkness (Bayley 1998).

2 We are grateful to the editors of this book for help with this chapter, especially Steve Sabat. We also wish to thank James Phillips, Gerritt Glas, Claire McGoldrick, Consuelo Isaacson, and Stone Wiske for suggestions, examples, and corrections.

3 The French language provides a particular source of equivocation here, he observes, in that the French 'meme' means both self and sameness. In contrast, 'same' cannot be confused with 'self' in English or German.

4 In this analysis we recognize Kierkegaard, when he speaks of the relation of the self to itself: '. . . in relating itself to its own self [it] relates itself to another' (Kierkegaard 1849, p. 146). We are grateful to Gerrit Glas for drawing attention to this echo of Kierkegaard.

5 Both tenets reflect the influence of Charles Taylor's writing on English-language philosophy.

6 Quante marks what seems to be a similar contrast using the language of *personality* or *biographical* and *persistence* senses of identity (Quante 1999). The personality or biographical sense of identity concerns 'the complex pattern of values, preferences, and beliefs, in which a person manifests who she is and wants to be' (Quante 1999, p. 366). Rather than speaking of personality or biographical identity, we shall employ Schechtman's language for the identity of identity politics and discourses of recognition. For further explication of characterization identity, see Radden (2004).

7 Acknowledgement of the part played in identity construction not by other people but by otherness (or Otherness) as a category is captured by Ricoeur through its phenomenological link with the experience of passivity. Such passivity includes, he says, three different experiences: that of the body in contrast to what is foreign to it, that of the self to what is intersubjectively foreign to it, that is, others, and the 'hidden passivity', which separates the self from conscience (Ricoeur 1992, p. 318). These are each extremely complex ideas and their full explication lies beyond the scope of this chapter, although for such explication the reader is directed to writing by Gerrit Glas (for example, Glas 2003).

8 A second emotional valence or attitude is the desire for authenticity. The definition of an authentic self is an elusive one, however, and the hallmarks of an achieved authentic identity are problematic, even controversial. Yet the impulse towards authenticity, and towards recognition and honouring of one's authentic or real self, does seem to be a culturally entrenched inclination. Although the ultimate coherence of this concept may be in doubt, the intensity and sincerity of people's yearning for it does not appear to be. This second kind of emotional valence has less bearing for the present investigation and we set it aside here, but readers interested in pursuing these ideas are directed to Jonathan Glover's 2003 Tanner Lectures (Glover 2003).

9 A compelling account of this progressive loss of self-awareness through early, middle, and late stages of decline, is found in David Shenk's work (Shenk 2002).

10 Documenting Iris Murdoch's voyage into dementia, Bayley points to the tenacity of a rudimentary sense of humour as a recalcitrant feature of the earlier person: 'Iris remained her old self in many ways . . . Humour seems to survive anything. A burst of laughter, snatches of doggeral, song, teasing nonsense rituals once lovingly exchanged, awake an abruptly happy response, and a sudden beaming smile . . . Only a joke survives, the last thing that finds its way into consciousness when the brain is atrophied' (Bayley 1999, pp. 34–5).

11 (Phillips 2004, personal correspondence.)

12 In the words of Michael Luntley: 'What is important to selfhood is not the stories you recall, but your *ability to update them*' (Luntley 2002, our emphasis).

13 This point in no way implies other analogies between the infant and the person with dementia.

14 The division of the self of narrative identity into narrator and narrative in Ricoeur is 'untimately unsustainable', in Phillips's words (Phillips 2003, p. 316).

References

Alcott, L. (2000). Who's afraid of identity politics? In: *Reclaiming Identity* (ed. P. Moya) pp. 312–44. Berkeley, California: University of California Press.

Baier, A. (1985). *Postures of Mind: Essays on Mind and Morals*. Minneapolis: University of Minnesota Press.

Baier, A. (1991). Who can women trust ? In: *Feminist Ethics* (ed. C. Card) pp. 233–45. Lawrence, Kansas: University of Kansas Press.

Bayley, J. (1999). *Elegy for Iris*. New York: St Martin's Press.

Benhabib, S. (1992). *Situating the Self: Gender, Community, and Postmodernism in Contemporary Ethics*. New York: Routledge.

Benhabib, S. (2002). *The Claims of Culture: Equality and Diversity in the Global Era*. Princeton, New Jersey: Princeton University Press.

Butler, J. (1997). *The Psychic Life of Power*. California: Stanford University Press.

Code, L. (1991). *What Can She Know? Feminist Theory and the Construction of Knowledge*. Ithaca: Cornell University Press.

Fraser, N. (1997). *Justus Interruptus: Critical Reflections on the 'Postsocialist' Condition*. New York: Routledge.

Gazzaniga, M. S. (ed.) (1979). *Neuropsychology*. New York: Plenum Press.

Glas, G. (2003). *Idem, ipse*, and loss of the self. *Philosophy, Psychiatry, & Psychology*, **10**: 347–52.

Glas, G. (in press). Person, personality, self and identity. a philosophically informed conceptual analysis. *Journal of Personality Disorders*.

Glover, J. (2003). *Tanner Lectures: Towards Humanism in Psychiatry. Lecture Two: Identity*. (Delivered at Princeton University, February 2003).

Jaworska, A. (1997). Respecting the margins of agency: Alzheimer's patients and the capacity to value. *Philosophy and Public Affairs*, **28**: 105–38.

Kierkegaard, S. (1849). [1954] *Fear and Trembling, and the Sickness Unto Death* (trans. W. Lowrie). New York: Doubleday.

Luntley, M. (2002). Keeping in touch: character and autobiography. (Abstract of a paper delivered at the conference *Dementia: Mind, Meaning and the Person*, Newcastle upon Tyne, UK, 2002.)

MacIntyre, A. (1984). *After Virtue*. Indiana: University of Notre Dame Press.

Meyers, D. T. (ed.) (1997). *Feminists Rethink the Self*. Oxford: Westview Press.

Nelson, L. H. (2001). *Damaged Identities, Narrative Repair*. Ithaca, New York: Cornell University Press.

Parfit, D. (1984). *Reasons and Persons*. Oxford: Oxford University Press.

Phillips, J. (2003). Psychopathology and the narrative self. *Philosophy, Psychiatry, & Psychology*, **10**: 313–28.

Quante, M. (1999). Precedent autonomy and personal identity. *Kennedy Institute of Ethics Journal*, **9**: 365–81.

Radden, J. (2003). Learning from disunity. *Philosophy, Psychiatry, & Psychology*, **10**: 357–9.

Radden, J. (2004). Personal identity, characterization identity and mental disorder. In: *The Philosophy of Psychiatry: a Companion* (ed. J. Radden), pp. 133–46. Oxford: Oxford University Press.

Ricoeur, P. (1990). *Soi-meme comme un Autre*. Paris: Editions du Seuil. (Based on the 1986 Gifford Lectures.)

Ricoeur, P. (1992). *Oneself as Another* (trans. K. Blamey). Chicago: University of Chicago Press. (All quoted passages are from this edition.)

Sandel, M. (1982). *Liberalism and the Limits of Justice*. Cambridge: Cambridge University Press.

Schechtman, M. (1996). *The Constitution of Selves*. Ithaca: Cornell University Press.

Shanley, M. L., Pateman, C. (ed.) (1991). *Feminist Interpretations and Political Theory*. Philadelphia: Pennsylvania State University.

Shenk, D. (2002). *The Forgetting: Alzheimer's: Portrait of an Epidemic*. New York: Anchor Books.

Taylor, C. (1989). *Sources of the Self: The Making of the Modern Identity*. Cambridge, Massachusetts: Harvard University Press.

Taylor, C. (1995). *Multiculturalism and 'the Politics of Recognition'*. Princeton, New Jersey: Princeton University Press. (An essay, with a commentary by Amy Gutmann (ed.).)

6 Can the self disintegrate? Personal identity, psychopathology, and disunities of consciousness

E. Jonathan Lowe

Introduction

We intuitively conceive of ourselves as strongly unified beings, at least from a psychological point of view. This idea sometimes finds philosophical expression in the doctrine of the *unity of consciousness*, taken as implying that conscious thoughts and feelings of the same person must be recognizable by that person as being uniquely their own thoughts and feelings and, as such, unmistakable for the thoughts or feelings of anyone else. However, a number of philosophers and psychologists have suggested that this intuitive view of ourselves is undermined by evidence arising from cases of dementia and other degenerative or pathological mental conditions. In this chapter, I mean to pursue the question as to how far we can or should take the concept of a unified self to break down in such cases and what implications, if any, such cases have for our ordinary conception of personal identity and human individuality. What such cases have in common is that they all exhibit various kinds and degrees of *alienation* of thought or feeling of a clearly delusional character. However, while I shall be considering some clinically well-documented psychopathological conditions in due course, I want to begin with a purely fictional example drawn from nineteenth-century English literature—partly because it is simple and vivid but also because it has frequently been cited by philosophers of mind on account of its implicit challenge to widely held conceptions of the nature of mental states.

Psychopathological alienations of thought and feeling

There is a well-known passage in Charles Dickens's novel *Hard Times*, in which Mrs Gradgrind is asked on her sick bed whether she is in pain, to which she replies, 'I think there's a pain somewhere in the room, but I couldn't positively say that I have got it' (Dickens 1969, p. 224). Her response is at once humorous and poignant, but prompts further reflection as to whether she could sincerely have meant quite literally what she said. Could someone really be aware of a pain in such a way as to be genuinely uncertain as to whether that pain was their own? If so, would their uncertainty turn on the issue of whether the pain was their own or *someone else's*, or instead on the distinct issue of whether the pain was their own or *belonged to nobody at all*? Or are both of these alternatives equally conceivable, in different cases? And if such questions can genuinely arise for someone in respect of a conscious feeling such as a pain, can they equally arise for someone in respect of a conscious *thought*? That is to say, could one be aware of a *thought* in such a way as to be genuinely uncertain as to whether that thought was one's own? And what light, if any, is thrown upon this philosophical question by empirical reports (see Stephens and Graham 2000) of such psychopathological phenomena as 'thought insertion' and the 'alien voices' that many sufferers from schizophrenia are said to experience 'in their heads'?

Before we can make headway with any of these questions, we need to be clear about the relevant sense in which, in such problem cases, a person is to be understood as *being aware of* a certain thought or feeling. For, clearly, there is a relatively uninteresting—and, for our current purposes, irrelevant—sense in which one could indeed 'be aware of' a thought or a feeling in such a way as to be genuinely uncertain as to whether that thought or feeling was one's own. To appreciate this, consider first the sense in which one is normally 'aware' of the thoughts and feelings of *other people*, namely, on the basis of observing their behaviour. If I see a large stone fall on someone's foot and then see that person scream and hop about clutching the foot, I will immediately realize that the person is in pain and, in this sense, *be aware of* their pain. Equally, if I hear someone say something in a language that I understand, evincing every sign of sincerity, I will immediately form the opinion that this person is expressing a certain thought and, in this sense, *be aware of* their thought. In both of these cases, I have what might be called a 'third-person awareness' of a certain thought or feeling—as it were, an outsider's awareness of it, as opposed to the sort of 'first-person awareness' of the thought or feeling that is characteristically possessed by the person who is actually *having* that thought or feeling. But, clearly, it is possible to have this sort of third-person awareness even of one's own thoughts or feelings.

Imagine the following scenario. Walking down the poorly lit corridor of a strange house, I stub my toe on an obstacle and feel a sharp pain. I clutch my foot and, by a rueful grimace, give expression to the thought that I should have looked where I was going. At the same time, I look up and to my astonishment see at some distance in front of me a person behaving in exactly the same manner. I momentarily form the judgement that that person, too, feels a sharp pain and has a rueful thought, before I suddenly realize that I am just seeing myself in a mirror. For that brief moment, I had a third-person awareness of my own thought and feeling—while simultaneously, of course, also having a first-person awareness of them. For a moment, I saw and made a judgement about myself just as another person would have done who had observed my behaviour. Clearly, though, given that it is possible to have such a third-person awareness of one's own thoughts and feelings, it is possible to be aware *in this way* of a thought or a feeling and yet be genuinely uncertain as to whether or not that thought or feeling is one's own. For instance, in the sort of scenario just described I might, owing to my temporary confusion, be momentarily uncertain as to whether I was really seeing another person or just seeing a reflection of myself in a mirror.

While the example itself may not be uninteresting, I persist in maintaining that it reveals only a relatively uninteresting sense in which one could be aware of a thought or feeling in such a way as to be genuinely uncertain as to whether that thought or feeling was one's own. It is an uninteresting sense precisely because it is one which we have no difficulty at all in understanding. What is interesting, because perplexing, is the question of whether one could have a *first-person* awareness of a thought or feeling and yet be genuinely uncertain as to whether that thought or feeling was one's own. The presumption is that Mrs Gradgrind had just such an awareness of the pain she thought to be 'somewhere in the room'. Similarly, it is presumed that those suffering from 'thought insertion' and the delusion that goes with it (that is, the belief that alien thoughts really are being inserted into their minds) are aware of the supposedly inserted thoughts in a first-person way—as it were, 'from the inside'—and not in the way in which one is typically aware of another person's thoughts on the basis of their audible speech. The schizophrenic's 'voices in the head' may, on the other hand, fall within the sphere of auditory hallucination, rather than being 'heard' in the non-auditory sense in which we 'hear ourselves think', when we engage in 'interior monologue'. The latter phenomenon seems, instead, to fall within the sphere of auditory *imagination*.

What is perplexing about Mrs Gradgrind's supposed condition is that it is hard to see how one could *have* a 'first-person awareness' of a pain, or any other conscious mental state, without thinking of it as being inalienably *one's own*. After all, the very point of using the term 'first-person awareness' in this context is to capture the distinctively self-reflexive character of this sort of awareness. To be aware *in this sort of way* of a thought or feeling is, it might be said, almost by definition to be aware of it as one's own. It is to be aware of the thought or feeling in that distinctive way to which we give linguistic expression by saying '*I* am thinking such-and-such' or '*I* am feeling thus and so'. What is perplexing about Mrs Gradgrind's putative condition is that she is supposed to have been aware of a pain in this sort of way and yet was *not* disposed to give expression to her awareness by saying, with complete confidence, '*I* am in pain'. And, although Mrs Gradgrind's case is a purely fictional one, it would seem—as I have already mentioned—that there are real-life cases that resemble Mrs Gradgrind's, involving individuals suffering from certain degenerative or pathological mental conditions. These, to characterize them quite generally, are cases in which individual subjects apparently have difficulty in identifying their own conscious thoughts or feelings as their own, or feel somehow 'alienated' from their own conscious thoughts or feelings.

Stephens and Graham on the phenomenology of thought insertion

Before proceeding further, I want to say a little concerning an interesting proposal advanced recently by Lynn Stephens and George Graham, in their attempt to account for the peculiar phenomenology of 'thought insertion'. They suggest that when this occurs, a thought is experienced as being part of one's own psychological history but that one does not feel that one is the *agent* of the thought. Thus, on their account, the subject has a normal first-person awareness of one of their own thoughts—recognizes it as occurring in their own mind—but is disposed to judge (delusionally) that *someone else is thinking the thought*: that, as it were, someone else has 'projected' the thought into the subject's mind (see Stephens and Graham 2000, p.157). And it seems that there is an inverse of this condition, in which subjects feel that they themselves are 'broadcasting' their thoughts to other people. If Stephens and Graham are right, then, the phenomenon of thought insertion indicates that there is *not*, in fact, such a tight connection as might have been supposed between what I have been calling 'first-person awareness' of a thought and the propensity to judge that one is, oneself, *thinking* that thought; that one is the *agent* of the mental episode in question. One lesson that they themselves draw is that delusional conditions like this should not be conceived as being indicative of any breakdown of 'ego boundaries'—that is, as being indicative of the deluded subject's inability to distinguish clearly between mental episodes which belong to their own psychological history and those that do not.

However, I have some doubts about the viability of Stephens and Graham's model, for it seems to presuppose at least the intelligibility of the idea of one subject's *thinking a thought in another person's mind*—given that, according to the model, deluded subjects are supposed to conceive of themselves as being victims of such activity carried out by other people. (For other criticisms of their account, see Hoerl 2001.) It is strongly arguable that the grammatical structure of sentences of the form '*S* is thinking a thought' is misleading, because 'think' in this context is not genuinely a transitive verb and the noun phrase 'a thought' here has the status of an 'internal accusative'. If that is correct, one cannot coherently regard a thought as being a *product* of an act of thinking, but only as *being* an act of thinking. Of course, one can still distinguish between an act of thinking and its *content*—*what* is thought, in the sense of what proposition is being entertained. (This, confusingly, is what Gottlob Frege (Frege 1956) called a 'thought'—a *Gedanke*—so let us set aside his usage for present purposes.) But, according to mainstream philosophical opinion, a thought-*content*—that is, a *proposition*—is not a psychological item belonging to the mental history of any particular thinking subject: rather, it is something objective and mind independent that is intersubjectively accessible to any number of different thinking subjects.

Now, if all of this is right, then it apparently *cannot* make sense, after all, to suppose that one subject might 'think a thought in another subject's mind', for the act of thinking must belong to the first subject and there is no *product* of that act that can be conceived as belonging, instead, to the second subject's mind—although, of course, various indirect *effects* of that act might well be mental episodes in another subject's psychological history. Thus, *pace* Stephens and Graham, thought insertion and the delusional beliefs associated with it cannot plausibly be modelled on what might be called the delusion of *usurped agency*, when a subject feels that another agent is, say, moving one of the subject's own limbs independently of the subject's own will. For it seems that there is nothing in the case of thought insertion that could be taken to correspond to the movement of the subject's limb, as 'belonging' to the subject but supposedly 'brought about' by another agent.

Of course, because the person experiencing thought insertion is in a *delusional state*, it would be inappropriate to insist that victims of it must be deploying a coherent concept of what thinking is in attempting to report upon the phenomenology of their condition. Even so, I surmise that Stephens and Graham themselves would agree that it is preferable, if possible, to appeal to *intelligible* models of such delusions and that they suppose their own model to be an intelligible one. However, this raises further and difficult questions concerning the analysis of delusional phenomena quite generally which I cannot go into here—in particular, the question of whether delusional states of mind can be considered to stand in any kind of rational relationship to other cognitive states of the deluded subject.

It might also perhaps be urged on behalf of Stephens and Graham's model of thought insertion that its crucial feature, which it could retain even in the absence of any distinction between an act of thinking and its 'product', is that the subject feels 'passive' with respect to one of their own thoughts. However, as they themselves acknowledge, this is a phenomenon that we all experience from time to time, without being subject to any sort of delusion, when we experience a thought—which we fully recognize as being 'our own thought'— popping unbidden into our minds. The problem about characterizing the phenomenology of thought insertion is to account for the deluded subject's sense that a certain thought, which in fact belongs to the subject, is not really *their own thought*, but somehow someone else's, even though the subject is aware of the thought with the same intimacy and immediacy with which anyone is normally aware of their own conscious thoughts. Presumably, the deluded subject must conceive of their *awareness* of the supposedly 'inserted' thought as belonging to their own psychological history, but it seems to me that the peculiarity of the phenomenon—to the extent that I have any grasp at all of what it might be like to experience it—is that the thought in question itself seems to the subject to belong to *someone else's* psychological history, part of which has somehow intruded into the subject's sphere of consciousness. But this is not consistent with Stephens and Graham's model, which I therefore feel constrained to reject.

Another point worth mentioning is that Stephens and Graham's model, even if it worked for the delusions associated with thought insertion, could not readily be extended to accommodate Mrs Gradgrind's putative delusion, which involves a *feeling*—a bodily sensation—being experienced as possibly not the subject's own: the problem being, of course, that we feel perfectly 'passive' with respect to feelings that we do nonetheless recognize as being unmistakably our own. It is true that Mrs Gradgrind's case is a purely fictional one and I do not know whether any properly documented clinical condition even approximates to it. However, it is not clear to me that there is anything in the nature of mental states or our awareness of them that makes Mrs Gradgrind's putative case any more mysterious than that of thought insertion, nor any reason why an account of the phenomenology of thought insertion should not be expected to be capable of extension to cases like hers, should they turn out to occur.

Philosophical theories of selfhood and personal identity

If our interest in such delusional cases as these is to advance much beyond mere morbid curiosity, we need to reflect now on what they might be thought to teach us about ourselves and about the nature of human personality and individuality. To this end, we should first reflect on what we do or should understand by such terms as 'person', 'self', and 'I'. We can perhaps do no better than to start with John Locke's famous definition of the term *person* in his *Essay Concerning Human Understanding*: a person, he says, is a

> thinking intelligent Being, that has reason and reflection, and can consider it self as it self, the same thinking thing in different times and places. (Locke 1975, p. 335)

There is a good deal packed into this definition and some of it might be queried, such as the emphasis on rationality. But one thing that, in my view, it does correctly insist upon is that to be a person it is not sufficient merely to be a sentient or even a thinking creature. A person must be capable of self-reflection and, at least to some degree, self-knowledge. There are many animals that show signs of feeling, intelligence, and even rationality but which apparently lack any awareness of themselves in the sense intended by Locke.

Of course an animal may be 'aware of itself' in the sense that it may, for example, be aware of one of its limbs as being wounded and act in an appropriate self-directed manner by, say, licking the wound. But there may be no grounds to suppose that the animal is aware of itself in a 'first-person' way as a subject of thought and feeling. Even if it has thoughts, it may have none that could only find appropriate linguistic expression with the aid of the first-person pronoun. I am not implying, here, that creatures that lack an ability to express their thoughts in language must therefore be incapable of having 'first-person thoughts' about themselves—although that is a possibility that cannot lightly be dismissed, I am just pointing out that to qualify as a person a subject of thought and feeling must at least be capable of having such first-person thoughts and that many intelligent animals apparently lack this capacity. It is well known, for example, that chimpanzees are rare amongst non-human primates in being able to 'recognize themselves' in mirrors, at least to the extent that they will attempt to rub paint marks off their foreheads, which they can see only by looking at their own mirror images. But even this does not establish that chimpanzees think of themselves self-consciously as being the subjects of their own thoughts and feelings, for it is far from clear that chimpanzees even possess the rudiments of a so-called 'theory of mind', that is, that they think of other chimpanzees, let alone themselves, as being subjects of mental states of thought and feeling. In point of fact, an ability to recognize oneself in the mirror is clearly not even a necessary condition of self-consciousness, even for a person who is not visually impaired, as there are well-documented cases of 'mirror self-misidentification', in which self-conscious subjects suffer from the delusion of thinking that they see another person when they look into a mirror (see Breen *et al.* 2000).

It is instructive at this point to compare Locke's definition of a person with David Hume's. Hume famously said, in the *Treatise of Human Nature*,

> When I enter most intimately into what I call myself, I always stumble on some particular perception or other . . . I can never catch *myself* at any time without a perception, and can never observe any thing but the perception,

and then goes on to affirm that a person is:

> nothing but a bundle or collection of different perceptions, which succeed each other with an inconceivable rapidity, and are in a perpetual flux and movement. (Hume 1978, p. 252)

A little later he remarks that,

> the true idea of the human mind, is to consider it as a system of different perceptions . . . which are link'd together by the relation of cause and effect, and mutually produce, destroy, influence, and modify each other. (Hume 1978, p. 261)

One striking feature of Hume's account is that he apparently identifies a person with a *mind*, rather than with some sort of being that *has* a mind but also has a body. Another is that he apparently considers a mind, person, or self to be nothing more than a 'bundle of perceptions', that is, a collection of ever-changing thoughts and feelings, tied together by nothing more than certain causal relations in which they stand to one another.

Such a view of the self, it might seem, need find nothing perplexing in Mrs Gradgrind's supposed condition, which it might represent as one in which a certain 'perception'—the pain of which she was vaguely aware as being 'somewhere in the room'—was so loosely tied to others constituting Mrs Gradgrind's mind at that moment as to be only questionably a member of the same 'bundle'. However, the very fact that Hume's view appears to accommodate Mrs Gradgrind's case so comfortably is indicative, I think, of its gross inadequacy. Hume himself was to acknowledge this inadequacy in the appendix to the *Treatise*, in which he notoriously remarks that,

> upon a more strict review of the section concerning personal identity, I find myself involv'd in such a labyrinth, that, I confess, I neither know how to correct my former opinions, nor how to render them consistent. (Hume 1978, p. 633)

Part of the problem with Hume's official view of the self, as articulated in the main text of the *Treatise*, is that he has no way of accommodating the distinction discussed earlier between 'first-person' and 'third-person' awareness of conscious mental states. Setting aside delusional cases like that of Mrs Gradgrind, to have a first-person awareness of a conscious mental state is to be directly aware of that state as being one's own—that is, as belonging to one's own mind. Now, for Hume, for a mental state to 'belong to one's own mind' is just for that state to be one of a certain bundle or collection of mental states tied together by certain causal relations. But *which* such bundle is the bundle that constitutes *my* mind? Hume cannot answer that it is the bundle whose members *I* am directly aware of in the distinctively first-person way. For he has already declared that I myself am nothing but that very bundle. By eliminating any notion of the self as a being that *has*, or is the *subject* of, its mental states and can recognize itself as occupying this role, Hume has obliterated the very distinction between first-person and third-person awareness that makes Mrs Gradgrind's supposed condition an object of perplexity and curiosity.

Perhaps, however, we can go some way towards reconciling the contributions of Locke and Hume to our understanding of the mind. Hume does indeed seem to have articulated an inadequate, because impoverished, conception of what it is to be a *person* or *self*. In this regard, Locke's account seems preferable, although perhaps still objectionable in some respects. On the other hand, maybe Hume has adequately characterized a certain *kind* of mind—the kind of mind that is possessed by creatures that lack a distinctively first-person type of awareness and consequently do not qualify as persons or selves. Perhaps the minds of sentient and intelligent but non-self-reflective creatures, including non-human primates, are indeed 'Humean' minds. For a conscious mental state to 'belong' to such a mind is just for it to be appropriately causally related to other such states and for the mind to 'belong' to a certain animal is just for those mental states to be appropriately causally related to physiological states of that animal.

What, then, should we say of ourselves—and what should we say of individuals like Mrs Gradgrind or those suffering from psychopathological conditions relevantly similar to hers? Are we—are they—Lockean persons or animals with Humean minds (cf. Sacks 1985, p. 28 and Brennan 1989)? Could we—could they—somehow be both, perhaps at different times? Could we say that personhood stands at one end of a spectrum of conditions, which is occupied at the other end by mentality of a purely Humean sort? That, certainly, would be preferable to saying that personhood itself is a matter of degree— that an individual can be either more or less fully a person. For to be a person, on the Lockean account, is at least to possess a capacity for first-person awareness of one's own conscious mental states. But one either possesses this capacity or lacks it—and it is not the sort of capacity that comes in degrees, like the capacity to do long division or to solve crossword puzzles.

Any creature that can comprehendingly raise the question of whether or not it, itself, is a Lockean person or an animal with a Humean mind thereby demonstrates itself to *be* a Lockean person, for it thereby demonstrates that it can 'consider it self as it self'. Because I am raising the question now, I know at present that I am a Lockean person. But perhaps we want to say that one's capacity to raise this sort of question and have this sort of self-knowledge is, or could be, a fluctuating one. One is tempted to say, perhaps, that in certain conditions—either of temporary mental impairment through the influence of drugs, or of permanent impairment through neurological degeneration—I might no longer be able to raise this sort of question and so might, at least for a while, no longer qualify as being a Lockean person but at most as having a Humean mind. However, there is an obvious and immediate difficulty with any such proposal. If *I* am a Lockean person, how could *I* continue to exist while possessing no more than a Humean mind? Should we not rather say that in the supposed conditions of mental impairment, *I* cease to exist and all that remains is a Humean mind, which is not *my* mind nor that of any person? Clearly, everything here turns on the question of what sort of being or entity it is that the word 'I' should be taken to denote when it is being used correctly and comprehendingly.

With respect to this question, we are perhaps still in no better position to provide a cogent and compelling answer than René Descartes was at the beginning of the *Meditations*, when he was convinced with absolute certainty that he *existed*, but was still completely in the dark as to *what* he was. As he puts it, 'I do not yet have a sufficient understanding of what this "I" is, that now necessarily exists' (Descartes 1984, p. 17). On the face of it, this is an extremely strange predicament to be in: to know with complete assurance that a term that one is using refers to *something* and yet to be quite unsure as to what *kind* of thing it refers to. Here it may be objected that Locke has told us quite clearly what sort of thing 'I' denotes: it denotes a *person*, which is a

> thinking intelligent Being, that has reason and reflection, and can consider it self as it self, the same thinking thing in different times and places.   (Locke 1975, p. 335)

But the problem is that this only tells us what a person can *do*, not what kind of thing can do that. Descartes believed that only an immaterial entity, the soul, could do what a person must be able to do to qualify as a person. But perhaps— indeed, very likely—he was wrong. Perhaps an organic brain or nervous system, or the central processing unit of a computer can do those things. In which case, entities of those kinds could qualify as persons, at least while they could do the things in question.

And yet, there is a seeming difficulty in any such suggestion and one which Descartes himself foresaw. This is that material things, including brains and computers, are not strongly unified entities in the way in which persons or selves seem to be. These material things are composed of many parts, which can be removed, replaced, and reorganized to varying degrees, as a consequence of which an unavoidable vagueness attaches to questions concerning the existence and persistence of such objects. There is no precise number or combination of nerve cells that would have to be destroyed for my brain to cease to exist. Indeed, it is impossible to say without being at all arbitrary precisely which nerve cells currently compose my brain. But, plausibly, no such vagueness attaches to *me* and my continuing existence. It could never be an open question—to me, at least!—whether or not *I* still exist. For just so long as I can so much as raise the question, I still exist. And, as we saw earlier, the capacity to raise such a question is not the sort of capacity that comes in degrees.

Unities and disunities of consciousness

What, if anything, could explain the 'strong unity' of the self—and is not the existence of such strongly unified selves precisely what is put into question by the sorts of pathological cases that we have been considering? Many philosophers, Locke included, seem to think that this strong unity consists in the so-called *unity of consciousness*. However, it is not always entirely clear what philosophers mean by the phrase 'unity of consciousness'. According to one widespread view, which seems to have been held by Locke amongst others, a mind exhibits unity of consciousness at any given time just to the extent that any conscious state belonging to that mind at that time is experienced as being 'co-conscious' with any other conscious state belonging to it at the same time. In other words, in such a mind there is never any 'bifurcation' or 'splitting' of consciousness.

Here I should remark that the technical term 'co-consciousness' is, unfortunately, subject to more than one use, because it is sometimes employed to characterize the supposedly parallel 'streams of consciousness' apparently exhibited in cases of multiple personality disorder, in which the various different 'alters' are said, in this sense, to be 'co-conscious' subjects somehow 'inhabiting' the same physical body (see, for example, Braude 1991, p. 106). So I must make it clear that henceforth what I mean by describing mental states as being 'co-conscious' is precisely that they *do* belong to the same 'stream of consciousness' and thus that a 'unified consciousness' in the sense now being considered is one which always consists of a single undivided 'stream'. (As for multiple personality disorder itself, interesting condition though it is, I shall say no more about it in the present chapter (but see Radden 1996)).

Now it is in fact rather doubtful whether any of us really possesses a 'unified consciousness' in the foregoing sense most (let alone all) of the time (cf. Wilkes 1988, pp. 145–57). We seem very often to be able to 'divide' our consciousness by consciously attending to two or more different matters at once, without bringing all of them together within the scope of a single act of attention. A familiar example is that of driving while simultaneously engaging in a conversation. Subsequently, one may be able consciously to recall some visual feature of the route taken and also something that one's interlocutor said at that point in the journey, without consciously recalling the events in question as having been experienced simultaneously. Of course, we cannot 'catch ourselves in the act' of dividing our attention—for this would require us to *attend* to what we were doing, thereby nullifying the division. This is doubtless why the phenomenon seems so elusive and, to some, even non-existent: but conscious recollection may reveal such divisions to have occurred, as in the example just described.

Even if it is disputed, as it may be, whether we can really ever divide our *attention*—if attention is thought of on the model of a searchlight which, as it were, can focus only upon one thing at a time—it remains plausible that we may experience conscious states at a time that are not, *at that time*, in the 'focus' of our attention. For example, one may not have been attending to a continuous humming background noise for a while, but when it suddenly stops one *notices* its ceasing and thereby becomes retrospectively aware that one was, all along, vaguely conscious of its presence. In such a case, it seems, there is a lack of co-consciousness between one's consciousness of the sound and one's conscious awareness of whatever it was that one was attending to at the time.

However, be all this as it may, unity of consciousness in the foregoing sense is *not* in fact threatened by examples like that of Mrs Gradgrind, for there is no suggestion that her awareness of the pain 'somewhere in the room' was somehow 'separate' or 'dissociated' from her awareness of other conscious mental states that she was able to identify confidently as her own. Disruptions to the unity of consciousness in the foregoing sense only present difficulties for theories of the self that attempt to explain the strong unity of the self in terms of this sort of unity of consciousness. This may pose a problem for Locke's theory, but not one for either Hume's or Descartes'. For Hume, the self does not possess strong unity in any case, because it is just a bundle of perceptions tied together by more or less loose bonds of causation—though, of course, this very notion reveals the inadequacy of his theory. For Descartes, the self does indeed possess strong unity, but for him this arises not from the unity of consciousness in the foregoing sense but from the simple or non-composite nature of the immaterial substance that, on his view, the self turns out to be.

There is, however, another sense that can be attached to the phrase 'unity of consciousness', one which is often associated with the name of Immanuel Kant and which in that context usually goes under the more grandiose title of the 'transcendental unity of apperception'. This is the sense in which different conscious mental states of the same person are all experienced by that person as belonging to the same 'I' or self. As Kant himself puts it, in a memorable phrase, 'It must be possible for the "I think" to accompany all my representations' (Kant 1929, p. 152). (Kant and his followers would add that the 'transcendental self' should not be thought of as any sort of empirically detectable object that persists identically over time. However, this claim is not only dubiously intelligible but also threatens to trivialize the notion of unity of consciousness with which it is associated—so I shall not presume its truth in what follows.) Locke, it has to be said, likewise seems to have subscribed to this notion of the unity of consciousness, for he famously urged that 'It . . . [is] impossible for any one to perceive, without perceiving, that he does perceive' (Locke 1975, p. 335)—and 'perceive' here is clearly being used by Locke in a very broad sense to include *thinking*. However, this is not, of course, incompatible with saying that Locke also subscribed to the notion of the unity of consciousness as involving 'co-consciousness', for it is perfectly possible—if somewhat implausible—to contend that the two notions necessarily go hand in hand. Be that as it may, whenever, henceforth, I speak of unity of consciousness in the 'Lockean' sense, I shall exclusively mean unity of consciousness in the co-consciousness sense.

Now, the other or 'Kantian' notion of the unity of consciousness is, it would seem, perfectly compatible with the phenomenon of divided attention, or lack of 'co-consciousness' between conscious states of the same person. On the other hand, unity of consciousness in this second sense plausibly cannot serve to explain, because it already seems to presuppose, the unity of the self. Moreover, it is this sort of unity of consciousness that is difficult to reconcile with cases like that of Mrs Gradgrind, because she seems to have conscious states of which she is aware in something like a first-person fashion but which she does not recognize as being unmistakably her own. In other words, although she experiences the pain as having an immediate felt quality much like one of her own pains, she does not experience it as being unambiguously *hers*. Much the same applies, it would seem, in previously described cases of 'thought insertion', where subjects claim to be aware of conscious thoughts— in much the way in which they would be directly aware of 'their own' conscious thoughts—but regard them either as being the intrusive thoughts of other people or else thoughts which do not properly 'belong' to anyone.

Psychopathology and the metaphysics of the self

Can we then, extract any interesting lessons for the metaphysics of the self from the clinical data of psychopathology? Perhaps the first thing to emphasize in this connection is that one must always treat with caution the ways in which individuals suffering from pathological psychological conditions report their own symptoms. Such reports are, like all communications between people about their inner mental lives, doubly subject to interpretation (and therefore also misinterpretation): the interpretation of the reporter and the interpretation of the reportee. If someone is in a state of mental confusion, we should not expect them to be able to give a particularly coherent description of that state. And someone who has never been in such a state may find it difficult to understand a first-hand report of what it is like. Even so, it would be rash of philosophers to insist that it is simply unintelligible to suppose that a conscious mental state could be experienced by someone as being 'like' one of their own but as seemingly *not* one of their own. The question that should concern philosophers is what, if anything, the possibility of such a state of affairs should be taken to imply for the nature of human minds and selves.

My own tentative verdict is as follows. First, I do not think that this sort of state of affairs, assuming it to occur, provides any support whatever for the Humean view of the *self*, which seems to me to be in any case hopelessly flawed, as Hume himself admitted. Nor do I think that it provides any support for the extravagant—but to some strangely alluring—view that personhood comes in degrees, or that the human self is somehow capable of undergoing gradual fragmentation. This is not to deny, as I made clear earlier, that Hume may have a satisfactory account of a certain *kind* of mind, that of non-self-reflective but otherwise sentient and intelligent animals. Indeed, a possible characterization of Mrs Gradgrind's putative condition is that, although she is a self-consciously aware person or self and consciously related to most of her own thoughts and feelings in the normal, first-person way, she also possesses some conscious mental states that she experiences only in the non-self-appropriating way in which non-self-reflective animals and very young human infants presumably do. And perhaps this sort of condition is much more widespread than one might suppose it to be while one is wide awake and contemplating such matters. Perhaps, indeed, we are all subject to it to some degree in states of semi-wakefulness—when, of course, we are in no fit condition to reflect upon the fact.

In my view, for reasons explained earlier, I do not think that 'pathological' cases like that of Mrs Gradgrind pose any threat to the notion of the unity of consciousness in the 'Lockean' sense—but I also think that this notion fails in any case to characterize the normal human condition, which seems to be replete with instances of divided attention or split awareness. What undoubtedly *is* threatened is the 'Kantian' notion of unity of consciousness, according to which all of our conscious mental states are directly apprehended by us as being states of the same self or 'I'. At the same time, however, it seems clear that the possible breakdown of the unity of consciousness in *this* sense in no way poses a threat to the notion that the self possesses a strong unity, because the latter sort of unity could not be explained by the former in any case.

As for the doctrine that the self is indeed strongly unified, I cannot see how to abandon it coherently, because I can make no sense of the suggestion that the question of my continuing or ceasing to exist is in any way infected by vagueness. The gulf between my existing and my not existing is as deep and as unambiguous as that between any two states of affairs could conceivably be. Nor is this claim at all obviously compromised by pathological cases in which subjects declare themselves to be 'dead'—Cotard's delusion (see, for example, Young 2000, p.64)—for, bizarre though such a thought may be, it is not straightforwardly tantamount to the thought that one does not *exist*. And, while it is true that some extreme sufferers from this delusion describe their condition as one of 'non-existence', it is not at all clear what they do or could mean by this.

Now, precisely *because* the gulf between my existing and my not existing seems so deep and unambiguous, I cannot see how I can coherently identify myself with my brain or any other materially composite part of my body, or with my body as a whole, for none of these things has strong unity—that is, the kind of unity that is possessed by something whose continuing existence is not infected in any way by vagueness. I do not think, however, that this forces me to agree with Descartes that what I essentially am is a simple immaterial substance or 'soul' (see Lowe 1996, Chapter 2). I prefer to remain agnostic and admit with all due humility that although I am as sure as I am of anything that I exist and am a strongly unified entity, I have no real grasp of *what* it is that I am (and if this is all that Kant intended by his talk of the 'transcendental self', then I am not necessarily at odds with him). Perhaps, in the end, this is what we really have to learn from the so-called pathological cases. And in learning this we learn, perhaps disconcertingly, that our own quotidian condition is not after all so very different from that of subjects who are customarily regarded as being abnormal almost to the point of incomprehensibility.

References

Braude, S. E. (1991). *First Person Plural: Multiple Personality and the Philosophy of Mind*. London: Routledge.

Breen, N., Caine, D., Coltheart, M., Hendy, J., Roberts, C. (2000). Towards an understanding of delusions of mis-identification: four case studies. In: *Pathologies of Belief* (ed. M. Coltheart and M. Davies), pp. 75–110. Oxford: Blackwell.

Brennan, A. (1989). Fragmented selves and the problem of ownership. *Proceedings of the Aristotelian Society*, **90**: 143–58.

Descartes, R. (1984). *The Philosophical Writings of Descartes, Volume 2* (trans. J. Cottingham *et al.*). Cambridge: Cambridge University Press.

Dickens, C. (1969). *Hard Times*. Harmondsworth: Penguin Books.

Frege, G. (1956). The thought: a logical inquiry (trans. A. M. Quinton and M. Quinton). *Mind*, **65**: 289–311. (Reproduced in Strawson, P. F. (ed.) *Philosophical Logic*. Oxford: Oxford University Press, 1967.)

Hoerl, C. (2001). On thought insertion. *Philosophy, Psychiatry, & Psychology*, **8**: 189–200.

Hume, D. (1978). *A Treatise of Human Nature* (ed. L. A. Selby-Bigge and P. H. Nidditch). Oxford: Clarendon Press.

Kant, I. (1929). *Critique of Pure Reason* (trans. N. Kemp Smith). London: Macmillan.

Locke, J. (1975). *An Essay Concerning Human Understanding* (ed. P. H. Nidditch). Oxford: Clarendon Press.

Lowe, E. J. (1996). *Subjects of Experience*. Cambridge: Cambridge University Press.

Radden, J. (1996). *Divided Minds and Successive Selves: Ethical Issues in Disorders of Identity and Personality*. Cambridge, Massachusetts: MIT Press.

Sacks, O. (1985). *The Man Who Mistook his Wife for a Hat*. London: Duckworth.

Stephens, G. L., Graham, G. (2000). *When Self-Consciousness Breaks: Alien Voices and Inserted Thoughts*. Cambridge, Massachusetts: MIT Press.

Wilkes, K. (1988). *Real People: Personal Identity without Thought Experiments*. Oxford: Clarendon Press.

Young, A. W. (2000). Wondrous strange: the neuropsychology of abnormal beliefs. In: *Pathologies of Belief* (ed. M. Coltheart and M. Davies), pp. 47–73. Oxford: Blackwell.

7 Keeping track, autobiography, and the conditions for self-erosion

Michael Luntley

Introduction

In this chapter I want to apply some ideas from recent work on self-consciousness to explore the following metaphysical issue: under what conditions would it make sense to say that severe dementia gives rise to a loss of self? I shall argue that on a broadly Kantian conception of the self there is a case for saying that the erosion of certain basic cognitive capacities central to autobiographical memory amounts to an erosion of the self. I suggest that it is an empirical matter whether or not severely demented patients display the relevant erosion of cognitive capacities. The argument shows, however, that the very idea of loss of self makes sense.

The basic cognitive capacities at issue concern the capacity for integrating ideas into an autobiographical unity, a unity that underpins our capacity to self-narrate. This requires an ability for temporal binding—treating an Idea at one time as bearing upon an Idea at another time. The simplest way in which this occurs is when a subject retains an Idea—a way of thinking of a thing, property or event—through time.[1] When a subject does this they keep track of the thing picked out by the Idea. Keeping track of things is one of the basic achievements of the self and, on the conception I exploit, it is a condition for the possibility of self-reference. Genuine self-reference is, on this conception, explained by self-consciousness conceived in terms of a set of cognitive capacities. The possibility I want to outline concerns the sort of breakdown in these cognitive capacities that amounts to a loss of self-consciousness and, thereby, a loss of self-reference. The breakdown at issue is the loss of the capacity to keep track of things.

This might seem to reverse the obvious order of dependence, for you might think that the ability to think of oneself is prior to the ability to think of other things. But on the conception of the self I exploit, the self is that which keeps track of things. More precisely, the self is the ground for the possibility of keeping track of things. The ability to think of oneself—to self-refer—depends upon the array of cognitive capacities for thinking of other things, for it is only with those in place that one has the capacity to think of oneself as an object, one thing among others.[2] The capacities for thinking of other things include, centrally, a capacity for temporal binding. On this conception, such capacities are conditions for the possibility of self-reference. The capacity for self-reference is explained in the light of these other capacities. When these capacities slip, especially the capacity for temporal binding, so too does the self. When the capacity for keeping track of things has been eroded there is nothing left to constitute a self. At that stage, self-consciousness and, thereby, self-reference is lost. The point is not that under such circumstances the subject fails to keep track of their own self, for on the conception I employ, the self is not something that is ever tracked. The self is always the tracker— the ground of the possibility of keeping track of things. So the erosion at issue in the case of severe dementia is not a failure to keep track of the self, but the failure to keep track of outer things. The self is not, on this conception, an inner thing that is tracked on analogy with outer things; it is the condition for the possibility of keeping track of outer things. When that goes, the self goes too.

The conclusion is counter-intuitive, for the sort of cases I envisage will include cases of patients who have some capacity for 'I' vocalizations. For example, a patient may have a capacity to utter sentences like, 'I am thirsty' but nevertheless have lost the capacity to keep track of things in the way required to manifest the cognitive capacities constitutive of self-consciousness and self-reference. Under such circumstances I suggest that despite the apparent self-reference involved in the language use, we can make sense of the idea that no genuine self-reference is available for such a language user. Whether it is right to think that is ever the case is an empirical matter.[3]

I shall outline the argument for this conclusion in the context of two competing conceptions of the self, which I shall call the Lockean and the Kantian models.[4] The Lockean model is a reductionist view of the self; for it is a conception on which the individuation of Ideas is taken as primitive and selves are defined over collections of Ideas. In contrast, the Kantian model treats the self as a condition for the possibility of certain basic cognitive skills, skills that critically underpin the achievement of keeping track of things. The self is, thereby, partly constitutive of the account of the ideas involved in such skills. On this conception, the self is not itself something that one tracks. For the Kantian, the first-person pronoun is not an expression the reference of which has to be achieved. It does not function like a demonstrative, let alone a name or description. There is such a thing as self-reference for the Kantian, but unlike all other forms of reference, it is not an achievement. For the Kantian, self-reference is fixed by the token-reflexive rule: any token of 'I' refers to whoever produced it. But that only fixes reference against a background of conditions for being a language user, someone capable of achieving, amongst other things, reference to objects. It is a condition for the possibility of achieving reference to other things that a language user manifests the cognitive skills that make up self-consciousness. When those skills are absent, the subject who utters sentences containing 'I' has lost the cognitive surround that makes it compelling to say that the token-reflexive rule alone suffices to fix reference. A laptop computer that was programmed to say 'I need a mains power source' when its battery ran low does not count as making self-reference just because it has produced a sentence with the first-person pronoun in it. The appropriate surround of cognitive skills is absent. The central hypothesis of this chapter is that we can make sense of circumstances under which things could be so bad for a severely demented patient that, notwithstanding their use of the first-person pronoun in sentences such as, 'I am thirsty', the appropriate cognitive surround, which warrants treating this as a case of self-reference, is absent.

The self and its Ideas

In this section I set up and review the difference between the Lockean and Kantian models of the self in a way that prepares for the argument I want to consider. For the Lockean, the self is not a thing over and above an enduring collection of Ideas. So, for the Lockean, the identity of Ideas is taken for granted and the self is treated as a function of ways of collecting Ideas. In contrast, on the Kantian conception, the self is that which provides the way of collecting Ideas into an inferential unity and this means that, for many types of ideas, the self is partly constitutive of the individuation of ideas. It is useful, as a first approximation, to represent the difference diagrammatically (Fig. 7.1).

The Lockean model has a collection of Ideas, which, taken together make up a self: Ideas are items with an identity and selves are defined over some function for collecting Ideas together into collections. The Lockean tends to assume that Ideas can be individuated as types of content. This is what makes them replicable in a way that generates the thought experiments of teletransportation, and so on, which have come to dominate much of the literature on personal identity.[5]

Once ideas are conceived independently of the subject for whom they are had, it becomes difficult to see how to find any principled way of rebundling them so that the collection identifies something recognizable as an enduring self. It is not just that the concept of a collection for the Lockean is independent

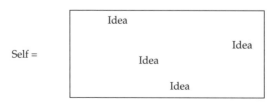

Fig. 7.1 Locke's view of the self

of the self, but it seems also to be independent of the notion of Ideas forming an inferential unity. The idea of an inferential unity is essential if Ideas are to have a role in the enterprise of making sense of the subject who has them. Inferential unity requires, at a minimum, that Ideas stand in normal logical relations to one another that can then be exploited in making sense of the bearer of Ideas. For example, if I think that it is raining and I think that it is cloudy then I know enough to think that it is raining and cloudy. The capacity to combine Ideas in simple inferences is essential if I am to be considered a subject apt for rational explication. It seems a plausible constraint on any bundling principle for Ideas that it deliver the notion that how Ideas fit together matters. And the idea of 'mattering' is difficult to understand independently of reintroducing a notion of subject, the self for whom Ideas matter. The intuition behind this thought goes back to Kant's notion of the transcendental unity of apperception.

The transcendental unity of apperception is the idea of the 'I' that accompanies all experience. Kant's insight was that experiences are not free-floating contents, they are contents that are *there for the subject*. Experiences are always had by a subject, the 'I' that accompanies them. A similar claim can be made for ideas. This produces a quite different image for thinking about the subject to the one in the Lockean tradition. It produces a Kantian way of thinking of the self as that in virtue of which Ideas are collected together. This can be represented as shown in Fig. 7.2. In this image, Ideas are only collected together in an inferential unity (represented by the dotted lines) insofar as they are had by the point of view of the self.

The central issue for the Lockean model concerns the principle by which Ideas are collected to form a unity and whether this does justice to the sense of a point of view that is needed to capture what it is like to be a self-conscious subject. Contemporary Lockeans tend to take the notion of unity-at-a-time as given and concentrate on the principle by which these collections are unified over time. The idea of a unity-at-a-time takes for granted a basic notion of a point of view—the Ideas available to a consciousness at a time. The Lockean then takes retention in memory as the principle to be appealed to in defining persons over time. That permits, however, degrees of retention and personal identity thus becomes a matter of degree, not an all-or-nothing affair. The more

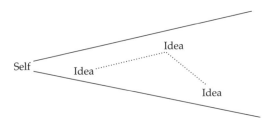

Fig. 7.2 Kant's view of the self

ideas I retain from an earlier self, the more I am similar to that self. For the Lockean, it is the identity of the ideas that matters, for identity of persons is defined over collections of ideas. *Prima facie*, the individuation of ideas identifies ideas as types of contents, rather than discrete particular contents.[6] Hence, of any given Idea, to individuate that Idea is to individuate something that is replicable many times over. This means that the replication of ideas and retention of a set of ideas by two subjects becomes possible, as does the retention of two previously separate sets of ideas by one subject. Hence, by Lockean principles, personal identity admits fusion and fission cases. Therefore, if personal identity is defined over a collection of ideas construed as items whose identity permits this sort of replication, there is nothing in that set to rule out the possibility of that set of ideas being, as it were, photocopied many times over so that the person that was me becomes multiply instantiated.

The Lockean model takes for granted the conception of the unity of Ideas that provides the collection of Ideas at a time, normally by assuming that these are the Ideas identified with states of a single brain. But that notion of unity does no real work for the Lockean other than to fix a starting point when considering how survival comes in degrees as later collections retain more or less of the initial set. The reason the assumed notion of unity does no real work is that what it picks out is a set of items (Ideas), the individuation of which treats them as items capable of replication. There is nothing in the idea of a unity-at-a-time that, for the Lockean, stops the possibility that that unity could be photocopied and thereby survive in many instantiations. The unity assumed here is a type of configuration of Ideas as types of representation.

It is easy to miss the difference between the Kantian and Lockean models. In describing Fig. 7.2, I have used the same concept, that of a 'point of view', which I said the Lockean appeals to in starting with their conception of a collection of Ideas that makes a unity-at-a-time. The difference between Lockean and Kantian is, however, large, for it is wholly unclear that the Lockean concept of a point of view appealed to for the notion of a unity-at-a-time captures the same thing as the Kantian concept. The Kantian concept of a point of view is of a collection of Ideas such that the way they fit together matters. The heart of the Kantian image is the thought that Ideas stand in inferential relations to one another and that they do so, in part, because of the way they are had for a self. It is because Ideas stand within the self's point of view that they come to stand in familiar inferential relations to one another. The challenge for the Lockean is to capture the thought that Ideas fit together in ways that matter, that they enjoy an inferential unity.

The unity of a point of view

The idea of the inferential unity of Ideas is fundamental to an account of thought. It seems impossible to conceive of a subject with a capacity for thought for whom Ideas do not enjoy inferential unity. And it is difficult to see how to account for that unity without granting the subject a use of 'I'. The idea that an impersonal account of such unity might work is often raised as an objection to Descartes' entitlement to his use of 'I' in formulating the cogito. But as Williams famously argued, Descartes was entitled to the 'I' in his statement of the *cogito*, for, as Williams remarks,

> The content of impersonally occurrent thought needs, it seems, to be relativized somehow; and there is no better way of relativizing it than the use of the first person. (Williams 1978, p. 97)

But once the subject is granted the use of 'I' they are then guaranteed a transparent unity of inference (Campbell 1997). It cannot be the case that a subject thinks

> I think that *P*

and

> I think that *Q*

and not find transparent and obvious that it follows that they should accept,

> I think that *P* and *Q*.

A subject who uses the first-person pronoun is guaranteed transparent inferential unity to their Ideas. So, use of the first-person pronoun ordinarily construed guarantees inferential unity, but that remark is only illuminating if we know what constitutes self-reference. We need an account of what constitutes the ordinary use of the first person. For the Lockean, there is no such thing as reference to a persisting substantive self and so, in the absence of a developed story about why self-reference is relativized to a time, the Lockean can hardly appeal to the phenomenon of use of the first-person pronoun to account for the unity of Ideas at a time.

An account is needed of what constitutes the inferential unity of Ideas. For sure, the Kantian will argue that Ideas enjoy an inferential unity because of the way they are had by a point of view, the point of view of a subject who uses the first person. But the Kantian will then go on and outline the assemblage of cognitive skills that underpin ordinary use of the first person. Before turning to outline the key aspects of this account for current purposes, let us be clear what it is that the Lockean fails to account for. That will then throw into perspective the way that the concept of a point of view that supports self-reference is grounded in the relevant basic cognitive skills that provide the required inferential unity.

You might think that the Lockean could avail themselves of the idea of the transparent unity of inference by treating self-reference at-a-time in Cartesian terms. By this I mean a conception of self-reference in which 'I' is treated as a term whose reference is secured by a quasi-perceptual act. This is to treat

'I' as akin to a perceptual demonstrative, like a special inward looking 'this'. The immediate problem with this suggestion is that 'this', unlike 'I', does not enjoy a transparent inferential unity. There is a substantive issue about the conditions under which inferences involving demonstratives are valid.

In general, we know that inferences of the form

a is *F*

a is *G*

_____

a is *F* and *G*

are valid. To say that this form is valid is to say that, in addition to the logical apparatus having their standard interpretation, each item of non-logical apparatus must make the same contribution to the determination of semantic value on each appearance. The notion of a valid form presupposes that we can individuate the non-logical apparatus in a way that preserves the identity of its contribution to the determination of semantic value of complex expressions. When the singular term is a demonstrative, it is a substantive issue to give such an individuation. There are many uses of 'this' that are syntactically identical without them playing the same semantic role. Given that it is a substantive issue to individuate the contribution demonstratives make to valid arguments, then any inference deploying demonstratives that appears transparent will only be so due to the obtaining of the relevant substantive conditions. That is to say, an account is required of the conditions under which

This is *F*

This is *G*

_____

This is *F* and *G*

is a valid inference. Russell's theory says that such conditions obtain when the subject of thought preserves acquaintance with the demonstrated object. This is why he insists that with genuine singular terms like demonstratives one has to argue quickly (Russell 1956, p. 203). Russell's view need not be endorsed as the final account of the matter, but it embodies a key insight.[7] Russell's insight is that the individuation of the semantic contribution of a demonstrative is dependent on the subject's point of view. That two uses of a demonstrative make the same contribution to the determination of semantic value of the sentences in which they occur is a matter of the thinking subject achieving and retaining an on-going acquaintance with the reference of the two uses. But that means that Russell's account cannot be deployed as a way of understanding the use of 'I' within the proposed Lockean unity-at-a-time on the model of a perceptual demonstrative, for Russell's account presupposes a substantive self who, as the achiever of acquaintance with the reference of a demonstrative, underpins the account of demonstrative reference. Russell's account of demonstratives is, therefore, already too Kantian to offer support to the Lockean.[8]

The Lockean's central problem is that they individuate Ideas such as to permit the very same Idea to be entertained independently of the identity of the Idea's owner. Clearly, there is a sense of 'idea' for which this seems appropriate. We speak of sharing ideas, of ideas being right for their time, of grasping another's ideas, and so on, but these are not the sorts of uses that one could expect to illuminate the rational economy of a subject's psychology. If a subject's point of view at-a-time is to be populated by Ideas individuated independently of the subject, an account is owed of how those Ideas come to be inferentially integrated. The starting point for the Lockean is, by definition, an individuation of Ideas that are not inferentially integrated in a way that makes sense of a subject's rational economy. That must be the case, for the Lockean individuation of Ideas allows for the possibility that the very same Idea could figure in two separate psychologies as when, for example, my Lockean consciousness is copied and divides into two. To achieve inferential integration within a subject's psychology there needs to be some account of how an Idea gets an individuation that accounts for it making the same contribution to the semantic value of complex expressions so that the Ideas together have a role to play in making rational sense of the subject.

In short, what is required is an account of how Ideas enjoy an inferential unity that makes rational sense of a subject's behaviour. Ideas need to figure in complex expressions such that ascription of beliefs and desires that deploy those complex expressions make overall rational sense of the subject. For this to be possible, the individuation of Ideas must be rich enough to show how the same Idea can figure in a sequence of complex expressions to make a valid inference. And that notion of valid inference must underpin our common sense notion of a subject being rationally explicable. Now, it is well known that many Ideas can only be individuated with respect to the subject, for example, demonstrative Ideas. As already noted, Russell's account of demonstrative Ideas is subject dependent. Many contemporary treatments are, in this respect, Russellian.[9] For such Ideas, the individuation is point-of-view-dependent. Such Ideas do not then survive independently of the subject's point of view. Such an individuation of Ideas is not then available to the Lockean.

For whom the inference tells

An individuation of Ideas that was subject dependent would provide items that were suitable to figure in the sort of rational inferential unity that makes up a point of view. Of course, such an individuation does not guarantee that of any given Idea the subject implicated in its individuation inferentially unifies that Idea with all others within their point of view. Subjects are not that rational. But a subject-dependent individuation of Ideas provides Ideas that are suited for inferential unification, it provides the conditions for the possibility of inferential unity. Whether such unity is actually achieved is another matter. What the Lockean model appears to lack is any account of how it is so much as possible that Ideas enjoy inferential unity. In contrast, with the Kantian model what we have is a thesis about the role of the 'I'—the self for whom inference tells—in the case of Ideas the individuation of which is subject dependent. In short, given the subject dependence of demonstrative Ideas, there is for the Kantian a simple account available of what underwrites the possibility of inferential unity for such Ideas. The account says that the inferential unity of demonstrative Ideas is due to an analogue of Kant's thesis of the transcendental unity of apperception. The thesis is that it is a condition on the possibility of valid demonstrative inference that the inference be accompanied by the 'I think'. Call this the accompaniment thesis:

> **Accompaniment thesis**: Where some singular term 'a' figures in a sequence that constitutes a valid inference, adding an 'I think' to each sentence in which 'a' occurs manifests the role the self plays in individuating the semantic contribution of 'a', for it provides the canonical representation of the form of the inference.[10]

It is important to be clear of the force of this thesis. The 'I think', the accompaniment of which provides the canonical representation of the argument form, is not what we might call an introspective 'I think'. If that were the case, the thesis would commit us to the view in which the 'I' is a referential term whose reference is secured by some type of inner demonstrative pointing. In contrast, what the 'I think' indicates is the existence of the acquaintance relation between subject and object thought about. The 'I think' manifests the existence of this acquaintance link. That is the basic substance to the demand of the accompaniment thesis. It is not enough merely for the subject to be consciously employing a demonstrative and so to be able to assert reflectively the 'I think'. The subject must have achieved an acquaintance with the demonstrated object. The thesis might be more accurately formulated in terms of the accompaniment of 'I attend to', for what the 'I think' picks out is something that is not transparent to the subject—the achievement of acquaintance with the object and whether or not I attend to something does more naturally require success on my part in picking it out.[11] With this clarification in place, I leave the thesis in its simpler formulation that echoes Kant's unity of apperception thesis.

To see why the accompaniment thesis holds of demonstratives, consider the case of a simple demonstrative inference,

(1) This is F

This is G

This is F and G.

The individuation of the demonstrative Idea that repeats in both premises and conclusion is subject dependent. The point is normally made in terms of what is required in order to individuate the sense of the demonstrative, for only then will one have an account in which the demonstrative term makes the same contribution to the determination of semantic value in each premise and the conclusion. The point is fundamentally Russellian and of a piece with Russell's conception of the role acquaintance plays in an account of meaning. It is the point that the individuation of Ideas is indexed to the subject's point of view. In Russell's hands this amounts to the claim that a demonstrative term gets to have a stable semantic value attached to it by virtue of the subject's on-going acquaintance with the object that is the term's semantic value. If this is right, then adding the 'I think' to each line of the inference makes manifest the role the self plays in ididividuating the semantic contribution of 'this'. Of course, there is a simpler representation of the form of the inference that might be thought a better candidate for manifesting its canonical form, namely that the inference is valid just in case it is of the form

a is F

a is G

---

a is F and G.

That, of course, captures well enough the syntactic form of the inference in virtue of which it is valid. But we know that with demonstrative terms a syntactic individuation is inadequate for individuating the concept of the repeatable contribution—the Idea—that the term needs to make on each occasion of use. That is why, for demonstrative terms, the canonical form of the inference is represented by

(2) I think this is F

I think this is G

I think this is F and G.

The force of this can be seen by contrasting (2) with

(3) I think this is F

You think this is G

??????

As it stands, nothing follows from my thinking of a demonstrated object that it is F and your thinking of a demonstrated object that it is G, even if the demonstrated object is the same item. It might be thought that this just shows that in supporting the accompaniment thesis I am appealing to a primitive and unexplained notion of a self implicated in the 'I think'. That is to mistake the direction of the dialectic that I set up at the beginning of this chapter. The 'I think' accompanies the sentences in the inference to render its validity in a canonical form not because it deploys a primitive notion of referring to a self; rather, all that the 'I think' serves to manifest is the existence of an on-going point of view, an acquaintance between thinking subject and object thought about. The accompaniment of the 'I think' is legitimate just in case there is an on-going acquaintance between subject and object. What I am taking as primitive is the notion of a point of view, something that is both subject and environment dependent in its characterization. For there to be an 'I think' there needs to be, in the demonstrative case, both the subject and the object thought about. The subject just is that which endures insofar as the cognitive capacities deployed in the inference endure; that is to say, those cognitive capacities required to support an enduring acquaintance with the demonstrated item.

The inference takes time to execute, so the acquaintance with the term's semantic value must be something that can endure. Acquaintance is dynamic, it has extension in time. How does the 'I think' come to have endurance? Again, the simple and obvious answer is that the 'I think' endures just in case there is an on-going acquaintance between the subject and the demonstrated object.

Consider a slightly different case. Consider the inference

(4) That is F

This is G

_____

This is F and G.

On the face of it, (4) is not a valid inference. But consider the scenario in which the subject is acquainted with an object that is out of reach and thinks that it is F. Then, as they move so that the object becomes close to hand they retain their acquaintance and think of the object that it is G. They then conclude that this very same object is both F and G. There is a case here for saying that there is an on-going dynamic sense for the demonstrative terms employed in (4) that makes this a valid inference just because there is a single recurring Idea expressed first with the term 'that' and then with 'this'.[12] If the subject fails to retain acquaintance with the demonstrated object during movement, then there will be no enduring Idea and no valid demonstrative inference expressed by the sentences deployed at (4). There might, of course, be other descriptive-based inferences.

For present purposes, I do not need to argue that the accompaniment thesis applies to all singular terms, although it is tempting to endorse a fully Russellian position in which, in effect, it is a condition on something being a genuine singular term that the accompaninent thesis applies. The plausibility of this more general thesis can, however, be briefly outlined. Consider a case involving proper names. Suppose I say

George Bush is F

and you say

If George Bush is F, Dick Cheney is G

and a third speaker says

Dick Cheney is G.

Is that a valid inference? The question is, of course, odd. We would need to know much more before agreeing that a valid inference has taken place. For all we know these utterances might have taken place in the correct temporal sequence but on different continents! In such circumstances there would fail to be the appropriate inferential unity to the Ideas, there would be no account available of how my utterance could bear upon yours such as to make the third utterance a conclusion. A first stab at what is required in order to see the above sayings as part of a common inference would be to require that they are all made as part of the same conversation. Then, of course, it would make sense to think that an inference was taking place for, ordinarily, use of the same syntactic item in a shared conversation is normally taken as use of the item with a common on-going sense. It is highly irregular, in the middle of a conversation about George Bush to start talking about another person, also called 'George Bush', without signalling that that is what one is doing. You cannot expect people to keep track of what is being said if you do that. You forfeit the idea that there is a unity to the Ideas being shared in the conversation. If membership of a common conversation is along the right lines in getting an account of the circumstances under which use of proper names counts as expressing Ideas with an inferential unity, that would seem to reinforce the above argument for the accompaniment thesis. It is difficult to see how to fill out the idea of membership of a common conversation without reintroducing some reference to the capacity of the individual members of the conversation to exhibit a capacity for awareness of such membership. If so, there is still an 'I think' that accompanies the use of the proper name, an 'I think' that signals the awareness of contributing to a shared linguistic activity.

I do not need to argue the point any further, for enough has already been said to reveal the depth of the difficulties that face the Lockean account of Ideas and self-reference. Consider again the extreme case in which three speakers in three distant locations utter the sentences about George Bush that would, were they party to a common conversation, enjoy an inferential unity that rendered the utterances part of a valid inference. In such a scenario it seems absurd to suppose that the three disjointed utterances could count as components of a valid inference. Nevertheless, that scenario is no worse than the situation that obtains with a Lockean account of Ideas.

According to the Lockean, the individuation of Ideas is subject independent. This means that the individuation of an Idea permits the possibility that the very same Idea can be replicated in different contexts and different subjects. The threat to a proper identity relation for persons in the Lockean philosophy arises precisely because Ideas are individuated in a way that allows them to be replicated many times over independently of the notion of a subject's point of view. So, whether or not I make it to survive the next 20 years, an Idea currently in my memory can survive as the very same item regardless of my fate. Twenty years from now my body might survive but my consciousness only bear a similarity relation to me now, rather than the identity relation. A more extreme scenario would be one in which my body does not survive but the Ideas, or some subset of them, that I currently have are copied into a different physical basis for memory. In that case, I appear to have left the scene but my Idea could carry on. But if the Lockean permits these radical notions of Idea identity independent of self-identity, then insofar as the Ideas matter, there is nothing about the Ideas as such, even when they all appear in just my mind, that makes the Ideas at play in the George Bush inference hang together in an inferential unity. For the Lockean, Ideas intrinsically do not hang together, for they are intrinsically individuated in a manner that permits their continuing individuation regardless of their bearing or not on each other. The Lockean has, in effect, a radical atomism about the individuation of Ideas. They simply do not get it together.

The argument does not close the case, but let me summarize the picture that I have been recommending as a Kantian account of how Ideas get to enjoy inferential unity. For the Kantian, a condition on the unity of inference is the possibility of the relevant Ideas being accompanied by the 'I think'. Ideas bear inferentially on one another because they fall within a subject's point of view, the view of the subject who thinks 'I think'. The 'I think' is not, however, a primitive. The position I have been recommending does not require a prior and primitive capacity to self-refer. The capacity to refer to other things is an achievement. It is an achievement that requires an ability to attend to things and retain that attention so that Ideas can bind over time and engage inferentially with one another. The capacity to self-refer is not an achievement, for the self picked out by 'I' is just that which holds Ideas over time and whose capacity for keeping track of things makes Ideas bear inferentially upon one another. On this broadly Kantian conception, there is such a thing as self-reference, but it is not primitive. Rather it is explained in virtue of a subject's capacity to keep track of things and thereby provide the basic temporal binding of Ideas required for Ideas to enjoy inferential unity. Therefore, if a case could be made for a subject who lacked such basic capacities, the case would thereby have been made for a subject who no longer could self-refer. For such a subject, the self would be eroded. When the capacity for keeping track of things goes, the tracker goes. And that is the self on the Kantian conception.

Dementia errors

Patients with severe dementia are prone to make errors that indicate a failure of temporal binding with very simple Ideas. It is an empirical matter whether any subjects make errors as basic as the ones I want to discuss, but in theory there is no reason to suppose they could not. I want to illustrate the sort of breakdown in temporal binding that *prima facie* amounts to loss of self.

The sort of case I have in mind is that of a patient who has lost the ability to hold together the basic narratives of daily life. For example, consider a normal subject who is thirsty at time t_1. They have a desire for a drink at t_1. Suppose now that a few minutes later they have a drink. At that later time a normal subject will be able to integrate their Ideas over time and amend their beliefs and desires in the light of their keeping track of events. A normal subject will be prone to endorse the validity of simple inferences like:

(5) I was thirsty
    I have had a drink
    _____
    I am not thirsty now.

This does not involve a keeping track of the self, but it does involve an ability to keep track of various basic needs and sensations and the way that these change given the way things are going in the environment. In varying degrees, this sort of keeping track of needs, sensations, and environmental circumstances is eroded in dementia patients. The inability to keep track of things comes in degrees and it is an empirical matter to test any given patient's ability to keep track of their own needs and sensations and how things are going.

We can consider a range of cases from patients whose capacity for temporal binding is trapped within discrete time frames to patients who show no capacity for basic temporal binding. The former might be the patient who needs to work out afresh each day who their daily visitor is, but who manages nevertheless to retain short narratives over the course of an afternoon's visit. The latter might be the patient who never really seems to keep track of who their visitor is, let alone when they last had a drink (minutes ago). Of course, such patients may make considerable use of the first-person pronoun. They may make all sorts of pronouncements such as, 'I am thirsty', 'I have not eaten', and so on. What interests me is the possibility of the patient who, despite such articulations, fails to achieve any significant temporal binding with these claims.

On the Kantian model that I outlined above, being a successful user of 'I' does not require an inward reference, a keeping track of something that has to be achieved. On the Kantian model, being a successful user of 'I' requires the capacity for outward reference, a keeping track of items in the environment and how they bear upon the state of things including one's own body. I claimed that keeping track of an object is an achievement, an achievement of the self, the 'I' that accompanies inferences that exploit temporal binding. The self is not itself something that one keeps track of. There is no temporal binding for the self. The self is the condition for the possibility of the temporal binding of

Ideas of objects and events in the environment. If a patient cannot achieve that sort of temporal binding, then there is nothing else, on the Kantian model, for successful 'I' use to consist in. The failure to keep track of objects and events in the environment, if severe enough, can amount to a failure of self.

Indeed, matters are worse. The severely demented patient who has lost the capacity for temporal binding is no better off than the Lockean self subject to fusion and fission, for they lack any principled way of bundling Ideas into inferentially integrated sets. Severe dementia can reduce a subject to a Lockean self. As we saw earlier, a Lockean self is no self at all. It is a reductionist conception on which selfhood has been eroded.

The above sort of case raises challenging metaphysical issues regarding our attitude to severely demented patients. Patients who fail to bind their Ideas about their food, drink, and so on over even short periods of time show a considerable forgetfulness. It is a forgetfulness that amounts to a failure to bind Ideas over time. Their ideas literally do not add up. When that happens, there is no acquaintance relation that individuates Ideas over time. The acquaintance relation manifests the way Ideas of objects are bound over time by a self, not because the acquaintance relation presupposes a primitive prior reference to the self, but because the self just is that which is made manifest by the existence of temporally extended acquaintance relations. This is what is made manifest by the accompanying 'I think'. When Ideas fail to bind, it signals no self.

It is tempting to suppose that the patient who fails to keep track of their own bodily states such as hunger, thirst, and so on is simply a self with a massive forgetfulness. On the sort of Kantian conception that I have been recommending that cannot be right. The supposition amounts to an attempt to secure self-reference with 'I' while acknowledging a forgetfulness with respect to hunger, thirst, and other bodily states. So, with the

> I am thirsty

the idea is that the patient has a self-reference even if they have lost track of their bodily states. But on the Kantian conception, there is no such thing as securing the use of 'I' independently of securing an ability to keep track of various basic features of the environment. For sure, there is nothing to rule out the possibility of a subject who fails to track their bodily states but nevertheless tracks a sufficient range of other environmental happenings to warrant a use of 'I' in self-reference. But my hypothesis was to consider a demented subject whose forgetfulness was so complete that there is nothing, not even their own bodily states, that they are able to track. In such circumstances, there is no way of maintaining self-reference against a backdrop of quite general failure to keep track of things. The only way to maintain self-reference under such circumstances would be by adopting a non-Kantian account of 'I', most likely a Cartesian one in which 'I' functions as an inner demonstrative.

Although the metaphysics are challenging, the above argument does not entail dramatic consequences for our moral attitudes to demented patients.

The self, whose erosion I have suggested is a possibility that can be conceived, is not necessarily the self that matters in considering the moral treatment of subjects. Even in the extreme case of a demented patient with an eroded self on my conception, there would still be a case for considering the sentient subject, the subject of pain, comfort, and so on, if such things matter for our assessment of the moral standing of a subject. The loss of self is compatible with remaining an object of moral concern by being a subject capable of experiencing pain, comfort, distress, and so on. The argument canvassed does mean, however, that there is a real sense in which the loss of self can precede bodily death and the end of sentience in the case of severely demented patients. This does not entail that such a subject is suddenly worth something less in our moral considerations, but it does suggest that we might need to consider afresh our cognitive attitude to such subjects.

It means that our cognitive attitude to such subjects should acknowledge the scope for saying that when they say 'I am thirsty' they are profoundly wrong. The possibility canvassed is not just that the carer might be better placed to judge the truth of the patient's thirst, for that is, after all, a possibility that can obtain with non-demented subjects. The point is that the patient is not placed to make a judgement at all. For such a patient there is no judgement taking place, because there is no self as judge—the self that tracks, attends to, and makes acquaintance with things.

Endnotes

1 I use a capitalized 'Idea' for a specific thought component—a sense.

2 Social constructionists will think this obvious because they hold that the capacity for self-reference is dependent on the capacity to refer to other subjects. It is not that sort of social dependency of self-reference that concerns me, but a more primitive dependency on the capacity to refer to things, objects, events, and processes outside of the subject.

3 I was led to think about these matters in response to my own reaction to the empirical data when, on reflecting on a relative's dementia, I was struck by the sense that there was a point to the thought their self had been lost before life was lost.

4 The philosophical territory I draw upon is rich and extensive. I simplify much in applying ideas from contemporary work on self-reference to bear upon the issue of what, if anything, we should say about the possibility of self-reference in severe dementia patients. Applying complex philosophical ideas to issues that affect policy matters is always tricky but I hope that the scholars whose work I draw upon will find their ideas still recognizable in this context.

5 *Locus classicus* Parfit (1986) and, for a recent corrective to the use of thought experiments, see Wilkes (1988).

6 The assumption that ideas are individuated as types of content is very contentious. It is one of the many points where the thinking behind the Lockean model breaks down. I return to this point below.

7 Apart from anything else, Russell's account is contentious precisely because he treats 'I' on a par with demonstratives or, at least, he says insufficient about the matter to distinguish an account of 'I' from a theory of demonstratives.

8 If I am right to insist on the Kantian character of Russell's insight, that places further pressure on the coherence of Russell's position that the genuine singular terms are 'this', 'that,' and 'I', for it is unclear that these three can be treated in the same way. Of course, Russell changed his mind about this triumvirate, later relegating 'I' from the set of genuine singular terms.

9 There is also 'Russellian' in sense of direct reference theorists, but their preoccupation is generally that of the formal semanticist, rather than an account of the inferential unity suitable for making rational sense of behaviour.

10 The canonical representation is simply that representation that most fully and transparently reveals the principles of individuation for the semantic elements involved. In this case, the claim is that the individuation of the relevant elements is dependent on the existence of the acquaintance relation between subject and object.

11 Recall that the reason why there is a transparent unity of inference with 'I' is precisely because with 'I' there is no achievement of acquaintance, for 'I' does not function as an introspective demonstrative.

12 For more on the idea of dynamic thoughts cf. Dokic (1997).

References

Campbell, J. (1997). The structure of time in autobiographical memory. *European Journal of Philosophy*, **5**: 105–18.

Dokic, J. (ed.) (1997). *European Review of Philosophy, Volume 2. Cognitive Dynamics*. Stanford: Centre for the Study of Language and Information (CSLI).

Parfit, D. (1986). *Reasons and Persons*. Oxford: Oxford University Press.

Russell, B. (1956). The philosophy of logical atomism. In: *Logic and Knowledge* (ed. R. C. Marsh), pp. 175–283. London: Allen and Unwin.

Wilkes, K. (1988). *Real People: Personal Identity without Thought Experiments*. Oxford: Clarendon Press.

Williams, B. (1978). *Descartes: the Project of Pure Enquiry*. London: Allen Lane Press.

8 The discursive turn, social constructionism, and dementia

Tim Thornton

Introduction

The structure of this chapter is as follows. In the first section, I characterize discursive psychology as, in part, an attempt to sidestep a worry about the privacy of meaning, which may have advantages in approaching dementia. I stress the importance of a constitutive claim it makes and show how social constructionism might underpin that constitutive claim.

In the central philosophical section of the chapter I outline objections to the constructionism that often underpins the discursive turn. Constructionism has been defended through an interpretation of Wittgenstein but there are, in fact, Wittgensteinian reasons to be suspicious of it. I go on to suggest that constructionism can still be present in interpretations of Wittgenstein that explicitly aim to avoid social constructionism.

In the final section I suggest an alternative approach to fill out the constitutive claim, which invokes the irreducible role of rationality rather than social construction. I suggest that this can be used to help interpret the speech and actions of dementia sufferers. But I suggest that, although false, a constructionist approach to meaning may play a positive heuristic role in making sense of dementia sufferers—even though it carries with it a danger of abuse.

A discursive approach to the mind has a number of attractions. Centrally, it places meaning in the public world. This helps sidestep a worry that might otherwise arise about the privacy of meaning and a version of the problem of other minds. The discursive view thus makes a phenomenon, which we generally take for granted outside, perhaps, clinical circumstances, more explicable. In general we can know or have 'access' to other people's meanings. We do generally know what other people mean. If meaning, by contrast with a discursive approach, is thought of as a matter of an internal state of mind then substantial further work has to be done to show how this could be shared. The discursive approach, instead, starts with a picture of meaning as essentially sharable and thus no such subsequent explanatory work has to be done.

A discursive view also helps place meaning in nature. This is a point to which I shall return. But, preliminarily, it helps to show that meaning is a perfectly natural aspect of the world that fits into an everyday conception of reality. But—and this will become an important point—it does not do this by relating it to a more basic natural scientific world view. At its best, it is a form of naturalism without being a form of reductionist naturalism.

In mental health care, especially dementia, a discursive view encourages a person-centred interpretational approach exemplified in the work of Steven Sabat and the late Tom Kitwood rather than the 'defectological' view in which 'the afflicted person is defined principally in terms of his or her catalogued dysfunctions' (Sabat 2001, p. 10).

In the case of dementia, a discursive approach *may* have a fourth further attraction. This depends on a connection between the discursive turn and constructionism, which will be outlined in the next two sections. By 'constructionism' I mean the view that meanings are constituted by on-going linguistic moves, rather than the on-going linguistic moves being governed by antecedent meanings. If the discursive approach is also constructionist then the following possibility arises. On the assumption that meanings are constructed in on-going conversations, this need not imply that all parties in the conversation take on equal conversational work in their construction. And thus it might seem that there can be compensation where one party is no longer equally able to take part through, for example, the onset of dementia.

Now there is an everyday sense in which this seems perfectly plausible. It is a matter of phenomenological fact that one can work to make sense of utterances that are not initially clear. But on a constructionist view this flows from a deep feature of meaning: the fact that it is of its very nature to be invented piecemeal. The work is not one of detection of meaning but co-creation. Whilst I do not want to cast doubt on the phenomenological fact just mentioned, I do intend to dispute this explanation of it.

Nevertheless, if it is to be a genuine alternative to the cognitivist orthodoxy, the discursive approach has to make a stronger claim than that meanings are *caused* by social factors and constructionism is one way to discharge that obligation. So, if not constructionism, then what? In the final section I shall highlight the fundamental distinction between a broadly discursive approach and cognitivism and outline its implications for thinking about meaning in the context of dementia.

The discursive turn and its contrast with cognitivism

In this section I shall outline the discursive approach to psychology or psychiatry, contrasting it with cognitivism; outline the importance of the distinction between constitutive and causal accounts of the role of social factors; and describe the connection between the discursive turn and social constructionism.

Discursive psychology is the name of a family of approaches taken by different authors, which share the central assumption that psychological phenomena can be investigated through the analysis of 'discourse'. The focus on discourse, as opposed to language, marks the fact that 'discourse is to be treated as a social practice which can be studied as a real-world phenomenon rather than a theoretical abstraction' (Edwards and Potter 1992, p. 15). Thus the focus is on actual utterances rather than the structure of rules or grammar that make up a language. Discursive psychology is based on the central idea that 'some central psychological phenomena are related in participants' discourse' (Edwards and Potter 1992, pp. 1–2). But, as I shall describe, this is not supposed to be merely a heuristic device but a radical theoretical perspective.

Edwards and Potter explicitly contrast their own approach in *Discursive Psychology* with a 'cognitivist' approach:

> A contrast is drawn between cognitivist approaches to language, where texts, sentences and descriptions are taken as . . . realizations of underlying cognitive representations of . . . [the] world; and the discursive approach where versions of events, things, people and so on, are studied and theorized primarily in terms of how those versions are constructed in an occasioned manner to accomplish social actions. (Edwards and Potter 1992, p. 8)

Whilst cognitivism takes utterances to be expressions of mental states, construed as underlying representations, a discursive approach inverts the priority and instead regards psychological phenomena as explicable in terms of the social phenomena of language use, action, and so on.

It will be useful to define cognitivist approaches a little more carefully. They can be illustrated by looking at computational theories of the mind described in standard textbooks on cognitive psychology. In his *Explorations in Cognitive Neuropsychology*, Parkin says

> Cognitive psychology can be defined as the branch of psychology which attempts to provide scientific explanation of how the brain carries out complex mental functions such as vision, memory, language and thinking. Cognitive psychology arose at a time when computers were beginning to make a major impact on science and it was perhaps natural that cognitive psychologists should draw an analogy between computers and the human brain. The computer analogy was used frequently to draw up a model of the brain in which mental activity was characterised in terms of the flow of information between different stores. (Parkin 1996, p. 3)

A key element of this approach is that for information (or 'content' as it also known) to be processed there have to be bearers of that information (or content). Thus the mind or brain is populated with states or 'representations' (as in the quotation from Edwards and Potter above) that carry meaning or *encode* content (for the latter phrase see Bolton and Hill (1996)). In other words, a computational approach to the mind presupposes a medium of computation: a system of inner states or representations. Thus states of mind are constituted, according to this view, by internal information bearing states of the brain or nervous system. In other words, they are constituted by factors within the skull. Utterances and other 'outer' behaviour are merely evidence of the inner states that cause them. I shall take this to characterize a cognitivist approach. A discursive approach, by contrast, inverts the priority of mind and linguistic behaviour presupposed by cognitivism.

One advantage of this kind of approach from a philosophical perspective is that it undercuts a worry about the privacy of meanings and mental states that might otherwise exist and which is encouraged by a cognitivist approach. If mental states are construed as internal states of a person, then a number of problems arise. First, there is the problem of other minds: how do we know what mental states others are in if all we have to base our judgements on are outward appearances? Second, how do we know what others mean if meanings are, again, internal matters? But third, if our own mental states are also internal states, how can they reveal the outer world? Why are we not trapped within a 'veil of perceptions'?

The discursive turn, by contrast, sidesteps the problem of connecting inner states to the world—and thus accounting for intentionality—by placing meaning firmly in the public realm. Broadly, if meaning is constituted in public interactions then the challenge to bridge a gap between the inner and the outer, the private and the public, falls away. The materials on which an account of meaning is to be based are always already outer and public.

These problems are mentioned by Harré and Gillett in *The Discursive Mind*:

> Obviously the things that fix the meanings of words cannot be hidden inside the respective heads of different people or else we would each be uncertain all the time what anybody else was talking about. Thus it is hard to say what I could mean by claiming that my thoughts are true, and my utterances meaningful, if I am trapped within them and at their mercy (and they are hidden inside me). The problem runs very deep because others cannot get outside their veils of perception either. This entails that none of us knows what the world is really like, nor what others think, nor whether anything we think is actually true, nor what anyone else means by the words they use, nor indeed what I mean by the words I use. Clearly, we have to find some way to make sense of the fact that we *can* aim to think true thoughts and express them in a common system of signs. This is an even more pressing need when we consider the fact that thoughts are communicable. (Harré and Gillett 1994, p. 43)

A discursive approach thus has a fundamental advantage concerning the metaphysics and epistemology of mind. But if it really has these advantages it must be genuinely distinct from the alternative, which, following Edwards and Potter, I shall call cognitivism. It must amount to a *constitutive* rather than a merely *causal* claim about the connection of mind and discourse. Even a cognitivist can accept, for example, that mental states or meanings are caused by social factors. They can take a wider view of the influences on psychological phenomena than one that restricts itself to what happens within the skull. But that is consistent with also holding, as cognitivists typically do, that such effects are mediated by what happens within the skull.

To be genuinely distinct, the discursive approach must involve a claim that psychological phenomena are not merely caused by social factors but also constituted by them, rather than constituted by factors within the skull. This is suggested by Harré and Gillett:

> In this sense, the psychological is not reducible to or replaceable by explanations in terms of physiology, physics, or any other point of view that does not reveal the structure of meanings existing in the lives of the human group to which the subject of an investigation belongs.   (Harré and Gillett 1994, p. 20)

By claiming that the psychological is irreducible, they suggest a stronger claim than the mere causal role of social factors. They summarize their view thus:

1. Many psychological phenomena are to be interpreted as properties or features of discourse, and that discourse might be public or private. As public, it is behaviour; as private, it is thought.

2. Individual and private uses of symbolic systems, which in this view constitute thinking, are derived from interpersonal discursive processes that are the main feature of the human environment.

3. The production of psychological phenomena, such as emotions, decisions, attitudes, personality displays, and so on, in discourse depends upon the skill of the actors, their relative moral standing in the community, and the story lines that unfold.   (Harré and Gillett 1994, p. 27)

Whilst this characterization is not completely clear, it contains a good indication of a constitutive view. Psychological factors are construed as aspects of discourse itself. Thinking comprises private discourse, that is, 'individual and private uses of symbol systems', but this is, in turn, derived from interpersonal processes. Psychological phenomena are not merely produced *by* discourse—as a cognitivist might agree when, for example, anger, construed as an inner state, is caused by harsh words—but produced *in* the discourse. The idea of 'private uses' or the claim that 'discourse . . . as private . . . is thought' is not completely straightforward, but, nevertheless, the approach summarized looks to be genuinely distinct from a form of cognitivism.

So far I have highlighted the central role that public utterance plays in discursive psychology and contrasted it with cognitivism. I have stressed the claim that it has to be a constitutive rather than a causal account of the mind if it is to be genuinely distinct from cognitivism. This leaves, however, the question of how that constitutive claim is unpacked. What exactly is the constitutive claim? How does discourse constitute psychological phenomena?

The most common answer to this question adopted by the discursive turn is a form of social *constructionism*. If psychological phenomena, including mental states and meanings, are constructed by utterances then this both explains the constitutive connection and also underpins a clear distinction between discursive psychology and cognitivism. (On the latter view, by contrast, utterances are merely evidence of pre-existing underlying states that do not depend constitutively on them.) The constructionist view of discursive psychology is expressed in the following passages.

> In this view, our delineation of the subject matter of psychology has to take account of discourses, significations, subjectivities, and positionings, for it is in these that psychological phenomena *actually* exist. For example, an attitude should not be seen as a semipermanent mental entity, causing people to say and do certain things. Rather, it *comes into existence* in displays expressive of decisions and judgments and in the performance of actions.   (Harré and Gillett 1994, p. 22, latter emphasis added)

> In keeping with the discursive approach to psychology, this study is based on the principle that meanings are jointly constituted by participants in a conversation. From the discursive point of view, psychological phenomena are not inner or hidden properties or processes of mind which discourse merely expresses. The discursive expression is . . . the psychological phenomenon itself . . . Personhood can be an interpersonal discursive construction, a property of conversations . . . The mind is no more than, but no less than, a privatized part of the 'general conversation'. Meanings are jointly constructed by competent actors in the course of projects that are realised within systems of public norms.   (Sabat and Harré 1994, pp. 145–46)

> Rather than seeing such discursive constructions as expressions of speakers' underlying cognitive states, they are examined in the context of their occurrence as situated and occasioned constructions whose precise nature makes sense, to participants and analysts alike, in terms of the social actions those descriptions accomplish.   (Edwards and Potter 1992, p. 2)

The broad thrust of these accounts of the discursive approach is that it is based on the constitution of psychological phenomena in utterances and other social actions and these construct the phenomena in question. The constitutive claim that helps distinguish a discursive approach from cognitivism is underpinned by a constructionist claim. If psychological phenomena are constructed in, for example, on-going conversations, then they cannot be constituted by states within the skull.

There is a further characterization of constructionist forms of discursive psychology that will be useful later. It is best described through a contrast, again, with cognitivism. A cognitivist approach aims to fit meaning and mental states within a broadly natural scientific account of the world in general and psychiatry and mental health in particular. It is thus a form of naturalism in its reductionist form. The problematic and puzzling phenomena of meaning are to be shown to be natural and thus not, in fact, puzzling by relating them to paradigmatically natural phenomena. The puzzling phenomena are explained in more basic terms and thus reduced to them. Of course, it is a matter of decision what the paradigmatically natural phenomena are. Jerry Fodor, for example, selects the catalogue *physicists* have been compiling 'of the ultimate and irreducible properties of things' (Fodor 1987, p. 97). But the aim of making sense of puzzling phenomena, of making them natural, takes the form of an explanation in more basic terms, whichever they may be.

Given that it resists the reduction of psychological phenomena to what lies within the skull, discursive psychology seems to stand opposed to that picture. Indeed, Hosking and Morley make this point explicitly:

'Social constructionism' (as we see it) refers to a loose concatenation of theoretical frameworks that emphasise both the constructive powers of human minds and their origins in conversations, conventions, and cultural traditions ... Such frameworks have developed from long-standing philosophical traditions, and they provide a background to at least two contemporary debates: one that contrasts psychology as a natural science with psychology as a moral science, and one that contrasts individual psychology with collective psychology. Often, but not always, those who see psychology as a natural science want to reduce social psychology to individual psychology. Often, but not always, those who see psychology as a moral science see psychology as concerned with reasons rather than causes and with forms of self-expression that are constituted in conversations, unique to certain times and places. (Hosking and Morley, 2004, pp. 318–19)

Hosking and Morley thus suggest that social constructionism—and by implication a constructionist form of discursive psychology—stands opposed to the reductionist naturalism that grounds cognitivism. Whereas cognitivism aims to fit mind and meaning into a natural scientific account, social constructionism aims to deny that and, possibly, to see psychology as a moral science rather a natural science. Whilst I agree that this is an important aspect of a broadly discursive approach, I shall argue in the second section that constructionism in fact shares some aspect of the reductionist naturalist approach and that discursive psychology is better purged of that reductionist aspiration.

If the discursive turn is underpinned by a form of social constructionism then, whatever its methodological fruitfulness in empirical investigation, it is a radical and counter-intuitive account of the mind. This prompts the question, is it tenable? One key influence on social constructionist accounts of meaning has been a family of interpretations of Wittgenstein to which I shall now turn to assess this question.

Wittgenstein and constructionism about meaning

In this section I shall briefly summarize a familiar argument for a social constructionist view of meaning drawn from Wittgenstein (for a longer treatment see Thornton (1998)). I shall set out some central philosophical objections to constructionism about meaning. Finally, I shall also critically examine a more recent implicitly constructionist reading.

Wittgenstein's discussion of rules, which lies at the heart of his *Philosophical Investigations*, has been taken by a number of authors to support a form of social constructionism about meaning. Rules and meanings are connected because meanings are normative. To understand the meaning of a word is to understand how to use it *correctly*. It is to understand the rule that prescribes its correct use. So an account of understanding rules in general will shed light on understanding meanings. The analysis will also have consequences for mental content—the 'meaning' of mental states—because that is also normative.

The problem that Wittgenstein introduces at the start of the discussion of rules follows from two features of understanding:

> But we *understand* the meaning of a word when we hear or say it; we grasp it in a flash, and what we grasp in this way is surely something different from the 'use' which is extended in time! (Wittgenstein 1953, §138)

> . . . isn't the meaning of the word also determined by this use? And can't these ways of determining meaning conflict? Can what we grasp *in a flash* accord with a use, fit or fail to fit it? And how can what is present to us in an instant, what comes before our mind in an instant, fit a *use*? (Wittgenstein 1953, §139)

Understanding a rule (such as the circumstances for the correct application of a word or for the equally open-ended continuation of a mathematical series) can be both manifested over time but also expressed at a particular time, when one grasps how to go on, perhaps saying 'Now I've got it!' If understanding has these two aspects, what is it that connects them?

Later in *Philosophical Investigations*, Wittgenstein describes a related puzzle concerning the intentionality of mental content more generally:

> A wish seems already to know what will or would satisfy it; a proposition, a thought, what makes it true—even when that thing is not there at all! Whence this *determining* of what is not yet there? This despotic demand? (Wittgenstein 1953, §437)

Again the question is what connects a state at one time with the worldly feature it is about (and even a feature that does not exist)?

The most promising approach to the question seems to be to sketch a mental mechanism that connects an initial experience, or state, of grasping a rule with its subsequent correct application. Wittgenstein, however, considers and rejects a number of plausible mechanisms. None can support the normative connection between understanding a rule or the meaning of a word and its correct application. (Similarly, no mechanism can connect an intentional mental state and what it is about.)

Saul Kripke, in an influential account of these sections, highlights Wittgenstein's criticism of theories that implicitly rely on an act of interpretation. It is tempting to think that understanding consists in something coming before the mind's eye, something like a symbol or picture. If, however, understanding were to consist in entertaining an inner symbol then it would do so only under a particular interpretation of that symbol. But—if understanding is a form of interpretation—the correct interpretation of the symbol would also have to be codified in a further inner symbol, which would, in turn, require further interpretation. And thus a vicious regress begins. It is vicious because the first symbol only has any meaning under an interpretation specified by the completed infinite series of further interpretations.

Kripke reinforces this argument by postulating a sceptic who challenges us to justify our normal pre-philosophical claim to know which arithmetic rules we have followed in the past, specifically addition. He postulates a sceptical alternative: a deviant version of addition that differs only in cases not so far considered. The challenge is to show that we have always added in the past rather than used the deviant function. The problem is that any previous statement we may have made of the rule, or any finite behavioural evidence for it, or any mental images that might depict it, can be interpreted in more than one way: in accord with both addition and the deviant rule (which differs only in cases so far not considered). Thus it seems that we cannot defeat a sceptical challenge to our claim to understand what rule we have followed in the past. But nothing is different about the present case. Kripke concludes that this undermines the very idea of determinate meanings:

> There can be no such thing as meaning anything by any word. Each new application we make is a leap in the dark; any present intention could be interpreted so as to accord with anything we may choose to do. So there can be neither accord, nor conflict. This is what Wittgenstein said in §202 [sic]. (Kripke 1982, p. 55)

In its place he deploys a form of social constructionism:

> It is essential to our concept of a rule that we maintain some such conditional as 'If Jones means addition by "+", then if he is asked for "68 + 57", he will reply "125" ' . . . The conditional as stated makes it appear that some mental state obtains in Jones that guarantees his performance of particular additions such as '68 + 57'—just what the sceptical argument denies. Wittgenstein's picture of the true situation concentrates on the contrapositive, and on justification conditions. If Jones does *not* come out with '125' when asked about '68 + 57', we cannot assert that he means addition by '+'. (Kripke 1982, pp. 94–5)

Kripke's suggestion is that whilst rules cannot prescribe their correct applications, there can be the appearance of rule-governed behaviour, and thus of meaning, providing that there is a community. The community provides a negative standard by which on-going practice can be judged. As long as they are not criticized by the community a subject can be considered to be following a rule. Thus something like correctness is constituted by the on-going judgements of the community.

Kripke is not the only philosopher to offer an explicitly constructionist view of meaning. Although he criticizes Kripke's sceptical argument, Crispin Wright also deploys a form of constructionism. According to Wright,

> One of the most basic philosophical puzzles about intentional states is that they seem to straddle two conflicting paradigms: on the one hand they are

> avowable, so to that extent conform to the paradigm of sensation and other 'observable' phenomena of consciousness; on the other they answer constitutively to the ways in which the subject manifests them, and to that extent conform to the paradigm of psychological characteristics which, like irritability or modesty, are properly conceived as dispositional . . . It seems that neither an epistemology of observation—of pure introspection—nor one of inference can be harmonised with all aspects of the intentional. (Wright 1991, p. 142)

Intention is only one example of a general phenomenon which also includes understanding, remembering, and deciding. In each case, the subject has a special non-inferential authority in ascribing these to themselves which is, nevertheless, defeasible in the light of subsequent performance. Wittgenstein's attack on explanations of such states shows that they cannot be modelled on a Cartesian picture of observation of inner experiences (because such inner states cannot prescribe what should satisfy them). But if understanding, intending, and the like are to be modelled on abilities instead, as Wittgenstein seems to suggest, how can the subject have special authority in ascribing these to themselves in the light of the attack on substantial explanation?

Constructivism appears to provide a solution to this problem. The basic idea is to deny that there is any inner *epistemology* and to devise a constructivist account of intention instead:

> The authority which our self-ascriptions of meaning, intention, and decision assume is not based on any kind of cognitive advantage, expertise or achievement. Rather it is, as it were, a *concession*, unofficially granted to anyone whom one takes seriously as a rational subject. It is, so to speak, such a subject's right to declare what he intends, what he intended, and what satisfies his intentions; and his possession of this right consists in the conferral upon such declarations, other things being equal, of a *constitutive* rather than descriptive role. (Wright 1987, p. 400)

All other things being equal, a speaker's sincere judgements constitute the content of the intention, understanding, or decision. They *determine*, rather than *reflect*, the content of the state concerned. The meaning of a word or the content of an intention is constituted by the on-going judgements a speaker makes. Elsewhere, Wright talks of meaning as being 'plastic in response to speakers' ongoing performance' (Wright 1986, p. 289).

Although constructionist interpretations of Wittgenstein have been influential, there is mounting reason to doubt that they are a satisfactory interpretation. The central philosophical objection to constructionism about meaning is that it fails in its main aim. It attempts to explain a problematic concept—in this case meaning or content including, centrally, its normativity—in simpler terms. In this aim it is a form of reductionist naturalism like cognitivist accounts of meaning. Having found the notion of understanding a rule (which prescribes correct use) or forming an intention (which prescribes what should satisfy it) puzzling, it attempts to rebuild that notion from more basic ideas. Kripke aims to capture an ersatz notion of the normativity of rules using the idea of (absence of) communal dissent. We are justified in ascribing accord with a rule to a subject providing that they have not disagreed with the community. Wright aims to capture the normativity of mental content such as the content of intentions using a subject's on-going avowals or judgements.

There are two main problems with the approach. First, neither Kripke nor Wright succeeds in recapturing the pre-philosophical notion that such judgements answer to something and that has radical and implausible consequences. To take just one key problem, without the notion that there is something that it would be correct to assert in a circumstance, we lose the right to think of states or affairs or facts that are independent of judgement. If so, such constructionism leads to a crude idealism.

Second, the approach is inconsistent in that both Kripke and Wright appeal to notions of meaning or content in their attempt to explain it. Kripke appeals to dissent, Wright to individual judgement. But both of these notions require prior grasp of norms: the norms governing the meaning of 'no', perhaps, and those governing the content of individual judgements that are supposed to 'unpack' or construct the content of intentions, respectively.

It is also important to keep in mind how constructionism falsifies everyday phenomenology. As McDowell asserts,

> But suppose I form the intention to type a period. If that is my intention, it is settled that only my typing a period will count as executing it. Of course I am capable of forming that intention only because I am party to the practices that are constitutive of the relevant concepts. But if that is indeed the intention that—thus empowered—I form, nothing more than the intention itself is needed to determine what counts as conformity to it. Certainly it needs no help from my subsequent judgements. (Suppose I forgot what a period is.) So there is something for my intention to type a period, conceived as determining what counts as conformity to it autonomously and independently of my judgements on the matter, to be: namely, precisely, my intention to type a period . . . This is common sense, not platonism. (McDowell 1998, p. 315)

This criticism of a constructivist account turns, however, on the absence of an alternative. If Kripke's reading of Wittgenstein were correct then a merely ersatz version of meaning might be the best that were possible. Thus the criticism that constructionism does not succeed in capturing our pre-philosophical notions of meaning only has bite if there is an alternative interpretation of Wittgenstein's negative view.

But in fact there is. As McDowell convincingly argues, Wittgenstein's critical arguments are directed not against meaning itself but against a particular philosophical explanation of it. Crucially, such explanations form what we might call the Cartesian 'master thesis'.

> We get a more radical divergence from Kripke, however, if we suppose that the thrust of Wittgenstein's reflections is to cast doubt on the master thesis: the thesis that whatever a person has in her mind, it is only by virtue of being interpreted in one of various possible ways that it can impose a sorting of extra-mental items into those that accord with it and those that do not.
>
> It is really an extraordinary idea that the contents of minds are things that, considered in themselves, just 'stand there'. We can bring out how extraordinary it is by noting that we need an application for the concept of accord, and so run the risk of trouble from the regress of interpretations if we accept the master thesis, not just in connection with grasp of meaning but in connection with intentionality in general. An intention, just as such, is something with which only acting in a specific way would accord. An expectation, just as such, is something with which only certain future states of affairs would accord. Quite generally, a thought, just as such, is something with which only certain states of affairs would accord.   (McDowell 1998, p. 270)

Thus the assumption that understanding is a form of interpretation is an instance of the master thesis that the mind is populated with items that merely *can be interpreted* as relating to the world. Rejecting that thesis, a thesis held by cognitivist approaches to the mind, also undermines the attraction of a social constructionist approach to meaning and mental states. Thus it undercuts the argument for a social constructionist form of discursive psychology.

Whilst Kripke's and Wright's explicitly social constructionist interpretations of Wittgenstein have faced most criticism, some form of constructionism can appear even in interpretations that are explicitly critical of social interpretations. A very recent account by Michael Luntley—who explicitly criticizes social interpretations of Wittgenstein—implicitly subscribes to a form of constructionism (Luntley 2002, 2003).

Starting with the assumption that language depends on patterns of use, Luntley asks, 'which comes first—seeing the similarities or the patterns?' and goes on to defend—on Wittgenstein's behalf—the former answer. The idea of seeing similarities is introduced by considering Wittgenstein's discussion of 'family resemblance' concepts such as games. Wittgenstein suggests that there is nothing common to all games but merely

> a complicated network of similarities overlapping and criss-crossing: sometimes overall similarities, sometimes similarities of detail.   (Wittgenstein 1953, §66)

Games form a family of resemblances but there is nothing common to them, 'no set of necessary and sufficient conditions' (Luntley 2002, p. 273). Thus to apply the concept 'game' requires that one sees the similarities between one instance and others despite the absence of an explicit general rule. Luntley suggests that rather than showing this concept to be in poor health, the more general Wittgensteinian lesson is that seeing similarities underpins patterns of language use in general, outside family resemblance cases.

> To say that seeing the similarities between things is primitive is to say that the normative patterns of correct use of words emerge from the activity of seeing similarities. (Luntley 2002, p. 275)

The challenge to this interpretation, however, is to avoid the Scylla and Charybdis of platonism and constructionism. Luntley rejects the view of patterns of use as transcendent (platonism). But I think that his alternative account is a form of constructionism and thus undermines the normativity it is supposed to describe.

One clue to this comes from an analogy deployed to explain how 'patterns of meaning are real structures in the ongoing practices of judges' (Luntley 2002, p. 283). Luntley considers the contrast between two ways of building a wall-following robot. On a standard artificial intelligence approach, everything about identifying and mapping walls is encoded in a robot's database and rules are specified as to how the robot is to act relative to its perceptual intake. On a situated robotics approach, by contrast, the robot is designed to veer to one side with a temporary steer to the other side activated by contact with its bumper. This second robot will follow any wall in its vicinity although no representation of the wall is encoded in it. The environment plays a 'constitutive element in cognition' (Luntley 2002, p. 284).

The analogy is imperfect—not least because it concerns a causal rather than normative behaviour—but Luntley suggests that it provides a model of how coupling with the environment generates patterns:

> Patterned behaviour does not have to be driven by a rule for the pattern. Patterns emerge from choice couplings with the environment (Luntley 2002, p. 285).

Nevertheless the account which takes the seeing of similarities as basic, and patterns as emergent, faces difficulties with the idea that we do not await subsequent judgement to determine the extension of concepts. One way of putting this is that we are not free to see just any similarity. This point is emphasized in the passages of *Philosophical Investigations* where Wittgenstein discusses the case of a pupil instructed to continue the plus two arithmetic series but who on reaching 1000 continues 1004, 1008, and so on. His interlocutor says

> 'But I already knew, at the time when I gave the order, that he ought to write 1002 after 1000.'—Certainly; and you can also say you meant it then; only you should not be misled by the grammar of the words 'know' and 'mean'. For you don't want to say that you thought of the step from 1000 to 1002 at that time (Wittgenstein 1953, §187).

Equally, the interlocutor did not consider the similarities he would have seen at that point. He did not give them thought. But he still meant the pupil to continue with 1002. That is what he *would* have said but, also, that is what he *should* have said. The judgement of similarity at that point is already, so to speak, determined by the rule in question. Luntley's attempt to give priority to the seeing of similarity as more basic than the pattern that emerges fails to sustain the normativity of the pattern. Neither should be regarded as more basic. In grasping a rule one grasps the pattern as a whole.

The analogy from situated robotics will not help in this case because there is no equivalent to the wall and thus the difficulty of a coupling and emergent story of norms or patterns is more exposed. (Having rejected platonism, Luntley cannot subscribe to the mathematical series itself as comprising a platonic 'wall' to couple with.) But even in the case of empirical, as opposed to mathematical, judgements the same basic point applies: the attempt to privilege individual judgements over patterns (no less than the converse priority) will falsify the phenomenology of guidance by norms. Whilst concept application is prompted by the environment—and thus the discourse, so to speak, the actual usage emerges from coupling—the normative pattern does not await to emerge from such piecemeal judgements but acts as a standard of correctness. Constructivism, even when shorn of its social aspect, still fails as an interpretation of Wittgenstein.

Dementia and the heuristic role of social constructionism

In the first section, I attempted to characterize discursive psychology, to stress the importance of the constitutive claim it makes and to show how social constructionism might underpin that constitutive claim. In the second section, I outlined an influential resource for constructionist accounts of meaning: Wittgenstein's discussion of rules. But I argued that constructionist interpretations of Wittgenstein are neither tenable accounts of meaning and mind, nor exegetically plausible.

In this final section I shall return to the question of what, if not constructionism, might underpin a constitutive claim and thus underpin a difference between discursive psychology and cognitivism. I shall also look to the role of social constructionism in thinking about dementia.

A clue to the former question lies in the passage quoted earlier:

> In this sense, the psychological is not reducible to or replaceable by explanations in terms of physiology, physics, or any other point of view that does not reveal the structure of meanings existing in the lives of the human group to which the subject of an investigation belongs. (Harré and Gillett 1994, p. 20)

Constructionism is one reason for denying that the psychological is reducible: that no lower level description will capture 'the structure of meanings existing in the lives of the human group'. But on the assumption that constructionism is not a coherent approach to mind and meaning, what other reason might there be for denying the reduction?

The alternative suggested by recent philosophy of mind and language is the role that rationality plays. Borrowing from the accounts proposed by Dennett and Davidson, inspired among others by the later Wittgenstein, discursive psychology could take its subject matter to be the rational pattern in human speech and action, a pattern that has no echo in underlying physical and neurological descriptions.

Both Davidson and Dennett argue that the ascription of meanings and mental states is essentially tied to an interpretative strategy: Radical Interpretation and the Intentional Stance respectively (Davidson 1984, pp. 207–25; Dennett 1987, pp. 13–35). By describing the strategy, they provide insight into the nature of the states—mental states and meanings—it describes. Dennett compares and contrasts it to two other strategies: the 'physical stance' and the 'design stance'. The former is based on physical laws; the latter on the assumption that a system will behave as it is designed to. The Intentional Stance, in turn, is based on predicting that a system will behave in accordance with the dictates of rationality applied in context.

Davidson approaches mind and meaning by considering the conditions for the possibility of making sense of the speech and action of others from scratch: the Radical Interpretation of a marooned anthropologist. Arguing that the ascriptions of beliefs and of meanings (to native speech) form an interdependent whole with only one source of evidence (correlations between utterances and worldly features), he argues that interpretation requires a rational Principle of Charity to constrain it. The thought experiment, however, also captures our own epistemic predicament even though it may not seem like that. Thus both Dennett and Davidson argue that minds and meanings both form essentially rational patterns and are essentially tied to the public realm of speech and action because of their essential connection to an interpretative stance. It is of their essence to be detectable from a third-person point of view. That claim marks a contrast with cognitivism where that connection is merely contingent.

But the contrast is more pronounced if there is also reason to think that the pattern of meanings in the lives of humans is not reproduced as a physiological pattern within their skulls. Such an isomorphism would suggest a possible reconciliation of cognitivist and discursive approaches with distinct, but equivalent, subject matters. An argument for this stronger contrast is, however, already implicit in the discussion of Wittgenstein above. No internal physiological state can have the normative properties of meaning. Davidson adds to this Wittgensteinian claim a parallel argument based more closely on rationality than normativity. He claims that any such parallelism would require that rational connections could be mapped onto a nomological pattern, but as they answer to distinct constitutive principles this is unlikely (see also McDowell 1998, pp. 325–40).

There is, then, a different way of underpinning the constitutive claim needed to distinguish a discursive turn from a form of cognitivism, which admits that social factors can cause mental effects. The constitutive claim can be underpinned by a view of meaning that ties it to a rational pattern in human lives without the need to argue, in agreement with the concomitant crudity of the constructionist claim, that the pattern is constructed *de novo* in on-going judgement.

A non-constructionist version of the discursive approach also adopts a different version of naturalism. I suggested at the start that cognitivism is a form of reductionist naturalism because it aims to fit minds and meanings into nature by reducing the mind to a mechanism characterized in information processing terms. I suggested in the second section that constructionist versions of discursive psychology also subscribe to a form of reductionist naturalism. They take the notion of meaning, especially its normative properties, to be problematic and attempt to reconstruct them from something more basic and less philosophically puzzling. Dennett and Davidson's 'stance stance' approach to mind and meaning also deserves to be called a form of naturalism. They aim to show how minds and meanings fit unproblematically into nature. But they attempt no reduction. Connections are made to interpretation and to rationality but no concept is taken to be more basic. Thus, properly understood, discursive psychology can be taken to contrast with reductionist naturalism after all.

Two final points are worth making, which bring the discussion back to dementia. First, whilst not a true account of the nature of psychological phenomena itself, a social constructionist version of discursive psychology can nevertheless be heuristically fruitful especially in the area of dementia. This point can be most easily made via an analogy with social constructionism in the history and philosophy of science.

Roughly speaking, social constructionism in the philosophy of science takes natural scientific or physical facts to have the same status that discursive psychology grants to underlying cognitive or mental representations; and it takes the social negotiations that comprise the practice of science to play the role of discourse for discursive psychology. At its most radical, it takes natural facts themselves to depend upon, or be constituted by, social facts. A less radical view simply ascribes no explanatory role to natural facts. Whatever the merits of that metaphysical picture—which at its most radical is a form of idealism—it concentrates analysis on the details of the complex practices that are central to an informed account of the history of science.

Whilst it is not necessary to think that these practices constitute, as opposed to reveal (when all goes well), natural facts, adopting that assumption motivates very clear scrutiny of those practices. This has given rise to much interesting history and sociology of science in marked contrast to earlier Whig history. The connection is encapsulated by Barnes's argument that reality is a poor explanatory principle because it is what every party in a scientific dispute has in common (Barnes 1996). Barnes therefore suggests that to explain how scientific disputes are resolved, and thus present and past scientific views established, one needs to look to other, social, factors. Barnes's argument is, however, too quick. Whilst all parties in a dispute may be said to share access to reality in some broad sense, a detailed account of how aspects of the world are revealed in experiment to one but not to another researcher could well mark a difference in the degree of access to that overall reality.

In fact, in recent analysis of science it is hard to draw firm lines between those who invoke almost exclusively social factors (perhaps Barnes (1996), Bloor (1976), and Woolgar (1988)), those who describe instruments and other black boxes without taking a view as to their genuine reliability (for example, Shapin and Schaffer (1985) and Latour (1987)), and those who espouse a form of naturalized epistemology that aims to capture the details of scientific practice without giving up everyday realism (Kitcher 1993). But, especially in cases of on-going or only recently resolved disputes (for example, Collins and Pinch 1993), a more social constructionist approach helps avoid a simple Whiggish explanation of the adoption of a theory just because that theory was true.

To return to discursive psychology, the same point about methodological fruitfulness appears to apply, especially in the case of dementia. If one thinks that psychological phenomena are constituted in or by public utterance then that should be the object of careful scrutiny by psychologists and psychiatrists. In the paper by Sabat and Harré, 'The Alzheimer's disease sufferer as a semiotic subject', for example, a very careful empirical examination of the utterances of Alzheimer's sufferers reveals that despite impairments, subjects are still capable of meaningful utterance and of conversations that are patterned in rational structures (Sabat and Harré 1994). The revelation is made all the more dramatic by editing out delays in conversations and presenting the results— like the transcriptions of traditional discourse analysis—as detailed transcripts of conversations. Alzheimer's sufferers are found to be sensitive to meaning in three senses: acting on intentions, interpreting events, and evaluating events. Careful attention to utterances and actions reveals a rational pattern of meaning.

In that paper, the empirical and interpretative results are presented within an explicitly social constructionist framework. But there is, in fact, no need to adopt that view to investigate or interpret their findings. The non-constructionist alternative sketched above would fit just as well because it takes meaning to be essentially available to public view. Even if meaning is not *constructed* in on-going conversation, attention to that conversation may be crucial, if there is reason to think that there is an essential connection between possession of a mind and the possibility of third-person interpretation. In fact, in Sabat's more recent book, *The Experience of Alzheimer's Disease: Life Through a Tangled Veil*, the same empirical and interpretative findings are presented without mention in that context of social constructionism, which is instead reserved for treatment of the construction of selves and even there merely serving as a heuristic device (Sabat 2001).

Nevertheless, taking meaning to be *constructed* in discourse may serve as strong motivation for inspecting the details of utterance. In this, constructionism contrasts favourably with a cognitivist approach. As Wittgenstein comments,

> If I am inclined to suppose that a mouse has come into being by spontaneous generation out of grey rags and dust, I shall do well to examine those rags very closely to see how a mouse may have hidden in them, how it may have got there and so on. But if I am convinced that a mouse cannot come into

being from these things, then this investigation will perhaps be superfluous. (Wittgenstein 1953, §52)

Social constructionism at least provides reason for inspecting the details of utterance (the grey rags and dust) even if it provides a strictly false account of meaning.

The second, and final, point concerns my suggestion that one attraction of the idea of the co-construction of meaning in conversation is that, in cases of dementia, one participant might take on more of the burden. Without some limits, however, whatever the attraction of that position, it cannot be true and threatens abuse. To take an example from the other end of life: it would allow the sincere ascription of youthful authorship of the 'round robin' letters sometimes written in the UK 'as from' small babies around Christmas. Such ascription would simply require a generous interpretation of babies' still limited behavioural repertoire by doting parents through which the meaning and thus authorial intention would be constructed, rather than revealed. There would be no further issue of whether this accurately tracked antecedent communicative intentions. Whilst in the case of such round robin letters no abuse is risked, in the case of dementia the construction of meaning by one party in a conversation would carry that risk. Sabat gives one such example:

> In many cases, caregivers often do attribute intention to the afflicted person in that caregivers may believe that he or she is acting deliberately to annoy them, when in fact the annoying behaviour is due to cognitive impairment. If the afflicted person's recall memory is severely affected, he or she may ask the same question repeatedly. This is hardly due to an intention to annoy anyone. It is of utmost import that caregivers identify the circumstances in which intention is present and healthy and not meant to annoy. (Sabat 2001, p. 222)

This practical example suggests a genuine danger of thinking that meaning is constructed in conversation rather than answering to speakers' intentions: there are in principle no standards by which to judge the caregivers' interpretation. This is not merely an epistemological problem: knowing what the sufferer means. That is also a real problem. But the risk of abuse is increased if one gives up on any notion of aiming to get right what speakers or sufferers actually mean. It is only by keeping a firm grip on what is meant by subjects that their wishes can be respected. It is better to keep a firm grip on the idea that to be able to be a semiotic subject requires some capacity to express genuine intentions and meanings than to adopt a sentimental attachment to the construction of meaning.

On the more modest account sketched above, meaning is not constructed piecemeal in conversations. But the benchmark for being, in Sabat's phrase, a semiotic subject, a subject who can respond to and use meanings, is set at the level of what is open to another person. It thus behoves analysts to search hard for signs of a rational pattern in speech or action because it is that, on this view, which reveals the mind at work.

References

Barnes, B. (1996). *Scientific Knowledge: A Sociological Analysis*. London: Athlone.

Bloor, D. (1976). *Knowledge and Human Imagery*. London: Routledge.

Bolton, D., Hill, J. (1996). *Mind, Meaning and Mental Disorder*. Oxford: Oxford University Press.

Collins, H., Pinch, T. (1993). *The Golem: What Everyone Should Know About Science* Cambridge: Cambridge University Press.

Davidson, D. (1984). *Inquiries into Truth and Interpretation*. Oxford: Oxford University Press.

Dennett, D. (1987). *The Intentional Stance*. Cambridge, MA:,MIT Press.

Edwards, D., Potter, J. (1992). *Discursive Psychology* London: Sage.

Fodor, J. (1987). *Psychosemantics: The Problem of Meaning in the Philosophy of Mind*. Cambridge, Massachusetts: MIT Press.

Harré, R., Gillett, G. (1994). *The Discursive Mind*. London: Sage.

Hosking, D. M., Morley, I. E. (2004). Editorial: Social constructionism in community and applied social psychology. *Journal of Community and Applied Social Psychology*, **14**: 318–31.

Kitcher, P. (1993). *The Advancement of Science*. Oxford: Oxford University Press.

Kripke, S. (1982). *Wittgenstein on Rules and Private Language*. Oxford: Blackwell.

Latour, B. (1987). *Science in Action: How to Follow Scientists and Engineers Through Society*. Cambridge, Massachusetts: Harvard University Press.

Luntley, M. (2002). Patterns, particularism and seeing the similarity. *Philosophical Papers*, **31**: 271–91.

Luntley, M. (2003). *Wittgenstein: Meaning and Judgement*. Oxford: Blackwell.

McDowell, J. (1998). *Mind, Value and Reality*. Cambridge, Massachusetts: Harvard University Press.

Parkin, A.J. (1996). *Explorations in Cognitive Neuropsychology*. Oxford: Blackwell.

Sabat, S. R. (2001). *The Experience of Alzheimer's Disease: Life Through a Tangled Veil*. Oxford and Malden, Massachusetts: Blackwell.

Sabat, S. R., Harré, R. (1994). The Alzheimer's disease sufferer as a semiotic subject. *Philosophy, Psychiatry, & Psychology*, **1**: 145–60.

Shapin, S., Schaffer, S. (1985). *Leviathan and the Air Pump*. Princeton: Princeton University Press.

Thornton, T. (1998). *Wittgenstein on Language and Thought*. Edinburgh: Edinburgh University Press.

Wittgenstein, L. (1953). *Philosophical Investigations*. Oxford: Blackwell.

Woolgar, S. (1988). *Science: The Very Idea*. Chichester: Ellis Horwood.

Wright, C. (1986). Rule following, meaning and constructivism. In: *Meaning and Interpretation* (ed. C. Travis), pp. 271–97. Oxford: Blackwell.

Wright, C. (1987). On making up one's mind: Wittgenstein on intention. In: *Logic, Philosophy of Science and Epistemology: Proceedings of the 11th International Wittgenstein Symposium* (ed. P. Weingartner and G. Schurz), pp. 391–404. Vienna: Holder–Pichler–Tempsky.

Wright, C. (1991). Wittgenstein's later philosophy of mind: sensation, privacy and intention. In: *Meaning Scepticism* (ed. K. Puhl), pp. 126–47. Berlin: de Gruyter.

9 The return of the living dead: agency lost and found?

Carmelo Aquilina and Julian C. Hughes

The pain! The pain of being dead! . . . I can feel myself rotting.[1]

We are like the dead . . . we drift away from life, no longer fearing to die nor craving and striving for our place in the sun.[2]

Introduction

The above quotations are taken from two of the 'living dead'. The first is from a fictional zombie in the 1985 cult horror movie *The Return of the Living Dead*. The second is from a person with Alzheimer's disease who experiences a similar drift into a twilight zone between life and death. The similarities are more than superficial.

The 'living dead' in the film are animated corpses. We are terrified as observers because we can identify with the awful situation that these creatures are in. The zombies are simultaneously rotting corpses but they are still sentient, feeling beings who can perceive the agony of decay. This chapter will consider whether the 'living dead' are not just creatures of the imagination but might also be people with advanced dementia. People with dementia can be treated as already dead and as walking corpses to be both pitied and feared, despite their obvious signs of life. The fate of *self* in the face of this neurological disease and the effects of anti-dementia drugs in re-animating these 'living corpses' are described and some of the philosophical issues that arise are discussed.

The living dead—a prevalent public paradigm?

Forgetfulness and the loss of the 'self' in old age have a long history. An ancient Egyptian script laments 'oldness has come . . . the heart is forgetful and cannot recall yesterday' (Minios 1989). The Latin word 'dementia' was first used in first-century Rome and stems from the word 'demens' meaning 'out of one's mind'.

The term, but not the concept, has metamorphosed many times. 'Senile dementia' was defined by the French psychiatrist Esquirol in 1838. A case of dementia was described by Alzheimer in 1907 and the term 'Alzheimer's disease' was coined by his mentor Kraeplin in 1910. 'Alzheimer's' finally emerged as a vernacular term for dementia thanks to lobbying by both medical researchers and carers (Berrios 1994).

The loss of mind in 'dementia' reflects the common and distressing observation by relatives, carers, and doctors that 'self' is lost slowly as the illness progresses. The scientific and popular literature has largely reflected this concept with books such as *The Loss of Self* (Cohen and Eisdorfer 2001) or *Alzheimer's Disease: Coping with a Living Death* (Woods 1989). Films like *Iris*,[3] showing the deterioration of the author and philosopher Iris Murdoch, and media reports describing the illness of the late US President Ronald Reagan, have continued to reinforce the idea of the *annihilation of self* in people's minds.

This idea of dementia is so negative and powerful it makes dementia one of the more terrifying illnesses to envisage. Herskovits (1995) asserted that the concept of Alzheimer's disease was a 'monsterizing of senility'. As with cancer, the diagnosis of dementia is often not disclosed for fear of causing distress (Drickamer and Lachs 1992). People have asked for and been assisted in committing suicide when they fear or have had such a diagnosis (Post 1993). Caregivers often report that the person they are caring for is no longer the person they once knew.[4] Some relatives, when asked when they would like to give up the responsibilities of being a carer, mention the stage when the person they are looking after stops recognizing them. Other carers ask for no life-prolonging treatment to be given to their demented relatives, as prolongation of life is seen as cruel. Others will go further. In a recent case of 'mercy killing' the judge showed leniency—because it was acknowledged that the accused had 'tried to care for a woman, who ceased to be the woman you married' (BBC News 2003).

The effect of professional carers' attitudes to the person with dementia is equally pervasive. Tappen *et al.* (1997) noted how caregivers generally avoid communicating with patients with dementia because the patients are not able to have meaningful communication. The same research observed how,

> nursing home staff frequently avoid all but task-oriented communication with people in the latest stages of the disease on the assumption that the severely demented experience life as meaningless. (Tappen *et al.*, 1997)

Ekman *et al.* (1991) found caregivers spent less time with severely demented clients and Beck (1996) described how nursing students described their experience of nursing demented people in distressed and negative terms. On ethical grounds, there have been concerns about the effects of the anti-dementia drugs (where there is anecdotal evidence that the drugs increase the person's awareness of deterioration in a way that is upsetting), which has led some to suggest that when the 'intact self' deteriorates into the 'now self', the use of such drugs becomes questionable (Post 1997).

Mental prisoners—the significance of lucid periods

Nevertheless, there are some (including many in this volume) who argue against the mainstream view that loss of self is inevitable in dementia (Post 2000). Amongst the most persuasive voices have been those of carers. Franzen (2001), in his account of his father's Alzheimer's disease, wondered 'whether memory and consciousness have such secure title . . . over the seat of self-hood. . . . in the two years that followed the loss of his supposed "self" I can't stop finding it'. He tells of his father's occasional but memorable utterances that suggested 'an awareness of his larger plight and his connection to the past and the future'. Bayley recounted similar experiences, utterances, and behaviour by his wife Iris Murdoch, which suggested a 'terrible lucidity' (Bayley 1998, p. 179). He described how he could not help thinking from time to time that an 'inner world' survived, 'which Iris is determined to keep from me and shield me from' (Bayley 1998, p. 178).

Both authors based their belief partly on so-called 'lucid episodes'. Lucid episodes are defined by Normann *et al.* as:

> episodes in the care of patients with severe dementia where the patient unexpectedly speaks or acts in a way which surprises the carer because the patient seems to be much more aware of her or his situation and to function much more adequately than usual. (Normann *et al.* 1998)

Normann and her colleagues noted many instances of lucid episodes reported by the carers they interviewed as well as many anecdotes from other authors. Most episodes occurred spontaneously when the patient was the subject of individual attention, or were triggered by strong emotions in the context of, for example, music and prayer.

Gubrium (1986) describes carers talking about 'a person . . . humanity' still being present, which 'still has feelings'; the disease merely 'destroys the ability to appropriately express them'. Shenk (2003) summarizes this feeling by describing dementia as 'a sort of mental confinement—the sufferer is incarcerated within the collapsing neural structures'. The feeling that there is an inner self, which cannot communicate with the carer, may be comforting in the face of tiring and relentless caring responsibilities (Jenkins and Price 1996).

There is an 'I' in dementia

Sabat and Harré (1992) maintain that 'self' is shaped by language. The use of first-person lexicals (FPLs)—for example, words like 'I', 'me', 'myself', 'mine', and so on—are indications that the self persists in dementia.[5] Jonathan Swift's last recorded words before his death from dementia were 'I am a fool' suggesting that he was aware of the death of his intellect (Shenk 2003, p. 226).

Tappen *et al.* (1996) examined communication in people with moderate to severe dementia and found that FPLs were used freely, which showed they were aware of how their lives had changed. Few of those aware that their cognition had changed gave an explanation. A few people felt shame at what they had become; some expressed regret and some resignation at what had befallen them. Some of the people they observed, however, referred to themselves in the third person and others did not acknowledge that anything had changed.

Tabak *et al.* (1996) reported how people with dementia interacted with their reflections. The severity of the dementia in the people studied is not recorded but the majority recognized themselves, commented on their appearance, or touched themselves to improve their appearance. The aims of the study were therapeutic, but it would also suggest the persistence of *self* in dementia. When confronted by a mirror, a few people became angry or ignored their own image in the mirror, though some interacted with the reflection as if it were another person. Such 'mirror signs' in dementia are well known (Bentham and Hodges 2002) and might be taken to suggest a loss of self. However, the loss of FPLs and 'mirror signs' might simply reflect aphasia (loss of speech) and agnosia (loss of the brain's ability to interpret sensory input correctly), which prevent the self from communicating or interacting with the outside world.

Different selves

A social constructionist view suggests that the self persists in other ways. In a deeply impressive and sustained analysis of the perspective of those who experience dementia, as shown by their language and conversation, Sabat (2001) develops the social constructionist view of different selves. There is not only the self of personal identity (Self 1), which is typically expressed by first-person pronouns (that is, FPLs); in addition, there is the self of mental and physical attributes (Self 2). Some of these attributes will persist in dementia—characteristic physical attributes for instance—even if others change. A loss or change in a mental attribute may or may not be, for the person with dementia, a matter of shame and humiliation, but (in part at least) this will be determined by the social environment. Similarly, our socially presented selves, or personae (Selves 3), that is, the faces we present to the world, require 'the dynamic interplay of mutual recognition' (Sabat 2001, p. 295). In other words, in a sense much stronger than is the case for Self 1 and Self 2, any particular Self 3 (for each of us has many, for example, parent, child, colleague, neighbour) requires co-operation from other people. Thus, it is difficult for the teacher to maintain their social presentation or standing *qua* teacher if there is no recognition of this self by anyone else. Hence, in dementia, Self 3 is very vulnerable because it can too readily be undermined by the reaction of others.

Malignant society

This is what Kitwood meant by 'malignant social psychology', according to which malignant social processes, such as infantilization and disempowerment, cause dementia by depriving elderly and mentally frail people of their humanity (Kitwood 1990). It may be that confusion is demonstrated, not by the person with dementia, but by those who do not hear the meanings being conveyed and, hence, deny the dementia sufferer's standing as a semiotic subject (Sabat and Harré 1994). The social environment, the people around, can either construct or deconstruct the self with dementia (Sabat and Harré 1992). Feil (1993) encourages 'validation' of the demented person's communication. In interpreting and understanding the apparently incomprehensible language of the person with dementia she asserts that the observer can go 'behind their disorientation'; and she adds, 'a basic humanity shines through' (Feil 1993, p. xxv).

In an interesting review of the socio-cultural trends that have shaped contemporary thought about Alzheimer's disease, Herskovits (1995) indicates how a debate has arisen concerning the nature of subjectivity. At one extreme, according to which dementia is understood (purely) pathologically, the self disappears irretrievably as the dementia with its pathology worsens. At another extreme, the self can be maintained by the efforts of those around. This view of the self underpins Kitwood's definition of personhood as 'a standing or status that is bestowed upon one human being, by others, in the context of relationship and social being' (Kitwood 1997, p. 8). Taking this optimistic view of the self on dementia led Kitwood and Bredin (1992) to suggest the paradoxical idea that people with dementia should be considered as more authentic, honest, and healthy than non-demented folks. They argued that 'everyday life . . . is deeply pathological', whereas people with dementia 'may become an exemplary model of interpersonal life, an epitome of how to be human'.

This optimistic view is in sharp contrast to the conclusion of Fontana and Smith:

> We cannot help but wonder how much of what we have considered to be the last vestiges of the patients' self has not been in fact a process of 'filling the gaps' on our past. Perhaps, what is left, after the victims' self 'unbecome', are but the scarce remains we have attributed to them. (Fontana and Smith, 1989).

As Herskovits (1995) points out, much of this theorizing about the self in dementia fails to take seriously the views of people with dementia. In turn, this fails to take seriously the capacity of people with dementia to make meaning (Lyman 1998). The writings and work of Kitwood (1997), Sabat (2001), and others, such as the poet John Killick (for example, Killick and Cordonnier 2000) help to rectify this deficiency. Perhaps the optimistic answer to the question of whether we are simply 'filling the gaps' is supported by the case history that follows.

The return of the living dead

With the advent of anti-dementia drugs the debate about 'self' in dementia is renewed and intensified. When the drugs have an effect, they can ameliorate some of the symptoms. For many this effect is only partial and mild but in a few it can be spectacular and unsettling.

Mrs G was an intelligent woman who presented to psychiatric services with some word-finding difficulties (dysphasia), short-term memory problems, and frightening dreams. She was distressed and embarrassed by her symptoms and had stopped going to church as she felt God had let her down. Dementia of the Alzheimer's type was diagnosed. Her co-ordination then deteriorated. She had started tripping over things and her dysphasia had worsened. A year after her initial presentation she was experiencing complex visual hallucinations and reacted badly to an anti-psychotic drug aimed at stopping the hallucinations. Parkinsonian features, namely a fine tremor and muscle rigidity, were noticed. Dementia with Lewy bodies was diagnosed. Throughout that year her hallucinations became more prominent. She would see boys, dogs, and other animals in her flat. Despite a trial of various anti-psychotics she became totally preoccupied by almost constant visual hallucinations and her speech became unintelligible. She was admitted to hospital because her family were exhausted looking after her. On the ward she was weaned off all neuroleptic drugs and booked for permanent care in a nursing home. She remained incapacitated, sometimes crawling on the floor to remove imaginary objects. After a few months her family decided to take her home, because there were no vacancies in any nearby nursing homes. The plan was that her husband would provide 24-hour care. Two years after her first presentation, at an out-patient clinic, an anti-dementia drug (one of the cholinesterase inhibitors) was prescribed. She was by then mute, not interacting with either the doctor or her husband. A month after starting the anti-dementia drug, however, the entry in the medical notes read:

> She has shown a remarkable improvement in her mood, interest, concentration and her ability to take in information. Perhaps the most remarkable improvement of all has been the improvement in her fluency and she was able to speak reasonably well to me about things we had talked about at our last clinic appointment.

Five months later, she continued to show 'remarkable' improvement in that her mood was much brighter, she continued to speak clearly, could do some housework, and walked along the seaside. Soon Mrs G was helping her husband with crossword puzzles and telling the doctor proudly, 'I am teaching myself to control my own individual life', which her husband still felt he had to translate by saying that she was fighting her illness. At a later appointment when her husband again insisted on telling the doctor about her problems she turned to him angrily saying 'Whose side are you on—me or the blinking doctor's?' Mrs G went on to have a long period of relative good health with lucidity, but increasing distress at her continuing hallucinations and physical decline. When her medication was stopped because of side-effects, her memory and language quickly declined. She was re-admitted to hospital a year later, lost her ability to speak again, and died peacefully.

The first author (CA) was the doctor prescribing the anti-dementia drug. When the patient came to clinic, it was not just remarkable that she was able to speak clearly and lucidly, *but that she was able to describe to him what had been discussed with her husband at the previous appointment when she had been mute and unable to interact.* The effect of this was to cause the author a mixture of emotions. One emotion was amazement at such a quick and significant improvement. Another was embarrassment at not having tried to speak to her during the previous clinic appointment. The final emotion was disquiet at the feeling that, like her, other people with severe dementia might be imprisoned and aware of what is happening whilst no one around bothers to speak to them!

The above case is a most spectacular example of the possible effects of anti-dementia drugs. More commonly the effects of these drugs are not as impressive, but are no less important to carers. Both authors have heard many carers comment that the person on such a drug seems 'more like his (or her) old self'. More spontaneity, familiar acts (like hugging the wife or laying the table) and improvements in speech delight carers precisely because the 'old self' has surfaced again. This is not to say that the restoration of self-awareness is always regarded as beneficial (Hughes 2000). Some people regain awareness of their situation and become depressed or, more rarely, even suicidal. In such cases withdrawal of the anti-dementia drugs can reverse the changes to a more relaxed but more confused state. The point, however, is that the extraordinary effect of the drugs in cases like Mrs G (which is by no means unique) demonstrates that where the self may seem to have disintegrated, in fact it may persist.

What has happened to the self?

What should we say has happened to the self in such a case? Here are the possibilities.

A projective illusion?

Was the returned self simply an illusion that we wanted to see because we had such high hopes of the drug?

A resurrection?

Was Mrs G's self destroyed and did the drug reconstitute it?

An impostor?

Was Mrs G's self destroyed so that the person the drug seemed to reveal was not the same person that had existed before the illness?

A freed prisoner?

Was it that the returned self was always there and all the drug did was to allow Mrs G to break through her imprisoning walls?

Mrs G was able to speak about herself and the progress she had made. The self, seen after the initiation of the drug, was much more than a projection: she was no longer confused. Mrs G was able to talk about events happening when her 'self' had apparently been lost, so her 'self' could not simply have been destroyed. Because her self was not dead in this sense, it would not seem appropriate to talk of resurrection.

Psychoactive drugs are known to change people's behaviour, as in the 'remaking of self' ascribed to 'Prozac' (Kramer 1997). Was Mrs G different when she emerged from her confusion? Her family claimed that she was back to her old self. This is reminiscent of the experience of lucid episodes we described above, but on a prolonged scale. It certainly appears to discount the possibility that the 'new' Mrs G was an impostor.

The final possibility is that Mrs G's self was still intact, but that she had been imprisoned by her illness, which had not allowed her to communicate. A degree of self-awareness and ability to retain and recall information had been present when she was uncommunicative. Thus, she was able to recall details of the consultation in clinic before the anti-dementia drug started to work.

We may infer that in Mrs G's case, her Self 1 and Self 2 had been intact despite her dementia, even if she could not communicate them; and her Self 3 (in all its manifestations) was entirely eradicated by those around her except insofar as they saw her as the victim of dementia. The possibility that her self was intact counts against the idea that ascribing selfhood to her would be merely a matter of 'filling the gaps'. Moreover, her ability to remember and reflect on what had occurred when she was one of the 'living dead' suggests that the persistence of her selves was not simply a possibility: she, *her self*, really was alive and kicking.

'Inner' and 'outer' selves

We might wish, for the sake of simplicity, to understand the self according to two broad models:

(1) the private subjective experience of being self-aware, which is seemingly dependent on biological structures;
(2) the public observable aspects of self, which depend on psycho-social structures including social relations, culture, and language.

We shall refer to these selves as the 'inner' and 'outer' selves. The three Selves of the social constructionists can be seen as traversing the gap between the 'inner' and the 'outer'. Indexing my Self 1 by a personal pronoun requires a public utterance, but is taken to reflect an 'inner' process. I inwardly, as it were, point at my Self. Self 2 is, in any case, made up of physical ('outer') and mental ('inner') attributes. Whilst Self 3, although manifestly public, involves an 'inner' act: we see our Selves as parents, teachers, or philosophers. We shall concentrate on the language of 'inner' and 'outer', because we believe that this approach sheds light on a dilemma commonly raised by dementia.

In the remainder of this chapter we shall (1) further explore the language of 'inner' and 'outer' as it is used in connection with dementia; (2) gesture at a philosophical uncertainty that the distinction between 'inner' and 'outer' is real (hence our use of quotation marks, which we shall now do without!); (3) consider the possibility that the person, as a situated embodied agent, might finally lose personhood (and all claims to a self) because of a failure of agency. We shall argue against this idea on the grounds that human agency is *situated*.

Inner and outer selves in dementia

'Descartes' error', according to Damasio (1994), was to believe that the mind has a life of its own independent of the body (that is, dualism). It is easy to see how, if Descartes (1642) was right to assert that 'I am a thinking thing' (*sum res cogitans*), it might be claimed, when dementia has left the person denuded of thought or the capacity to think, that the death of the inner self amounts to the death of the person as a whole. The contrary (non-dualist) view, taken by materialists or physicalists, disagrees with Descartes that the mind and the body are separate. According to this view, the mind is *nothing but* the body (Armstrong 1968). Nonetheless, it again seems a fairly straightforward step to suggest that the profound neuropathological breakdown in dementia must entail the loss of the inner self. And, again, the loss of the inner self is equated with the death of the person. Hence, people with dementia are described as 'shells', as not being the persons they once were.

The inner self—what Locke called the 'thinking conscious self'—where psychological continuity and connectedness are located (Parfit 1984), is essential to the person because 'without consciousness there is no person' (Locke 1964, p. 218). In a similar way, Sacks sums up the central importance of memory eloquently:

> To be ourselves we must *have* ourselves—possess, if need be re-possess, our life-stories. We must 'recollect' ourselves, recollect the inner drama, the narrative, of ourselves. A man *needs* such narrative, a continuous narrative to maintain his identity, his self.   (Sacks 1985, pp. 105–6)

Damasio (2000) calls this narrative the 'extended self' with its access to autobiographical information on top of a simple awareness of the present. Just as the loss of collective memory destroys a people or culture, so the loss of memories of what has made the person unique will lead to the loss of the individual's 'self'. Dementia, by its attack on the inner self, whether one is a dualist or a physicalist, destroys the person.

It is certainly the case that people with dementia can be aware of the loss of their capacities and of aspects of their inner selves. Iris Murdoch spoke of herself 'sailing into the darkness' (Bayley 1998, p. 179) and Shenk quotes a patient as feeling 'your whole inside and outside' breaking down (Shenk 2003, p. 9). McGowan (1993) felt there was 'less of me every day than there was the day before'. At some stage in the illness (Post (1993) called it the stage when one forgets that one forgets), the person with dementia may reach a tranquillity born of unawareness, but the slide to that stage is usually not pleasant and is accompanied by a sense of inner capabilities being lost.

The decline of the inner self is accompanied by changes in the 'relational self' (Herskovits 1995). This outer self is manifested through interactions in the external world. It is therefore manifest both by the people who relate to the person with dementia, as well as by the changes in behaviour and language of the person with dementia. As we have discussed, it is typically the Self 3 that is regarded as the outer self, but aspects of the outer self are involved in Selves 1 and 2.

When we think of the outer self, the possibility of malignant social psychology is never far away. Jonathan Swift was attacked as a person and an author because of his behaviour during his dementia (Shenk 2003, p. 170). Ex-president Ronald Reagan was said to be his old self when he was able to give a familiar, fluent speech at his 83rd birthday party dinner but 'slipped into his unsettling new self' at his hotel after the dinner and later friends stopped visiting him when he could no longer recognize them (Shenk 2003, p. 21). The most striking example of how the relational self is stigmatized is the attack on the artist De Kooning. In 1995 a panel of art museum directors and artists concluded that De Kooning's works, painted after his dementia had started, were 'not fully realised works of art' (Shenk 2003, p. 205). Denying the value of an artist's work is a direct attack on his 'personhood' and is a testimony to the power of stereotyping. Once De Kooning was regarded in this way his standing as an artist, which contributed to both his Self 2 and Self 3, was undermined, as was therefore his selfhood. Thus the outer public self is as fragile as the inner, subjective self.

Having said this, the public (outer) self is also open to support from others. The narrative of the person, as remembered by their deeds, sayings, stories, and writings, can be preserved by other people in memory, or more publicly in written or other records. Jenkins and Price (1996) proposed that nurses should help carers to preserve personhood by,

> building a memory of the patient . . . a catalogue of shared events and celebrations . . . In these terms a person consists of a rich array of shared feelings, reminiscences, traits, and characteristics that extend beyond the response they can currently hope to receive from the patient.

In a similar way Kitwood was keen to emphasize the outer nature of selfhood:

> In dementia many aspects of the psyche that had, for a long time, been individual and 'internal', are again made over to the interpersonal milieu. Memory may have faded, but something of the past is known; identity

remains intact, because others hold it in place; thoughts may have disappeared, but there are still interpersonal processes; feelings are expressed and meet a validating response; and if there is a spirituality, it will most likely be of the kind that Buber describes, where the divine is encountered in the depth of I–Thou relating. (Kitwood 1997, p. 69)

Is the inner outer or the outer inner?

The suggestion made by Kitwood that the internal psyche might be made over to the 'interpersonal milieu' raises the possibility of confusion at a philosophical level between the inner and the outer. Talk of 'inner selves' and 'outer selves' in connection with dementia seems almost natural. We ordinarily accept, it seems, that there is a real distinction here. But how solid is the divide between the inner and the outer? Or is it somewhat leaky?

The distinction between inner and outer was one that exercised the philosopher Ludwig Wittgenstein and upon which he poured some scorn:

> . . . But now it is said: We can't be certain when a child really begins to hope, for hope is an inner process. What nonsense! For then how do we know what we are talking about at all? (Wittgenstein 1981, §469)

It is true that hope is a subjective experience, something we might routinely call inner. Wittgenstein, however, is pointing out that—in order for us to understand the whole concept of hope—it must also be a shareable and public phenomenon. Otherwise, as he suggests, we could never know what other people mean when they say they are hopeful. More than that, we can see hope dawning, just as we can see pain!

> If I see someone writhing in pain with evident cause I do not think: all the same, his feelings are hidden from me. (Wittgenstein 1953, p. 223)

Elsewhere Wittgenstein says

> When mein, gesture and circumstances are unambiguous, then the inner seems to be the outer; it is only when we cannot read the outer that an inner seems to be hidden behind it. (Wittgenstein 1992, p. 63)

The language of inner and outer is perfectly natural to us as human beings, but one of Wittgenstein's favourite themes was that language can bewitch us, fool us into thinking of the reality of the inner as if it had the concreteness of concrete.

> It is only in particular cases that the inner is hidden from one, and in those cases it is not hidden because it is the inner. (Wittgenstein 1992, p. 33)

If we think of someone with dementia we may wish to focus on the inner and conclude that it is missing: the inner self is dead. Or, we may conclude that the inner self is trapped in the outer shell: the defective body or dysfunctional brain. According to Wittgenstein's lights, however, both conclusions are fatuous. In one sense, *either* conclusion might be true: we know what they are both getting at. But in a more important sense (it could be argued) a human being with dementia is first and foremost a human being and, as such, is capable of characterization in terms of both inner and outer. They will still have gestures and behaviours, to which we should continue to react in a human way. It will then be perfectly natural to think of the human being as having some sort of subjectivity, but that is because they act in ways that fit with our shareable practices. We make sense of them in perfectly natural ways within this context.

> If I ask someone on the street for directions then I prefer a friendly answer to an unfriendly one. I react immediately to someone else's behaviour. I presuppose the *inner* in so far as I presuppose a *human being*. (Wittgenstein 1992, p. 84)

The *presupposition* of the inner is grounded in a world in which it makes sense to regard even an incoherent utterance or an uncertain gesture as meaningful, if made by a human being, precisely because this is what we do all the time in our interactions with other human beings. The only alternative is to regard the individual with dementia as not only devoid of subjectivity, but also as (in some sense) less than human—and that is hard to do, especially in the face of evidence from lucid episodes and cases like Mrs G's. Wittgenstein famously said 'The human body is the best picture of the human soul' (Wittgenstein 1953, p. 178).

Having a human body, therefore, just being the sort of beings that we are, leads to the pre-supposition of an inner reality. This suggests that we must act towards people with dementia, even in the severe stages, as if they are fully human, inner and outer, subjective and objective, private and public. Not to do so, on the grounds that the inner is dead or inaccessible, is to ignore the continuity between the outer and the inner.[6] So long as there is outward behaviour, it is reasonable to act towards the person as if they are a human being. Not to do so would be to undercut one's own standing as a person.

The divide between inner and outer is not leak-proof. Our inner states are manifest by outer behaviour. Our shared understanding of outer characteristics is a prerequisite of meaningful language. Outer behaviour, that is, requires shared (inner) understanding. To pursue the point made by Wittgenstein, we might say that the body *shows* the soul. The person with dementia, according to this line of thought, by virtue of their body (because the human body reflects the human soul[7]) should be treated humanely as befits any human person.

The importance of *situated* agency in severe dementia

In this next section we shall use the notion that persons are situated embodied agents (Hughes 2001) to focus on the idea of being a *situated agent*. This should not lead us, however, to ignore the importance of *embodiment*, which marks out our mode of being in the world.

> If human being is 'in-the-world', if human subjectivity is necessarily embodied, then my existence as a subject is not that of an 'inner object', accessible only to myself, but that of an object in the world who manifests his consciousness in his observable actions. (Matthews 2002, p. 97)

Hence,

> being an *embodied* agent itself involves being embedded in the world and links the inner self with the outer self. Indeed, being embodied—because of the way our bodies reflect our selves and also participate in the world—breaks down the distinction between the inner and the outer. (Hughes 2003).

One of the shocking things about talk of the 'living dead' is that it might suggest that those of us who are involved in looking after people with severe dementia are doing something gruesome. Perhaps we are looking after dead people. This would be terrible if it were true. Against this stands the idea of the 'relational self': the idea that *other* people are crucially important in maintaining, at some level, the personhood of people with severe dementia. But this could just be sentimentality. Perhaps it makes us feel better if we think that what we do makes a difference to the (so-called) 'empty shell' that used to be a person.

Mrs G, in the case we discussed above, was able to demonstrate her surviving personhood. Yet it is always open to someone to argue that at some stage in dementia the person will have gone. At some stage before biological life is over, the biography is really ended and there are no grounds for thinking that there is anything meaningful occurring within the outer shell. Consider, for example, the case of Mr A.

Mr A had a diagnosis of Alzheimer's disease made 8 years ago, but had shown symptoms of forgetfulness for 2 years before that. He was supported at home until 3 years ago when, following in-patient assessment, it was thought that continuing psychiatric nursing care was appropriate. Having initially been mobile but unsteady, Mr A is now immobile and requires to be hoisted. He exhibits no verbal communication. He sits all day in a beanbag, but requires to be moved to prevent pressure sores. He has to be fed and is at risk of choking. He is doubly incontinent. He is losing weight. He can be irritable during personal interventions. Mostly he just sits, stares, sleeps, and shows no emotion.

In line with the situated-embodied-agent view of the person (Hughes 2001), it can be argued that Mr A should be thought of as a person inasmuch as he is situated and embodied: that is, he is a human being, who shares with us a human form and, like us, he is situated in a huge variety of contexts, which are personal, historical, social, psychological, cultural and spiritual, and so on. The question is, however, whether it makes sense to say that Mr A is an agent? Albeit he is situated and embodied, but what does he do that is agentive?

Actually, one agentive thing has already been identified: he can be irritable during personal interventions. Such behaviour is not at all uncommon. Might it not mean something? Well, it could be argued, it is simply a reaction, a sort of reflex. It will mean something to others but is it clear that it means anything to Mr A himself? It could be argued that it is meaningful to the nursing staff, who sentimentally tend to the 'living dead' and fill in the gaps to create some meaning for themselves, irrespective of Mr A.

The notion of the 'body-subject' found in Merleau-Ponty (see Chapter 10 and Matthews 2002) suggests that our bodies are not objects that we can view like any other objects, as it were, outside ourselves. In the case of Mr A's irritability, for instance, the following seems to be relevant:

> Treating our body as part of our subjectivity . . . implies that not all aspects of our subjectivity—not all ways, for instance, in which we may be purpos-ive—need necessarily be fully 'conscious' in the sense of being objects of *explicit* awareness. For our bodies may have a purposive relationship to objects even if we do not cherish any *explicit* intentions for those objects. Reflex or instinctual actions, for instance, may be purposive but not consciously so . . . (Matthews 1996, p. 92, emphasis added)

Mr A's irritability demonstrates purpose, despite his lack of *explicit* inten-tion. What we wish to ask is whether, in the absence of '*explicit* intention', this sort of purposive act is enough to make Mr A an agent?

The notion of agency brings into play the notion of intention. However, in philosophical parlance the notion of 'intention' is complicated. At one level, the 'intention' I have whilst performing an action is the thing I am *explicitly* aiming at: it is the reason I might give for acting in this way. Let us call this *explicit* intention. At another level, the intentional nature of an action can be taken to imply that which the action, being of this type, itself aims at. In this sense, the intention of the action links to the meaning of the action. When an agent acts, they might have something explicit in mind; but equally it might be that the action itself aims at something. In either case, when an agent acts as an agent, there is something aimed at in the action, which is other than the agent and which contributes towards the action being the type of action that it is.

Let us try to imagine what it would be for a human being to act without any consideration of the first sort of intention (what for now we have called *explicit* intention) coming into play. Imagine someone sleep-walking for instance, such as Lady Macbeth trying to wash the blood off her hands. Is she still acting as an agent? Could she simply be an automaton?

One way to regard her as an automaton is to think of her as a biological machine. Perhaps we could give a causal account, in terms of biology, con-cerning why she moves in these ways; and similarly we could give a causal account, perhaps, to explain Mr A's reactions to certain personal interven-tions. There is also, however, a causal account in terms of psychology, with-out recourse to explicit intentions, to explain Lady Macbeth's movements.

As the doctor in *Macbeth* says:

> Unnatural deeds
> Do breed unnatural troubles, infected minds
> To their deaf pillows will discharge their secrets
> More needs she the divine than the physician.   (Shakespeare 1951, Act 5,
> Scene 1, 69–72)

Maybe there is a psychological explanation for Mr A's behaviour even in the absence of '*explicit* intentions' or '*explicit* awareness'. Similarly, there might be social causes. This is certainly possible in the case of Mr A. Perhaps the extent to which he appears as an automaton, acting without explicit awareness or intention, is only a reflection of the extent to which he is subject to a 'malignant social psychology'. However, we need to be aware of the dangers of this social constructionist approach. If Mr A's apparently agentive movements are actually only a reflection of social causality, then he is a type of automaton, albeit a socially constructed one.

To summarize, we can have purposive actions without *explicit* intentions. There will be *causal* statements to be made about the actions of an automaton in such an instance; but whether the actor in such cases is *simply* an automaton, rather than an agent, requires us to consider instead what *constitutes* human agency.

We wish to suggest that *explicit* intention may or may not feature in the acts of agents, but nevertheless agentive actions will, by their nature, be intentional, in the sense that they will have an aim and a contextual meaning. Apparently purposive action can be *caused* (biologically, psychologically, socially) without involving *explicit* intentions. If, however, we try to give a *constitutive* account of agency—what it actually *is* to be an agent—then the notion of something being aimed at, an intention in the sense of the act being meaningful, comes into view. But what also comes into view is the world with which the agent interacts. For, to be an agent is to be an agent in the world. Our actions cannot simply and solely be regarded as the final outcome of a causal chain; they have some sort of meaning in the world. This is a reflection of our embeddedness in the human world.

We reach this conclusion by ignoring the *causes* of actions and looking instead at what *constitutes* human action as the action of an agent. By doing this, however, we bring into play the embedding context of the world in which the person is situated as an embodied agent of this kind. Thus, our initial inclination to ask whether Mr A was an agent, as it were *separately* from the description of him as situated and embodied, was misconceived. We might think we can make this separation if we are looking at merely causal explanations of an action, but not once we think of what constitutes agency. Once the notion of intention is introduced (and accepting that intentions are not always necessarily 'explicit') the notion of the embedding context that gives the action a purpose or meaning follows. So, a purposive act is one that involves, if it is a human purpose, the human world of situated embodied agents.[8] Nevertheless, the embedding context cannot be just *any* embedding context, it must be an embedding context that is truly human. To be so it must square with the wider concerns and practices that shape human life. This judgement has its roots in the broader contexts of human action and the human world.

Lady Macbeth's actions are not just to be thought of causally. To *some extent* she does act like an automaton, but she cannot be regarded as a complete automaton, because her actions have meaning in a context. Similarly, Mr A's actions cannot be divorced from the context within which they can be understood and regarded as genuinely meaningful. There is a sense, then, in which we can act with purpose even in the absence of explicit awareness, or consciousness, by virtue of our nature as situated embodied agents.

Even if we do not 'cherish any *explicit* intentions' for particular objects, we may still have a 'purposive relationship' to them (Matthews *op. cit.*). The intentional nature of an action is, on this view, given by its embedding context. So, even in severe dementia the patient can still be regarded as a person.

In Paragraph 420 of the *Philosophical Investigations*, Wittgenstein (1953) tries to imagine that the people around him are automata, that they lack consciousness, even though they continue to behave the same as usual. He describes the idea as 'uncanny'. He says that if you go into the street and say to yourself that everything you see happening, such as children playing, is the result of automatism, then either these words will seem meaningless, or you will have a strange, uncanny feeling.

In remarks at the end of the *Philosophical Investigations*, Wittgenstein considers what it would mean to say that someone was not an automaton. He implies it would make no sense, in ordinary circumstances, to say this on its own. It might mean that the person does not behave like a machine, but we would only *say that* under certain circumstances. In ordinary circumstances it would not, of course, enter our heads that a person was a mere machine. A dedicated nurse looking after someone, like Mr A, with severe dementia would tend, we think, to say as Wittgenstein does in his discussion, 'My attitude towards him is an attitude towards a soul' (Wittgenstein 1953, p. 178). This would reflect the nurse's engagement with the person as a subject of concern, not simply as an object. Tending to someone with severe dementia is not a matter of sentimentality, but is a matter of our intersubjectivity, in which actions are not merely reflexes or instinctual (although they might be those things as well), but are meaningful in the context of an engagement between situated embodied agents. These are not the 'living dead'. They are the dying who live and who deserve our care and concern because of their continuing place as persons in the human world.

Endnotes

1 From the film *The Return of the Living Dead* (1985), MGM/United Artists, Scriptwriters, Dan O'Bannon, Rudi Ricci, and Russell Streiner. Script made into a novel of the same name by John A. Russo (Russo 1985).
2 Morris Friedell in Shenk 2003, p. 241.

3 *Iris*: screenplay in 2001 by Richard Eyre, based on Bayley (1998).

4 As in Tony Hope's case described by McMillan in Chapter 4 of this book (pp. 65–6).

5 For a contrary view see Chapter 7 in this book, by Michael Luntley.

6 The 'continuity' between inner and outer derives support from the externality of mind, discussed in Chapter 1.

7 This is a way of saying that we are *just this type of being*. But it is on account of what this entails that we go on to say beings of this type—even with dementia—should be treated humanly well.

8 The heavy emphasis placed on the embedding context in this section might lead to a macabre possibility. Perhaps Mr A is now a dead corpse, but the nursing staff continue, in some terrible delusional way, to 'fill all the gaps'. They still talk to him, wash him, dress him, and tend to him carefully. If this were the embedding context, would we have to say that Mr A was still a person, still a situated agent, because his personhood is held in place by others? The answer is, of course, that the scenario is preposterous. Why? Because this sort of behaviour simply does not fit into the broader patterns of practice that constitute normal life. Tending to a corpse, however tenderly, as if it were a living person, is simply madness. As we go on to say, any such practice must square with other practices. It is the overview that gives meaning. Still, in context, tenderly caring for a corpse does make some sense—but not if it were done as if the person were alive. That would be a form of madness. (JCH is grateful to Professor Ray Tallis for raising this point and to Professor Guy Widdershoven for discussing it with him. However, neither can be held responsible for the content of the thoughts expressed.)

References

Armstrong, D. M. (1968). *A Materialist Theory of the Mind*. London: Routledge and Kegan Paul.

Bayley, J (1998). *Iris: a Memoir of Iris Murdoch*, London: Abacus Books.

BBC News (2003). Mercy for dementia killer. (Available at http://news.bbc.co.uk/1/hi/scotland/3218311.stm (accessed on 23 February 2005).)

Beck, C. T. (1996). Nursing students' experiences caring for cognitively impaired elderly people *Journal of Advanced Nursing*, **23**: 992–8

Bentham, P., Hodges, J. (2002). Psychiatric and clinical cognitive assessment. In: *Psychiatry in the Elderly*, 3rd edn (ed. R. Jacoby and C. Oppenheimer), pp. 201–25. Oxford: Oxford University Press.

Berrios, G. (1994). Dementia: historical overview. In: *Dementia* (ed. A. Burns and R. Levy), pp. 5–20. London: Chapman and Hall.

Cohen, D., Eisdorfer, C. (2001). *The Loss of Self*. New York: W. W. Norton & Company.

Damasio, A. R. (1994). *Descartes' Error: Emotion, Reason and the Human Brain*. London: Picador.

Damasio, A. (2000). *The Feeling of What Happens: Body, Emotion and the Making of Consciousness*. London: Vintage.

Descartes, R. (1642). Meditations on first philosophy. In: *Descartes: Philosophical Writings* (ed. and trans. E. Anscombe and P. T. Geach, 1970), pp. 59–124. Sunbury-on-Thames: Nelson's University Paperbacks.

Drickamer, M. A., Lachs, M. S. (1992). Should patients with Alzheimer's disease be told of their diagnosis? *New England Journal of Medicine*, **326**: 947–51.

Ekman, S, Norberg, A. Viitanen, M., Winblad, B. (1991). Care of demented patients with severe communication problems. *Scandinavian Journal of Caring Sciences*, **5**: 163–70.

Feil, N. (1993). *The Validation Breakthrough: Simple Techniques for Communicating with People with Alzheimer's Type Dementia*. Baltimore: Health Professions Press.

Fontana, A., Smith, A. (1989). Alzheimer's disease victims: the 'unbecoming' of self and the normalisation of competence. *Sociological Perspectives*, **32**: 35–46.

Franzen, J. (2001). The long slow slide into the abyss. *The Guardian Weekend*, **15th December**: 15–29.

Gubrium, J. F. (1986). *Oldtimers and Alzheimer's: The Descriptive Organisation of Senility*. Greenwich, Connecticut: JAI Press.

Herskovits, E. (1995). Struggling over subjectivity: debates about the 'self' and Alzheimer's Disease. *Medical Anthropology Quarterly*, **9**: 146–64.

Hughes, J. C. (2000). Ethics and the anti-dementia drugs. *International Journal of Geriatric Psychiatry*, **15**: 538–43.

Hughes, J. C. (2001). Views of the person with dementia. *Journal of Medical Ethics*, **27**: 86–91.

Hughes, J. C. (2003). Ethics research in dementia: the way forward? In: *Focus on Alzheimer's Disease Research* (ed. E. M. Welsh), pp. 241–61. New York: Nova Biomedical Books.

Jenkins, D., Price, B. (1996). Dementia and personhood: a focus for care? *Journal of Advanced Nursing*, **24**: 84–90.

Killick, J., Cordonnier, C. (eds.) (2000). *Openings: Dementia Poems and Photographs*. London: Hawker Publications Limited.

Kitwood, T. (1990). The dialectics of dementia: with particular reference to Alzheimer's disease. *Ageing and Society*, **9**: 177–96.

Kitwood, T. (1997). *Dementia Reconsidered: The Person Comes First*. Buckingham and Philadelphia: Open University Press.

Kitwood, T., Bredin, K. (1992). Towards a theory of dementia care: personhood and well-being, *Ageing and Society*, **12**: 269–87.

Kramer, P. D. (1997). *Listening to Prozac*. London: Penguin Books.

Locke J. (1964). *An Essay Concerning Human Understanding* (ed. A. D. Woozley). Glasgow: William Collins/Fount.

Lyman, K. A. (1998). Living with Alzheimer's disease: the creation of meaning among persons with dementia. *Journal of Clinical Ethics*, **9**: 49–57.

Matthews, E. (1996). *Twentieth-Century French Philosophy*. Oxford: Oxford University Press.

Matthews, E. (2002). *The Philosophy of Merleau-Ponty*. Chesham: Acumen.

McGowan, D. F. (1993). *Living in the Labyrinth: a Personal Journey through the Maze of Alzheimer's Disease*. New York: Delacorte Press.

Minios, G. (1989). *History of Old Age: From Antiquity to the Renaissance* (trans. S. H. Tenison). Cambridge: Polity Press.

Normann, H. K., Asplund, K., Norberg, A. (1998). Episodes of lucidity in people with severe dementia as narrated by formal carers. *Journal of Advanced Nursing*, **28**: 1295–300.

Parfit, D. (1984). *Reasons and Persons*. Oxford: Oxford University Press.

Post, S. G. (1993). Alzheimer's Disease and physician assisted suicide. *Alzheimer Disease and Associated Disorders*, **7**: 65–8.

Post, S. G. (1997). Slowing the progression of Alzheimer's disease: ethical issues. *Alzheimer Disease and Associated Disorders*, **11 (Suppl. 5)**: S34–6 and Discussion, S37–9.

Post, S. G. (2000). *The Moral Challenge of Alzheimer Disease: Ethical Issues from Diagnosis to Dying*, 2nd edn. Baltimore: Johns Hopkins University Press.

Russo, J. A. (1985). *Return of the Living Dead*. London: Arrow Books.

Sabat, S. R. (2001). *The Experience of Alzheimer's Disease: Life Through a Tangled Veil*. Oxford and Malden, MA: Blackwell.

Sabat S. R., Harré, R. (1992). The construction and deconstruction of self in Alzheimer's Disease. *Ageing and Society*, **12**: 443–61.

Sabat, S. R., Harré, R. (1994). The Alzheimer's disease sufferer as a semiotic subject. *Philosophy, Psychiatry, & Psychology*, **1**: 145–60.

Sacks, O. (1985). *The Man Who Mistook His Wife for a Hat*. London: Picador.

Shakespeare, W. (1951). *Macbeth*. In: *William Shakespeare: The Complete Works* (ed. P. Alexander), pp. 999–1027. London and Glasgow: Collins.

Shenk, D. (2003). *The Forgetting: Understanding Alzheimer's—A Biography of a Disease*. London: Harper Collins.

Tabak, N., Bergman, R., Alpert, R. (1996). The mirror as a therapeutic tool for patients with dementia. *International Journal of Nursing Practice*, **2**: 155–59.

Tappen, R. M., Williams, C., Fishman, S., Touhy, T. (1996). Persistence of self in Alzheimer's disease. *Image: Journal of Nursing Scholarship*, **31**: 121–5.

Tappen, R. M., Williams-Burgess, C., Edelstein, J., Touhy, T., Fishman, S. (1997). Communicating with individuals with Alzheimer's disease: examination of recommended strategies, *Archives of Psychiatric Nursing*, **11**: 249–56.

Wittgenstein, L. (1953). *Philosophical Investigations* (ed. G. E. M. Anscombe and R. Rhees, trans. G. E. M. Anscombe). Oxford: Blackwell.

Wittgenstein, L. (1981). *Zettel* (ed. G. E. M. Anscombe and G. H. von Wright, trans. G. E. M. Anscombe). Oxford: Blackwell.

Wittgenstein, L. (1992). *Last Writings on the Philosophy of Psychology. Vol II. The Inner and the Outer* (ed. G. H. von Wright and H. Nyman, trans. C. G. Luckhardt and M. A. E. Aue). Oxford: Blackwell.

Woods, R (1989) *Alzheimer's Disease: Coping with a Living Death*. London: Souvenir Press.

10 Dementia and the identity of the person

Eric Matthews

Introduction

When we care for someone with dementia, or when we fear the possibility of becoming demented ourselves, it is easy to fall into thinking of dementia as a kind of 'living death'. We say things like 'She's not the mum I used to know as a child' or 'He's not the man I married': it is as if the person is no longer there with us, even though their body is still living and breathing. The person's body, as we might put it, is seen as still alive, but the person 'inside' the body is experienced as dead, or as good as dead. There is an obvious contradiction in saying that a person is both alive and dead at the same time, but it expresses as well as anything could the confusion in our feelings about the dementing person. They are not really dead, so that we cannot even grieve properly for them; but at the same time we feel we *ought* to grieve their loss, because it is *as if* they were dead. These feelings are not entirely irrational: there is an element, but only an element, of truth in this view, because awareness of oneself *as* a self, as the individual one is and memories of one's own past life as a person are crucial to our view of what it is to *be* a self, more crucial than physically looking the same. People do change physically as they get older and sometimes so radically that they are hardly recognizable as the person they once were; but even so we can soon identify them if they can recall past experiences that we have shared with them. But to say that continued self-awareness is 'crucial' in this sense is not the same as saying that it is *all* there is to being the self one is.

What we are expressing when we say such things is a particular view of personal identity. A view of personal identity is an account of what it is to be the individual person one is, what makes one the *same* person at different times, and so at what points one begins and ceases to be the individual one is—the points at which a person is born and dies. These are *philosophical* questions, with a long history of being discussed among philosophers; but they are also questions that go to the heart of human life and the way in which we relate to ourselves and to others. The view expressed has much in common with certain classical philosophical accounts of the self and self-identity and it is my contention in this chapter that a consideration of these classical accounts may help us to arrive at a clearer and perhaps even a more humane view of people with dementia. If we can see what is true and what is confused about them, we can perhaps develop a more adequate view of personal identity, which will make possible a better explanation of our tangled feelings about people with this condition and so help us to deal with them in a more sensitive way. As I hope will become clear by the end of this chapter, this is one case in which the apparently purely cerebral abstractions of philosophy can make a real difference to human relationships.

Locke and Parfit

But the way in which they can make a difference can be shown only by first engaging in a certain amount of philosophical discussion, which may seem, at first sight, to be extremely abstract and complex and to have little to do with real human issues. I must ask for patience and hope that that patience will eventually be rewarded. To begin with, I must say something about the philosophical tradition to which these accounts belong. Because space is limited, I shall choose to consider only two typical representatives of the tradition, one from the early modern period and one still alive and flourishing. The first figure to be considered was in some ways the originator of this way of thinking about personal identity, the seventeenth-century English philo-sopher John Locke. In Chapter xxvii of Book II of his greatest work, *An Essay concerning Human Understanding* (Locke 1964), the chapter entitled 'Of identity and diversity', which he added to later editions of his work, he sets out an account of what is involved in saying that something is the same thing now that it was (or will be) at some other time—in other words, what are the criteria of *identity*. But what interested Locke most of all was the particular case of *personal* identity. In his account we can find the outlines of the view of personal identity that I claimed above to lie behind the feelings we often have about people with dementia.

Locke states an important principle in Section 7, namely, that,

> ... to conceive and judge of it [identity] aright, we must consider what idea the word it is applied to stands for ... for such as is the idea belonging to that name, such must be the identity ...   (Locke 1964, II.xxvii.7)

We can call this 'Locke's principle' and express it more simply by saying that what we mean by 'identity' depends on what kind of thing we are talking about. So, following this principle, if we want to understand *personal* identity, the identity of a 'self', we must ask what kind of thing a 'person' or 'self' is. Is a person a kind of *thing* (or 'substance', to use Locke's term), like, say, a piece of gold? A piece of gold is simply a set of particles of matter of a particular kind; so it remains the same piece, he would argue, as long as it has (and only as long as it has) precisely the same physical constitution—it is made up of the same particles of matter. It ceases to exist, as that particular piece of gold, when it loses that physical constitution. Or is a person more like a living organism, like a tree, for example? The acorn and the mature oak tree do not share the same set of particles, but what unites them is the continuing biological life that is present in both of them: this particular oak tree is the one that has grown out of a particular acorn. It ceases to exist, as this oak tree, when it ceases to be biologically alive.

Locke argues that, if we think what we mean by the word 'person' (what idea the word stands for, as he puts it), then we shall see that the continuing identity of a person is not like that of either a piece of gold or a tree. What the word 'person' stands for, in its ordinary use, Locke contends, is neither a particular kind of substance with a certain kind of physical constitution, nor a particular kind of living organism. So what does it stand for? Locke's suggestion is that the word 'person' stands for

> . . . a thinking, intelligent being, that has reason and reflection, and can consider itself as itself, the same thinking thing, in different times and places; which it does only by that consciousness which is inseparable from thinking. (Locke 1964, II.xxvii.9)

That is, a thinking thing, or person, is identified, neither by its physical constitution, nor by its biological character, but by certain kinds of characteristically personal *activities* and *states*. The most characteristically personal activity, he is suggesting, is *thinking*: so, what makes a person the particular individual that they are, is that they can reflect on their own existence and so identify themselves as who they are. The root of our personhood, in short, is *self-consciousness*: thinking of oneself as 'me', identifying certain past activities as 'mine' as opposed to someone else's, and anticipating certain future situations as those which will involve 'me', rather than, or in addition to, other people. Self-consciousness is what enables a thinking thing, or person, to 'consider itself as itself'. And that is, therefore, the essence of our identity as the persons we are. As he goes on to say, 'For, since consciousness . . . is that that makes everyone to be what he calls self, in this alone consists personal identity' (Locke 1964, ibid).

Thus, for Locke, the essence of our personhood and personal identity lies in *thinking of ourselves as who we are*, in our consciousness of being 'me': I was the same person in the past to the extent that I am now conscious that that was me, that I can now remember what I did, said, felt, and thought then as something which *I* did, said, felt, and thought. I began to exist as the individual person I am when I began to become self-conscious in that sense (which does not, of course, coincide with when I began to exist as a biological organism, at conception, or as a particular set of physical particles, which have existed, presumably, as long as matter has existed). And I will go on existing as the person I am for as long into the future as I continue to be conscious of, and to remember, that identity. I will die, that is, cease to exist as the particular person I am, when and if I lose that sense of my own continuing identity. But that will not necessarily be when my body ceases to exist as a living organism. The living organism goes on existing as long as biological life continues, but there is nothing in Locke's definition of a person to imply that the time when biological death happens coincides with the time when I die as a *person*.

We should say a little more here about this point, that is, about Locke's specific distinction between my identity as a person and my identity as a biological organism of a certain species (what he calls a 'man' or we might prefer to call a 'human being'). The identity of a 'man', like that of any other animal (or like that of an oak tree), consists in

> ... nothing but a participation of the same continued life, by constantly fleeting particles of matter, in succession vitally united to the same organized body.
> (Locke 1964, II.xxvii.6)

That is, a human being remains the same biological organism as long as it remains alive. By Locke's principle about identity mentioned earlier, that implies that the idea of a 'man' is different from the idea of a 'person'. Hence, the person may go on existing even if the biological organism does not (this is the idea of personal immortality); and conversely (more important from our present point of view), the biological organism can exist, be alive, even if the person has ceased to exist as such. Thus, the Lockean view of the person provides a theoretical, philosophical basis for the intuition that someone with dementia, at least if it is severe enough to destroy all personal memories, is still biologically alive, but is no longer a person, and certainly no longer the person they once were.

Locke, as said earlier, initiated a tradition of thinking about personal identity, which has had many representatives over the intervening centuries. They have not usually agreed with Locke's analysis in every respect, but they share at least the essentials with him. Probably the most distinguished contemporary representative is the English philosopher Derek Parfit, who has developed this view in a number of articles and in his book *Reasons and Persons* (Parfit 1984). Parfit's view is significantly different from Locke's in a number of ways, which I will come back to shortly, but his similarities to Locke are more important from our present point of view. Parfit's arguments make considerable use of 'thought-experiments', mostly of a rather science fiction kind, in which we are invited to think of some rather bizarre (and sometimes physically impossible) circumstances and ask ourselves whether we should say that someone did or did not remain the same person in those circumstances. This is meant to help us to clarify the meaningful boundaries of application of the concept of 'personal identity'. But, as I shall argue shortly, and as we might expect given Locke's principle, the very way in which he interprets these thought-experiments implies that he is in fact *recommending* a certain view of what a person is, rather than simply describing the one most of us have already.

For instance, in *Reasons and Persons*, he uses the story of a 'teletransporter', a device like the one in *Star Trek* in which a person could be transported from one point to another, distant, point at the speed of light. Parfit's machine works by scanning the person's brain and body and then recording the exact states of all their cells. This information is then beamed to the distant receiver, where it is used to create an exact replica of the original person, complete with memories and self-consciousness. In the original and simpler form of the machine, the scanning process also destroys the person's cells at the starting point. Parfit assumes that in this case we would all accept without hesitation that what had happened was that the person who arrived at the distant destination was the self-same person as the one who had entered the scanner at the point of origin. (He also discusses for his own purposes a later version of the machine in which the scanner *does not* destroy the original cells, but that introduces complications that are irrelevant from our present point of view.)

We might well, and I certainly will in a moment, question Parfit's assumption that we should all readily accept that identity had been preserved in this situation. But suppose, for the sake of setting out his argument, we ignore such doubts for the moment. If we can, then it seems to follow from the thought-experiment that we do not think that personal identity depends in any way on having the same body. Our imaginary traveller, after all, is supposed to remain the same person at the end of the journey, but to have a different body made up of a totally different set of particles (though arranged in the same way as in the original). What is supposed to make them the same person? First, that they are an exact physical copy—in other words, he *looks like* the same person. But more important for Parfit is what he calls 'psychological continuity'. Roughly speaking, this is a combination of similar behaviour and the *continuity of memory* that Locke lays so much emphasis on. The person who arrives at the distant destination *thinks of himself* as the person who left the departure point and remembers the experiences had by that person before departure as *his own* past experiences.

So, Parfit thinks, we would all naturally conclude that it *was* the same person as the one who left the departure point; and this is all we would need to draw that conclusion. He even suggests that, if the scanning process destroyed the original person, it would be some kind of consolation to that person that their replica was going to survive. 'Dying when I know that I shall have a Replica', he says, 'is not quite as bad as, simply, dying'; and a little later, he suggests that being destroyed and Replicated is about as good as ordinary survival' (Parfit 1984, p. 201). The Replica, in Parfit's science fiction story, tells the dying original person 'that he will take up my life where I leave off. He loves my wife, and together they will care for my children. And he will finish the book that I am writing' (Parfit 1984, ibid).

This is, one might say, simply a story about a situation that is at least highly unlikely and may well be physically impossible. But Parfit thinks that, even so, if we can make sense of it in the way he suggests, it sheds light on what we mean by 'being the same person' in less bizarre situations. If we would all agree that the teletransporter has successfully transported the person to the distant destination (Mars, in the story), then that means that we regard an exact physical and psychological Replica of me as equivalent to me. I survive (or as good as survive) for as long as there is someone around who looks like me, behaves like me and thinks of himself as being me, and who seems to remember my past life in the way I do. And that means that all there is to being me is looking like me, behaving like me, thinking of myself as being me, and remembering my past life as *my* past life (not in the way we remember things happening to other people). A 'person' is simply a set of experiences and ways of behaving which are linked in these ways.

There are both similarities and important differences in this to Locke's view. It is similar in that it makes continuing to think of oneself as oneself and continuing to remember one's past life the essential things about survival. But if a surviving Replica is 'about as good as ordinary survival' (Parfit 1984, p. 201), then that changes the meaning of 'survival' and 'identity'.

We can see this better if we consider another case, similar in some ways but significantly different in others. Suppose I had an identical twin, who had shared my life with me, and so remembered most of the things which I also remember, and was emotionally very close to me. And then suppose that I was seriously injured in an accident and knew that I would die very soon. My twin brother, on the other hand, being uninjured, would live for many years after my death. Because he was so similar in looks and behaviour to me, many people seeing him would think it *was* me. He would preserve all my memories of my life, which had been mostly shared with him. And he might promise to look after my wife and children and to finish my book in the way I myself would want it finished. He might even, by some aberration of human psychology, be so carried away with all these continuities that he came to think of himself as actually *being* me. None of this, I think, would be much consolation to me: I would not think of his survival in these circumstances as 'about as good' as my own survival. I might appreciate his kindness in looking after my wife and children, but it would not be in any sense the same as *my* looking after them.

In this case, we can readily see that this is so: my twin brother is clearly *not* the same person as me, even if he has the same kind of continuity with my past self that Parfit's Replica is supposed to have. In other words, the kinds of continuity between me and my Replica, which Parfit speaks of, do not amount to *identity* in any strict sense. But, instead of taking this as a counter-argument to his position, Parfit uses it as the basis for a more radical statement of that position. He rejects the idea that what we call 'personal identity' is strictly *identity* at all. It is rather nothing more than 'psychological continuity' in the rather loose sense of 'continuity' indicated. Indeed, he argues that the question whether someone is, or is not, the same person as someone who lived in the past is not a matter of fact, something to which a straightforward 'yes' or 'no' answer can be given, but a matter for *decision*. The answer to questions about personal identity depends on whether we decide that there is sufficient 'psychological continuity' between that earlier person and this person now for us to say that they are one and the same person; and different people may have different ideas about what counts as 'sufficient' continuity. So presumably whether or not our loved one with dementia is judged to be the same as the person they used to be is a matter for us to decide: do they remember enough for us to say, 'Yes, they are the same person', or do they fall short by our standards? Some of us would say they were, some that they were not; but there is no 'right' answer to the question.

Parfit's arguments, as already mentioned, are based on the assumption that we would all readily agree to his interpretation of his thought-experiments. But the conclusions that he draws are so counter-intuitive as to cast doubt, to say the least, on that assumption. He is not simply reporting what we all mean by 'being the same person', but interpreting these bizarre situations in terms of a preconceived idea of his own about personal identity, one that is radically different from all normal ideas. (And perhaps, as some critics of his work have suggested, the sheer bizarreness of his imagined situations makes it easier for him to do this.) In our normal understanding, the survival of a replica of me is by no means the same thing as my survival, any more than the survival of my twin brother is. And whether or not someone's demented mother is still the same person is not a matter for rather arbitrary decision but something of deep emotional significance.

At first sight, Locke's account of personal identity does not seem to be liable to these objections. For Locke, either there is continuity of consciousness or there is not. If there is, the person is objectively the same; if not, she is not. But if we look more closely, we may see that Parfit has identified a problem in the position shared by Locke and himself. It is only because Locke does not recognize the problem of saying what counts as 'continuity of consciousness', we might say, that he can make survival an all-or-nothing matter, not a matter of degree. But there is a problem, as Parfit sees. If we try to rely on continuity of consciousness alone, without any other criterion to back it up, then it becomes hard to say when simply saying 'I am the same person' confirms that one is indeed the same and when it does not. Surely, being the same must have something to do with something more objective than a simple claim to be the same, something which would enable the claim to be independently verified. Probably this means that it is something to do with *physical* or *bodily* continuity. After all, why is the survival of my twin brother or my Replica not my own survival if it is not because my twin or Replica is *physically* distinct from me?

Important though the differences between Parfit and Locke may be in some respects, then, for our purposes they pale into insignificance compared to their essential similarities. And this is directly relevant to our concern with dementia. If our aged relative with dementia, who still looks so like she used to, nevertheless does not recall anything very much about her past life, then I do not see how, from Parfit's point of view any more than from Locke's, one could say that she was to be regarded as the same person. The key thing that they have in common is a certain view of what a 'person' is—that a person is to be identified in terms of self-consciousness and that identity has nothing to do with anything else, such as biological or physical continuity. My life as me, for both of them, begins and ends with the life that I recognize as mine and can recall as mine: if you like, with the life that I might record in my autobiography.

Criticisms of Locke and Parfit

As said earlier, there must be an element of truth in this view of the self and self-identity. Indeed, if there were not, it is hard to see why such intelligent and acute philosophers as Locke and Parfit should have found their accounts plausible (or why we should find it so natural to think of people with dementia as the same in one respect but not the same in another). We all tend to distinguish between *looking like* the same person and *actually being* the same and it sounds plausible to say that actually being the same is being able to share with other people *the memories which we have of the person's past life and of their relations with ourselves*. Our aged relative with dementia looks like the same person, but cannot share memories with us, perhaps cannot even recognize us. That is why we feel her state as a kind of living death. Nevertheless, there are serious problems with the view. To explore these problems will, I think, help us to see both the attractions and the limitations of this conception of dementia. In particular, I shall argue that there must be something more to being the person I am than simply thinking of myself as that person.

The first of the problems is a purely logical point, touched on already in the previous section, but expounded most clearly and effectively by an eighteenth-century philosopher, Bishop Joseph Butler, in the essay *Of Personal Identity*, which formed an appendix to his work *The Analogy of Religion*, published in 1736. Butler accepts that self-consciousness is what 'makes us aware' of our own identity. But he rejects the Lockean view that self-consciousness '*constitutes*' personal identity, that is, that it is continuity of self-consciousness that *makes* us the persons we are. There is a simple logical fallacy, Butler argues, in this view. As he puts it,

> ... one should really think it obvious, that consciousness of personal identity presupposes, and therefore cannot constitute, personal identity.   (Butler 1736)

Very simply, what Butler is saying is that one cannot be conscious of oneself unless there is already in existence a self to be conscious of. That would be rather like saying that knowing something makes it true. It is part of the meaning of the word 'know' that I can only know that Paris is the capital of France if it is already the case that Paris *is* the capital of France. My knowledge of the fact does not create the fact, it merely records something pre-existing. If that is so, and if, as Butler assumes, self-consciousness is knowledge of the self's existence, it cannot be self-consciousness that constitutes or creates the self.

Parfit, of course, would say that personal identity is not a matter of *fact*, something we can *know*, but one for *decision*. But that only sounds plausible if it is not a purely *arbitrary* decision. We would have to decide that someone now is the same person as someone who lived in the past on the basis of certain criteria—how much real 'psychological continuity' there is between the present person and the one who existed in the past. And, unless we are to allow unlimited claims to be the same person as someone who existed in the past, this must be *real* psychological continuity: I must *really* remember what that person did and experienced as something that I did or experienced (unless, that is, we are to accept Parfit's view of the self as a kind of construction; but we have seen how much that conflicts with our ordinary feelings about ourselves and others). The remembering, in short, must be *knowledge* of it as mine and so Parfit's account is open to very similar objections to those raised against Locke. If Butler is right, then, personal identity must depend on something other than continuity of consciousness. And, by Locke's principle, that means that the idea of a 'person' cannot be defined solely in terms of continuity of self-consciousness.

This is connected with other problems, which Butler also pointed out in his essay. First, I must have existed *before* I became self-conscious, because becoming self-conscious is only logically possible if there already existed a self to be conscious of. In more everyday terms, my life began, surely, when I was born (or perhaps when I was conceived) and both these events surely predate any self-conscious life I have had. If so, then my life as an individual must be logically independent of my self-conscious life. However important to my identity self-consciousness may be, it certainly cannot be the whole story. In much the same way and for much the same reasons, my memories of my own life must emerge from a pre-personal existence. I must first have existed as myself, but without consciousness or memories, in order for me then to be able to remember my own existence. Finally, as many people besides Butler have pointed out, no one is aware of their own existence all the time. Even the most dedicated narcissists at least have periods of dreamless sleep during which they are not aware of their own existence or identity at all, but still go on existing and being the persons they are. We do not die every time we lapse into dreamless sleep and then revive again when we wake up. If we did, we should be faced with the bizarre problem of what connected today's self with yesterday's, given that there was a gap in existence during the intervening night. Or would we be prepared to accept the possibility that a person's existence was as disconnected as a series of flashes of light with gaps between them? If we did, we would not go any way towards solving the problems about dementia, but we might find ourselves with all sorts of other problems about human life generally.

All these considerations suggest that personhood or personal identity cannot be reduced to self-consciousness and its continuity. Locke's principle, that in order to decide questions of identity we need criteria of identity based on what kind of thing we are talking about, remains valid. But the considerations set out above imply that we need a different idea of what a person is on which to base our conception of personal identity and continued personal existence. We need an idea of what makes a person the individual that they are, which includes more than continuity of self-consciousness. In the next few pages, I shall develop such a view of personal identity, based on the thought of the French phenomenologist, Maurice Merleau-Ponty (1908–1961) (see Merleau-Ponty (1962, 1965); see also Matthews (2002)).

Merleau-Ponty and the 'body-subject'

But first it is necessary to explain some of the background to Merleau-Ponty's account. To be a phenomenologist, for Merleau-Ponty, meant to attend to our actual concrete experience of the world first of all, rather than trying to construct a systematic general picture of the world deduced from pre-conceived abstract concepts. To put it differently, he wanted to question all the assumptions about our experience that we form on the basis of traditional science and philosophy by testing them against what we actually find the world to be like. In the case that interests us, if we want to understand what a 'person' or 'self' is, we should not attend to what science or philosophy say it *must* be, but rather to what we actually mean by these terms in our everyday experience. Our science itself emerges, after all, from that basic human experience, as we try to find rational explanations of what experience appears to show.

From that point of view, what we mean by a 'person' is an actual human being, with whom we can have certain kinds of dealings and relationships—someone like ourselves, to whom we can relate as 'another self', that is, with whom we can converse and cooperate (or equally whom we can refuse to talk to and can regard as an enemy). In order for us to be able to have these kinds of dealings with them, they must be biological organisms of our own species (or perhaps of other species like our own in relevant respects), be able to communicate with us, have feelings and attitudes like our own or at least intelligible to us, and so on. And this implies that, even from the first-person point of view, we must regard ourselves as such biological organisms of the human species who are able to communicate thoughts and feelings to others. In short, persons are a kind of biological organism, essentially embodied creatures, but a biological organism, which is capable of thought and reflection on their experience and of communicating these thoughts and so forth to other persons. Merleau-Ponty's view is often expressed by describing the human person as a 'body-subject' (though he himself does not seem to use this expression). The term obviously has two parts: 'body', referring to the fact that persons are essentially biological creatures; and 'subject', indicating that they are also creatures who are capable of thought, reflection, and communication.

The hyphen in the expression 'body-subject' indicates that these two elements in what it is to be a person are not separate from each other: that being embodied affects the nature of human subjectivity; while being connected with human subjectivity has a bearing on the nature of the human body. A person is not a 'subject' loosely attached to a 'body', as in Descartes's dualistic view of mind and body as separate and distinct things, but a unified being who expresses their 'subjective' thoughts, feelings, and so on, in bodily form—in speech, in gesture, in behaviour, in interactions with their environment, both human and natural, and so on. Subjectivity exists, on this view, not in some kind of 'inner world', divorced from everything physical. Subjectivity exists in these physical expressions—as for instance you are now reading my thoughts about persons. And conversely, even our bodily existence is 'intentional', that is, directed or purposive (whether or not that purpose is explicitly conscious). For instance, what is going on in my brain at the moment is directed towards formulating and conveying these thoughts in the words I am now writing. To understand my behaviour at the moment, you need to understand not only the mechanisms of brain function but also my purposes in behaving in this way. And even the mechanisms of brain function need to be understood in terms of the role they play in making it possible for me to express my thoughts in words. A person seen as a body-subject is thus neither simply a piece of biological machinery, nor a pure consciousness, but a unity of the two: a consciousness that expresses itself through bodily activity (above all, through speech and writing) and a body that is among other things a vehicle for expressing thought.

We obviously must exist first as biological organisms before we can even begin to think, so the 'body' element of the 'body-subject' clearly has priority in a certain sense over the 'subject' element. This is what makes it inadequate to think of personhood exclusively in terms of thought or consciousness. As Butler saw, consciousness can exist only if there is something for it to be conscious *of*; so consciousness depends on a preconscious existence. A 'person' cannot therefore be defined in terms of consciousness alone, because consciousness cannot exist on its own, and being the person we are cannot be equivalent simply to thinking I am that person. It is the other way around. I can think of myself as me only because I *am* me, and what I am, what makes me the individual I am, must extend beyond what I am explicitly conscious of. This conception of personhood clearly allows for the notions of development and of what might be called levels of individuality. Reflection on our existence logically presupposes that we first have some existence to reflect upon. And we know empirically that this is indeed how things are. We start life as infants, who do not engage in much reflection: but infants are already individuals, as any proud parent will say. They are distinct, not only physically, but in their ways of responding to the world around them. It is simply that their distinctive individuality is not at a very refined or sophisticated level, because that requires reflection, which in turn requires the development of language. Even when reflection does begin, it develops from an initially primitive point, becoming more sophisticated as the person has more experience and can build later reflection on earlier. And what may originally have been the result of conscious, or at least semi-conscious, thought—ways of doing things, kinds of response to situations, and so on—becomes 'sedimented', in Merleau-Ponty's phrase, that is, becomes gradually embedded in our unconscious habits.

In this process, our individuality becomes more refined—we gradually become the persons we are, in the sense of the complex and very distinctive individuals that adult human beings tend to be. Other people's sense of who we are as adults is at least as much to do with the unconscious, or not fully conscious, aspects of our way of doing things as with our explicit memories of our past existence. Our identity, from the point of view of others in our life, is essentially defined by our participation in communicative relationships with them, where by 'communication' is meant not only explicit expression of our conscious thoughts in language but also these kinds of wordless self-expression.

In this way, the concept of the body-subject implies first that personal life emerges from pre-personal bodily existence. We have an identity of our own from birth, but it becomes gradually more distinctive and in a sense 'more personal' as we accumulate memories of our experiences and reflect upon them and as in turn our conscious thought and reflection becomes incorporated in our unreflective way of living. In one sense, Locke and Parfit are right: the possibility of forming a more complex sense of our own identity by thought and reflection is central to our concept of what a human person is. Where they go wrong is in ignoring the many other features of our concept of a person, which form the background to this self-conscious life and which are important to the ways in which we treat persons. The other side to the notion of body-subject is equally important: not only does our existence as a person emerge from our embodiment, but also our bodily existence has to be understood as the expression of our individuality—at all levels—not just in the sophisticated communication of language and consciously recalled experience, but also even in such simple things as our body-language, our habits of behaviour, our characteristic mannerisms and gestures, and so forth.

Practical applications

Having set out the philosophy, we can now finally get back to more practical matters. What do all these abstract-sounding philosophical considerations have to do with the ways in which we think of, and treat, people with dementia? Most of all, they mean that we can no longer accept the simple description of dementia as a 'living death'. If we accept Merleau-Ponty's conception of the human person as a 'body-subject', it follows that we cannot simply identify persons, in the manner of Locke, Parfit, and others, with their self-consciousness, with their sense of themselves derived from reflection on their own life experiences. From this it follows in turn that we cannot say that a person ceases to exist as such once recall of their personal memories and the connected sense of who they are have been lost, as is presumed in (at any rate) the most severe cases of dementia. Something of their individuality survives even so. For on Merleau-Ponty's view a great deal more that is crucial to personal identity still remains in such a case. For us who care for them, all those elements in them that are not conscious or explicit will still remain the same. This will include anything that is due to genetic influences, as well as (probably more importantly) all that may originally have been conscious and reflective but has become 'sedimented' into habits. This is part of the tragedy of dementia: these surviving elements of the individual's personality are sufficient to make us feel that they are still here with us.

An example that comes to mind is that of an elderly woman with dementia I know of, who recalls little of her past life and is barely aware of where she is now. Nevertheless, one part of her past that she still retains is her ingrained sense of politeness, which is expressed in certain of her spontaneous ways of behaving. For example, she still recognizes, as seen in or inferred from her behaviour, if not in her conscious memory, the need to keep a conversation going—the importance of not allowing an uncomfortable silence to fall. This recognition leads her, amongst other things, to fill in with something to say even when she has lost the thread of what she was saying earlier. For those who have known her for a long time, this very familiar characteristic is a part of what makes her the person she is, a surviving fragment of a once much richer identity.

But it is *only* a fragment, and what she once was was indeed much richer. That is the other dimension to the tragedy of dementia. The person with dementia may seem to us to have lost a large part of what made them the distinctive complex individual that they have been. Much that is most distinctively individual about us, the things that really make us ourselves, as it might be expressed, are, as said earlier, the result of continuing reflection on our memories of our own life experiences. The fullest sort of individual identity is something we acquire gradually over the course of our development towards adulthood, which continues to change subtly even during our adult life, as we add fresh memories and fresh reflections on our past. It is this developed adult sense of self to which other adults respond, which they love or hate, when they think of an individual as most truly their unique self. Because it depends for its continued existence on recall, then there is a sense in which people with severe dementia have lost some of their identity as persons, so that they are 'no longer the people they once were'. This is the element of truth in the Locke–Parfit view, and it fully explains, in my opinion, the devastating sense of loss that those who love someone with dementia usually feel: they have indeed lost something precious about the person they love. The sense of loss is all the greater just because some elements of the person still survive. Severe dementia is a fate which, for those who love the demented person, is in some ways *worse* than death, because at least, when someone is literally dead, we can remember them as they were in the full richness of their individuality and are not presently faced with what we may see as a diminished version of them.

Nevertheless, it is important to emphasize that dementia, although it may be a fate worse than death, is not death. This is relevant from an ethical as well as a personal point of view. Some core elements of identity as the person they have been continue to exist. The person with dementia, even in the severest cases, is not, as it is sometimes insultingly expressed, a mere 'vegetable', a mere biological entity with no elements of the personal about them. Nor (slightly less insultingly) are they in the same category as, say, a cherished pet animal, whom we love and care for even though (and perhaps in part because) it lacks the characteristically human level of identity that depends on the ability to have and retain conscious experiences. The person with dementia is not even in the same position as a newborn child.[1] This is not only because, except in the most severe cases, they retain some elements of their conscious identity in a way that a child necessarily cannot; but also because there survives something of their adult individuality in the habits of behaviour in which it has become 'sedimented' in the course of their development to adulthood and beyond. These characteristic gestures and ways of doing things are what keep alive the sense of the individual they once were, even if the more sophisticated levels of that individuality have been removed.

This is important for the ways we treat people with dementia. We are not now, and perhaps will never be, in a position to 'cure' dementia, in the sense of restoring the lost continuity with the person's past life. But it does not follow that all we can do is to 'care for' the person, in the sense of keeping them clean and tidy and decently fed, clothed, and housed. Important though caring in that sense is, it is something we would want to do as much for the family pet as for our dementing grandmother and so does not respect the latter's specifically human dignity. What we can do, over and above such caring, is to help to keep a person's sense of self, and so of self-respect, alive longer. In part, this means reinforcing any remaining elements of conscious self-identity by talking to the person about our past shared life with them and encouraging their own reminiscences. This is something, of course, that is widely recognized and already practised by good carers. But we can also help to preserve the less conscious elements in a person's identity that have been discussed in this chapter. One way we can do this is by making their physical surroundings as familiar as possible, so retaining the physical links with their past, which help to support the sense of selfhood. We can try to make it possible for the person to stay in their own home, with appropriate care of course, for as long as it is practically and economically feasible (we should even be prepared to take some risks in order to do this, because it is part of human dignity that a person should be allowed to live their own life even if some risk may be involved). And when it is no longer feasible, and the person needs to be cared for in an institutional setting, every effort should be made to humanize that setting by including pictures, ornaments, items of furniture, and so on from the person's own home.

This certainly will involve some costs and some might object that it is a wasteful use of resources to incur such costs for people who are near the end of their lives and are incapable of making much contribution to society in return. But if we think that health care must have some kind of ethical basis and if we accept the arguments of this chapter that people, even with severe dementia, retain enough of their individual identity to be still human beings rather than 'vegetables', then there is surely an obligation to incur these costs in order to respect their human dignity. In ways like these, an adequate philosophical theory of personal identity, however abstract it may sound, can have very practical consequences for the ways in which we think about, feel about, and deal with people with dementia.

Endnote

1 And see further discussion of this point by Harry Cayton in Chapter 17.

References

Butler, J. (1736). *Of Personal Identity*. (Appendix to *The Analogy of Religion*, various editions; the appendix is most easily available in Perry, J. (ed.) (1975). *Personal Identity*. Berkeley: University of California Press.)

Locke, J. (1964). *An Essay Concerning Human Understanding* (ed. A. D. Woozley). Glasgow: William Collins/Fount.

Matthews, E. (2002). *The Philosophy of Merleau-Ponty*. Chesham, Buckinghamshire: Acumen Publishing.

Merleau-Ponty, M. (1962). *Phenomenology of Perception* (trans. C. Smith). London: Routledge and Kegan Paul.

Merleau-Ponty, M. (1965). *The Structure of Behaviour* (trans. A. L. Fisher). London: Methuen.

Parfit, D. (1984). *Reasons and Persons*. Oxford: Clarendon Press.

11 Meaning-making in dementia: a hermeneutic perspective

Guy A. M. Widdershoven and
Ron L. P. Berghmans

Introduction

In life, people are continuously engaged in processes of meaning-making. Such processes take place between the person and the world around. Meaning-making involves interaction with things, such as coffee cups, computer keyboards, television remote controls, cars, and bicycles. People know what these things are insofar as they are able to manipulate them and integrate them in their lives. Meaning-making also involves communication with other people. Through other people one comes to understand, by sharing stories, how situations are handled in the world. Meaning-making is already happening before any conscious activity is taking place: a person can drink coffee or use a keyboard without any preconceived thought and involve themselves in storytelling and gossiping without prior deliberation.

Dementia is tragic, because it threatens this process of meaning-making. When a person becomes demented, the interaction with objects and other people becomes problematic. A person may no longer understand what to do with an object, or lose control over its use, for example, when they are no longer able to find a key, or drive a car properly. Communication with other people may become difficult, because the person does not recognize them, or is unable to respond properly in a dialogue. Because dementia makes people appear to react awkwardly, others may become puzzled and frustrated with them. The result is a breakdown of a shared life-world. Insofar as things and other people are no longer part of a self-evident whole of actions and reactions, the demented person loses, to some degree, the previous ability of meaning-making. This is usually experienced as a fatal loss, both by the person themselves and by others in the person's surroundings.

However painful the process of dementia may be, the decrease of meaning-making is not a total loss. As long as they live, people remain able to respond to the world and to communicate with it. Until very late in the process of dementia, people are still able to manipulate objects and to react to others. An indication of the demented person's meaning-making can be seen in their emotions and moods. When a person is glad or annoyed, the situation is experienced as meaningful. Emotions and moods invite other people to take care of the person and to try and help them to deal with the situation.

However problematic, meaning-making remains the vehicle for people to orient themselves and to find their way in life. This holds not only for the demented person, but also for those who care for them. The changes in the process of meaning-making can make a person's behaviour seem strange for others. Caregivers may find it harder to handle the situation. Yet, they will not lose all control. The challenge for them will be to develop new ways of meaning-making in a situation that is less easy to handle then it used to be. In this respect, the task is the same for the demented person and for those who take care of them.

What processes play a role in meaning-making in dementia? In order to answer this question, we will make use of hermeneutic philosophy, especially the work of Heidegger and Gadamer. Hermeneutic philosophy analyses being-in-the-world as a process of understanding. It focuses on the importance of breakdowns as instances in which understanding is both frustrated and at the same time presents itself as a challenge. When one is no longer able to understand, the crucial role of understanding becomes clear; so too does the necessity to restore understanding by adjusting one's view and trying to establish a new common ground. In order to illustrate this idea, we shall present the case of an elderly woman in a nursing home, Mrs P, who is becoming demented. She has difficulties in finding her way and others have trouble in dealing with her and helping her. She has an advance directive, but is unable to make clear exactly what she expects from it. Next we shall discuss some basic notions from hermeneutic philosophy. We shall specifically discuss moods and understanding as characteristics of human existence, the hermeneutic circle and the role of breakdowns, dialogue as a fusion of horizons, along with play and ritual. We shall show that these notions can help us to understand what happens in the case and can inspire a new approach to it. Finally, we shall show that, from a hermeneutic perspective, new light can be cast upon the role of advance directives in dementia care.

The case of Mrs P

Mrs P is an elderly woman living in a nursing home. She is often said to be confused. Mrs P appears not to feel herself at home. She seemingly walks around aimlessly and hardly talks to other residents. She has a prior advance directive, which states that she wants her life ended if she is no longer competent and unable to take care of herself.

When a nurse talks to Mrs P about her wishes and shows her the advance directive, she is somewhat puzzled. She tries to read the document, but has trouble understanding what it says. Suddenly, she recognizes it, and says 'That is mine.' When asked whether she wrote the text herself, she answers in the affirmative. She is then asked whether she still upholds the view stated in the document. She answers 'Yes, certainly!' Then she remarks that the situation is 'not that bad yet'. When asked about what should be done if the situation should become worse, she displays mistrust of the staff, especially the physicians. She says that her former general practitioner refused to help her. The current physician in the nursing home is not much help either. No one does what she wants, she says bitterly.

The nursing home physician acknowledges that Mrs P's situation is difficult and thinks that something should be done about it. He starts a conversation with Mrs P. When asked how she feels, Mrs P says she is bored during the day. She is glad when it is 4 p.m., at which time she is allowed to return to bed. In bed, she is happy. She can think about all kinds of things and silently sing her own songs. The physician suggests to Mrs P that she could join group sessions in which residents take part in activities, such as doing needlework. Mrs P declines. 'Needlework is nothing for me!' she says emphatically. The conversation comes to a standstill. According to the physician, the situation is without prospect.

Moods and understanding as characteristics of human existence

Hermeneutic philosophy deals with the preconditions of understanding (the Greek word *hermeneusis* means the act of interpreting messages and texts). It was developed by Heidegger (1927) and Gadamer (1960). According to Heidegger, human existence is being-in-the-world. Being-in-the-world has two sides: finding oneself moved and moving oneself. Against Descartes, who defines *res cogitans* over against *res extensa* as an intellect without space and time, Heidegger stresses that human existence is always in space and time. Before mathematical thought is possible, human existence is positioned in space and time. Before being able to calculate, one is already oriented in and orienting oneself towards the world.

According to Heidegger, the first side of being-in-the-world, finding oneself moved, is related to the basic characteristic of being-in-the-mood. Heidegger illustrates this with the example of fear. Fear is not a result of calculating the consequences of a future evil. The object of fear is experienced as fearful before any calculation is being made. Fear is related to care. One fears if one experiences something one cares for as being endangered. Fear also shows that one is personally involved. Even if one fears for something external to one's own body (one's house or one's loved ones), the relation to oneself is at stake. Moods, such as fear, show that human existence implies finding oneself thrown into the world.

Heidegger relates the second side of being-in-the-world, moving oneself, to the basic characteristic of *understanding*. Understanding implies knowing how to handle things. It is oriented towards the future. Whereas being-in-the-mood is related to human existence as being thrown into the world, understanding is related to projecting and planning. Understanding means 'seeing as': one is able to see a cup as something to pour coffee in, a car as something to drive. Understanding is prior to seeing a thing as a meaningless object. One has to abstract the cup or car from the already known use and context if one wants to regard such objects as just meaningless.

The two basic characteristics of human existence, being-in-the-mood and understanding, are mutually related. Orienting oneself is based upon being oriented and results in a new orientation. To return to the example of fear: fear can motivate a person to flee and the act of fleeing can in turn result in a change of mood. (For instance, an intensification of fear may occur, when in fleeing one becomes aware of the pursuing danger more explicitly; or the opposite, a feeling of relaxation when danger is evaded through fleeing.)

When we look at Mrs P's case, we can recognize the two characteristics of being-in-the-world, distinguished by Heidegger. Mrs P clearly shows moods. She is annoyed and irritated by other residents, she is restless, she is angry (with an undertone of resignation) towards her physicians. These are all 'negative' moods. She does not seem to be happy and other people around her are not pleased to see her in this state. Yet she also has other, more 'positive', moods. The moment she starts talking about being in bed she becomes happy and relaxed. Obviously, she is able to feel comfortable and at peace there. Although her moods are not always easy for herself and for others, they show that the world has meaning for her and that she is moved by it.

The second characteristic, understanding, can also be seen in Mrs P's behaviour. She moves herself, albeit not always in direct and straightforward ways. She wanders about, which shows that she is looking for someplace else to be, or that she has nothing else to do, or that she is anxious. When addressed by others, she responds and is able to present her views. She is clear about her wish to go to bed and is able to get the staff to respond to this, because she is allowed to go to bed at 4 p.m., a rather early time of the day (even in nursing homes). Mrs P also knows how to handle the advance directive shown to her. She takes it in her hand and starts reading it. After some time, she is able to recognize it as hers. She also makes clear that she sees it as an important document, which she wants others to take into consideration.

The people who take care of Mrs P are also moved by and moving in the world. The nurse who discusses the advance directive with Mrs P is interested in her and in her advance directive. Although communication is not easy, he remains oriented towards Mrs P. He is able to manipulate the document and to encourage Mrs P to talk about it. In this sense, he knows how to handle the situation. The physician is also moved by Mrs P. He finds himself in a difficult situation, and does not know exactly what to do. In his reaction, mood and understanding clearly influence one another. The mood of frustration results in a lack of ability to solve the problem (perhaps the lack of ability to solve the problem results in frustration too) and this again fosters the feeling of hopelessness. Although the physician is able to have some conversation with Mrs P, the way in which the conversation evolves shows that the physician does not really understand Mrs P (and vice versa).

There appears to be a lot of meaning-making in the case of Mrs P. Both Mrs P and the people around her are being moved and move themselves. They show moods and understanding. Yet, the processes of meaning-making are not totally successful. Mrs P is not able to find rest most of the day; only in bed is she happy. The nurse does not know what to do with Mrs P's response to the advance directive. The physician feels frustrated and hopeless. How should these problems be dealt with? What can be done? These questions require a more in-depth analysis of the process of understanding, especially of the role of breakdowns.

The hermeneutic circle and the role of breakdowns

According to Heidegger, understanding is based upon pre-understandings. In order to make sense of a thing or a text, we already have to be able to handle it and to see it as a thing or a text. This implies that understanding never starts from scratch. If, in interpreting a text, one refers to what is actually there, this does not do away with the perspective one already has. Interpretation is never a matter of grasping what is there without any preconditions or preconceptions. On the contrary: every interpretation is based upon a primordial view, which is based upon one's knowledge of how to handle the situation.

Does this not bring us into a circle? We seem only to be able to understand, if we already understand. Heidegger acknowledges that there is a circle here. Yet, he stresses that it is not a vicious circle. In the process of understanding, preconceptions can prove to be fruitful. In pouring coffee into a cup, we can find that the result is in line with our expectations, so that we can have a cup of coffee. By practising, we can further develop our skills and learn more about the art of having coffee than before. The same holds for the interpretation of texts. Although we can understand a text only by having preconceptions, the process of interpretation can lead to a refinement of our preconceptions. This process is called the *hermeneutic circle*. According to Gadamer (1960), it has the form of a spiral.

In the process of understanding, pre-understandings are not always fruitful. When this experience occurs (where one's presuppositions are shattered) it is the experience of *breakdown*. When a tool breaks down, one comes to realize that certain presuppositions implicit in one's way of handling the tool are no longer valid. If the coffee we have just poured into our cup appears to be cold (a shocking experience for those who like their coffee hot), we have to conclude that something has gone wrong (for example, that the electric kettle we used does not work properly, so that we have poured cold water on the coffee filter). Shocking as it may be, this experience enables us to become aware of our presuppositions—and to change them. Because we are usually able to trust our pre-understandings, a change will not easily be brought about. Yet, the experience of breakdown can lead to drastic changes in our understanding of the world. Next to refinement through the hermeneutic circle, the necessity of change after a breakdown can lead to a growth of understanding. These two hermeneutic elements of change can also be seen in Kuhn's theory of scientific revolutions (Kuhn 1970). The growth of knowledge through application of existing pre-understandings is characteristic of normal science; major breakdowns are typical in a period of crisis, which can result in a scientific revolution. In a period of revolution, the scientists involved do not know their way about any more. This problem can be solved if leading scientists agree on a new position and a new set of pre-understandings is developed, which can serve as a basis for future research.

In the case of Mrs P, the hermeneutic circle and the phenomenon of breakdown are clearly present. Mrs P shows certain pre-understandings about her situation, which enable her to move around and to understand the words people say to her. Yet, her understanding is not always successful. When walking through the corridors, she does not really know what to do, until she is allowed to go to bed. When the nurse shows her the advance directive, she is at first puzzled. Whatever she might have expected, it was not her own written declaration of will. The confrontation shows aspects of a breakdown. It takes quite a while before she recognizes the letter as hers. This process of recognition takes the form of a hermeneutic circle: she gradually comes to understand that she herself wrote the advance directive. The result of this process of understanding, however, remains limited. She hardly sees the consequences of her declaration for her present situation. The conversation between Mrs P and the physician shows various breakdowns. When Mrs P says she feels bored and wants to go to bed, the physician is surprised to hear that she is not bored in her bed. On the other hand, when the physician suggests Mrs P might take up an activity during the day, Mrs P appears to be repelled by the idea of doing needlework. These examples show that Mrs P and the physician have different presuppositions about what is good in life and are shocked to see that their views are not shared.

Although the participants in the case of Mrs P have some productive pre-understandings and are at times able to develop these further, the elements of breakdown are abundant and appear difficult to solve. Mrs P does not really know what to do with her advance directive. She and the physician do not come to a joint understanding of the situation. The situation resembles the period of crisis in scientific revolutions. Many pre-understandings, taken for granted previously, do not work any more. There is a need for a fundamentally new way of dealing with the situation. How can a revolution in meaning-making be brought about in daily life? What is needed to change the breakdowns so as to arrive at a more productive way of dealing with the situation?

Dialogue as a fusion of horizons

A breakdown makes one experience that one's presuppositions are not in line with the presuppositions embedded in the tool one tries to use. This is apparent in the breakdown of an electric kettle. One of the presuppositions in using the kettle is that it will always function properly. Yet the machine itself is built in such a way that it has a limited period of proper functioning. Upon reflection, one realizes that any kettle might stop functioning properly at any moment, including this one. Yet this way of thinking is not at all relevant when one heats water. The expectation is that the kettle will work, not that—given its technical limitations—it might not work. However much we may be able to see the risk of a breakdown intellectually, in ordinary life we do not presuppose it as a real possibility. The latter would be the case only if the kettle tended to malfunction regularly, but that would imply that it would exemplify another presupposition related to proper functioning.

The mismatch in presuppositions inherent in a breakdown can be characterized as a divergence in horizons. Users of a tool act from their horizon of expectations. The tool presents another horizon. This divergence of horizons can also be seen in the process of interpreting a text. If the horizon of the interpreter and that of the text are different, the text will fail to be intelligible. A satire, for instance, will be misunderstood if one reads it as a factual statement and neglects the subtle reversal of roles and interpersonal relationships. This process of misunderstanding will continue until the reader sees what the text aims at. At that moment, the reader gets access to the horizon of the text. They will acknowledge that they had mistakenly taken their own horizon as the proper one. They will have to leave their horizon and enter into that of the text.

The process of becoming open to the horizon of the text does not mean that one simply steps out of one's own horizon. Given the fundamental status of pre-understandings, one cannot leave them totally behind. If understanding would be a matter of stepping directly into the horizon of the other (a tool, a text, another person), we would be back to the view of understanding as starting from scratch, a view which was criticized above. Hermeneutic philosophy is critical of objectivism (there is one good perspective, from which the matter under consideration can be fully grasped). Yet it does not imply relativism (perspectives are different and fundamentally alien to one another). Hermeneutics goes beyond the opposition between objectivism and relativism (Bernstein 1983). In dialogue, one can learn to understand the other, not by leaving one's own point of view behind, but by broadening one's perspective so that the viewpoints meet and merge. Dialogue involves a process of deliberation, which brings about moral learning (Emanuel and Emanuel 1992; Widdershoven 1999). Dialogue is a process of *fusion* of horizons, in which one does not remain what one was before (Gadamer 1960). Thus, in coming to see the text as a satire, the reader will still have to decide whether the reversal of roles succeeds in clarifying specific aspects of the human condition in general and the specific situation the text deals with in particular. Simply noticing the rhetorical style of the text is not the same as understanding it. The text does not aim to make the readers see it as a satire, but to make them share the implicit critique of the situation that is the object of satire. The fundamental problem of interpretation goes beyond a mismatch of styles. It deals with the question of whether the proposed view of the world in the text gives rise to a change in view of the reader. Such changes are not only a matter of opinion, but also have practical consequences. If the satire is convincing, the readers will change their view of the situation and act accordingly (for instance, by not voting for the political leader who is satirized).

In the case of Mrs P, horizons are divergent. One example of this concerns the advance directive. Mrs P's view of the document is not in line with the perspective embodied in it. At first she does not even recognize the text as a declaration of (her) will. After a while, she does recognize it, but she is unaware of its possible significance for the situation she is in. Therefore, the advance directive is of no support to her. The perspective embodied in the advance directive is not only alien to Mrs P, but also to her caregivers. The nurse is interested in Mrs P's view of the advance directive, but he does not intend to give the declaration a role in the process of care. This is also the case for the physician, who does not even discuss the advance directive with Mrs P. The horizons of the advance directive and that of the people present in the case do not meet.

Between the people in the case, there are also mismatches. The horizon of Mrs P on the one hand and those of the nurse and the physician on the other hand, are not in line. When the nurse and Mrs P are discussing the advance directive, the nurse wants to know Mrs P's current views concerning what is stated in the document. Mrs P responds that she still holds on to her former views and that she mistrusts the physicians. The nurse takes notice of these statements, but no corresponding action follows. The advance directive is not used in care planning; and nothing is done to deal with the mistrust of the physicians. As we saw, the conversation between the physician and Mrs P shows a divergence in what is seen as important in life. Mrs P wants to be happy in bed, whereas the physician stresses the need to be active. The two perspectives clearly do not meet.

When we take a closer look, there is dissimilarity between the two interactions: that between Mrs P and the nurse and that between her and the physician. The nurse is interested in Mrs P's views, but he does not take these into account in planning care. He listens, but does not act. He resembles a person smiling at a satire, but not changing his political preferences. The physician, on the other hand, is hardly interested in Mrs P's views. Yet, unlike the nurse, he wants to change the care process. He wants things to improve and makes various suggestions. These do not work, because they lie outside Mrs P's horizon. We may conclude that a fusion of horizons is lacking in both cases, for various reasons. The nurse recognizes that Mrs P has specific views, but he does not feel the need to understand her perspective. He takes the views of

Mrs P for granted, but does not integrate them into his own view of the world. The physician, on the other hand, wants to impose his own views on Mrs P, but does not understand that Mrs P thinks differently and is likewise not able to achieve a fusion between the two horizons.

What is needed in order for a fusion of horizons to occur? A hermeneutic approach would require that one both acknowledges that the perspective of the other is different from one's own and that one is also interested in bridging the gap between the two. These two aspects are crucial elements of a *dialogue* wherein people are open and prepared to learn from differences in perspective.

> To reach an understanding in a dialogue is not merely a matter of asserting one's own point of view, but a change into a communion in which one does not remain what one was. (Gadamer 1960, p. 379)

Such a dialogue is possible in dementia care (Widdershoven 1999; Widdershoven and Widdershoven-Heerding 2003). When we look at the approaches of the nurse and the physician in the case, a dialogue is, however, not easily establishable. A revolution is necessary before Mrs P will actually feel heard. The caregivers would have to be really interested in her and in her views on what counts as a good life. They should both be open to her and be prepared to change their own way of seeing and handling the situation. They would have to be able to take part in Mrs P's way of meaning-making and invite her to develop new ways of dealing with the situation. How can this be achieved?

Play and ritual

One might be tempted to think that a dialogical process of fusion of horizons is primarily a matter of argumentation and discursive deliberation. Although arguments and discussions can be a vehicle for mutual understanding, they are not the sole vehicle. Moreover, the working of arguments and deliberations should not be reduced to a matter of exchange of information and logical reasoning. The example of the satire shows that a process of convincing another person requires rhetorical means. Logical analysis can be rhetorically powerful, but it can also be counterproductive. Logic does not make rhetoric redundant; it actually requires the latter to be effective in a dialogue.

The fusion of horizons that Gadamer talks about requires an interplay between two parties. One can become open to another perspective only if one is invited to take part in it, in the same way as a person is invited to a dance. The invitation should neither be enforcing nor show a lack of engagement. A proper invitation is hard to resist, not because it is overpowering, but because it is polite and honourable to the person invited. The invitation is a prequel to the dance itself, showing a process of tuning, in which both parties respond to one another in a ritualistic way. During the dance, this process continues and makes the dancers feel part of a larger unity. The interplay is not merely a matter of tuning between individuals. The rhythm of the music and the example of others is important in bringing about a practice of joint movements.

Dialogue is first and foremost a process of *play* between parties, based upon *rituals*. Conscious forms of interaction are dependent upon such preconscious ways of aligning and tuning. The notion of play refers back to what was said before about being-in-the-mood and understanding. Play is being moved and moving at the same time (Gadamer 1960). That is not to say that argumentation and discussion have no content. It does mean, however, that the development of shared views is not a matter of finding the right content and then communicating it, but that what is right in content can only be established in and through a process of communication that is carried forward by means of play and ritual.

Play and ritual play an important role in dementia care. Joint activities, such as singing or eating, are central elements of nursing home life. Staff and residents may feel united when performing such activities. This is probably the reason why the physician suggested that Mrs P should join group activity sessions. Yet she did not feel tempted by these activities. This, however, does not mean that she is not open to play and ritual at all. She describes going to bed as a playful and ritualistic event. Being in bed, she sings to and by herself. That is why being in bed is meaningful to her. From a hermeneutic perspective, one could try and find other forms of play and ritual in which Mrs P can take part. These should not be imposed upon her, but should be offered in an inviting way. In order to communicate with Mrs P, the caregivers could try to move through the world together with her, see what she likes about being in bed and offer alternatives. In this way they would empower her and persuade her to try out new ways of behaving (Moody 1992). They should take her seriously, both in her bad and her good moods. They should help her to change situations she experiences as annoying and frustrating and further develop ways of acting that she experiences as pleasant and rewarding. Is it possible to develop joint rituals akin to her way of being in bed during the rest of the day? Is it possible to develop joint ways of dealing with things clearly important to her, such as her advance directive?

Advance directives as hermeneutic tools

Advance directives are not very common in dementia care. A minority of people execute advance directives, even after being educated about the possibility. Physicians, particularly those working with people with Alzheimer's disease, are not familiar with them. If asked how they would deal with an advance directive, the most common answer is that it should not be followed strictly, but be considered as one of the relevant elements in the process of decision making. Physicians think that advance directives can give an indication of the patient's values and that as such they can play a role, but they want to make the final decision themselves. Research has shown that people with advance directives get the same amount of life-prolonging treatment (such as resuscitation) as do those without such directives (Teno *et al.* 1994).

From a hermeneutic perspective, the hesitation of patients and physicians towards creating advance directives is understandable. The idea that advance directives can stipulate exactly what should be done in the future is not in line with a hermeneutic view of meaning-making (Widdershoven and Berghmans 2001). Suppose that an advance directive states that the person does not want to live any more if they are no longer able to recognize their family or friends. Does such a declaration tell the doctor exactly what to do? Can the physician execute the directive blindly? Will there not always be a need for interpretation of the directive in the light of the given circumstances? When can the doctor be sure that the patient no longer recognizes family and friends? Is this when their names have been forgotten? Or when they no longer seem to regard them as people who mean something to them in some way? How should we decide the latter? This example shows that an advance directive is always in need of interpretation. The doctor has to judge whether the present situation comes under the rule that is stated in the advance directive. Advance directives do not specify how they are to be executed, as rules do not specify how they are to be applied (Wittgenstein 1973).

From a hermeneutic perspective, written documents may play a role in healthcare, not as predetermined orders, but as tools that help to structure shared decision making. Heidegger's analysis of the crucial role of tools can be helpful here. People give meaning to the world by using tools: they can see through glasses and contact lenses, transport themselves with bicycles and cars, and think with pen and paper or keyboards and computer screens. These tools are prostheses; they are extensions of our body (Merleau-Ponty 1945). Tools and instruments do not stand between ourselves and the world; they are our entrance to the world. Merleau-Ponty mentions the example of a blind person's cane. The cane is not a source of information to be analysed, it is part of the sensory system and enables the blind person to walk as senses enable people who can see to walk. The cane is not external to the person's body; it has become part of their embodied identity. Tools are parts of rituals. They are used in a repetitive way and, in handling them properly, we have to use the right timing or tempo. Tools do not refer to the world, but make the world present, as a work of art makes the person depicted present. In this sense a tool is symbolic (Gadamer 1960, 1977).

If advance directives are to be relevant to decision making about the treatment and care of incapacitated people, they have to be used as tools. This means that the people who use them need to be familiar with them and need to have integrated them into their daily practices. They will have to be able to use the text as an aid to structure the decision-making process (Emanuel and Emanuel 1989), which requires that all the people involved (patient, family, and staff) get used to the text and learn how to handle it. This can work only if advance directives are treated not as isolated statements about a person's general preferences, but as instruments inviting all those who are concerned to become engaged in practices of meaning-making in relation to treatment and care (Widdershoven and Berghmans 2001).

How can Mrs P's advance directive be changed into a hermeneutic tool? This would require using it to order communication about living a good life. One should not focus only on what Mrs P has written in the past, but try to understand what this says about her present situation. This requires a hermeneutic circle between the text and Mrs P's present expressions and experiences. Can the text clarify Mrs P's present concerns (for instance her interest in privacy)? Can her present utterances throw new light on the text? The advance directive states what she thinks is important and can help to discuss what this means in the present situation. In such a discussion, all parties should be involved. Mrs P, the nurse, and the physician should be challenged to develop new routines and rituals together, based upon the advance directive and making it concrete in the present. Finally, the advance directive should not be seen as a set of rules to be followed, but as a symbol for Mrs P's view of a good life. The text should be treated as a token of her autonomy, requiring respect, and as a vehicle to further her autonomy.

Conclusion

People are continuously involved in processes of meaning-making. They interpret and try to make sense of what happens around them, so that they understand the world and know what to do. Processes of meaning-making are not the result of conscious calculations or decisions by the individual; they precede such activities and serve as their foundation. In dementia, meaning-making becomes problematic. Common ways of understanding often tend to break down. Perspectives, which used to be shared, may drift apart. From a hermeneutic perspective, the challenge is to find ways to reintegrate these perspectives once again. This requires a dialogical attitude, exemplifying both openness and preparedness to change. A fusion of horizons is not a conscious achievement brought about through the exchange of information. It is a realignment that occurs when people take part in joint movements and rituals and find themselves changing into a community. Such processes can be developed in dementia care by sharing everyday activities, such as eating or singing. They can be sustained by tools, which may help people to orient themselves in a common world. From a hermeneutic perspective, advance directives should not be seen as objective statements about prior wishes, to be executed when the moment has come, but as vehicles for joint meaning-making, before and during the experience of dementia. As tools, such documents can orient behaviour and symbolize shared practices of care.

References

Bernstein, R. J. (1983). *Beyond Objectivism and Relativism*. Oxford: Oxford University Press.

Emanuel, L. L., Emanuel, E. J. (1989). The medical directive: a new comprehensive advance care document. *Journal of the American Medical Association*, **261**: 3288–93.

Emanuel, E. J., Emanuel, L. L. (1992). Four models of the physician–patient relationship. *Journal of the American Medical Association*, **267**: 2221–6.

Gadamer, H.-G. (1960). *Wahrheit und Methode* [*Truth and Method*]. Tübingen: JCB Mohr.

Gadamer, H-G. (1977). *Die Aktualität des Schönen* [*The topicality of the beautiful*]. Stuttgart: Reclam.

Heidegger, M. (1927). *Sein und Zeit* [*Being and Time*]. Tübingen: Max Niemeyer Verlag.

Kuhn, T. S. (1970). *The Structure of Scientific Revolutions*. Chicago: Chicago University Press.

Merleau-Ponty, M. (1945). *Phénoménologie de la Perception* [*Phenomenology of Perception*]. Paris: Gallimard.

Moody, H. R. (1992). *Ethics in an Aging Society*. Baltimore: Johns Hopkins University Press.

Teno, M. J., Lynn, J., Phillips, S. R., Murphy, D., Youngner, S. J., Bellamy, P. *et al.* (1994). Do formal advance directives affect resuscitation decisions and the use of resources for seriously ill patients? SUPPORT Investigators. Study to Understand Prognoses and Preferences for Outcomes and Risks of Treatments. *Journal of Clinical Ethics*, **5**: 23–30.

Widdershoven, G. A. M. (1999). Care, cure and interpersonal understanding. *Journal of Advanced Nursing*, **29**: 1163–9.

Widdershoven, G. A. M., Berghmans, R. L. P. (2001). Advance directives in dementia care: from instructions to instruments. *Patient Education and Counseling*, **44**: 179–86.

Widdershoven, G. A. M., Widdershoven-Heerding, I. (2003). Understanding dementia: a hermeneutic perspective. In: *Nature and Narrative. An Introduction to the New Philosophy of Psychiatry* (ed. B. Fulford, K. Morris, J. Sadler, and G. Stanghellini), pp. 103–11. Oxford: Oxford University Press.

Wittgenstein, L. (1973). *Philosophical Investigations*. New York: MacMillan.

12 I am, thou art: personal identity in dementia

Catherine Oppenheimer

Introduction

As a non-philosopher, I find it difficult to think of personhood in the abstract; all my experience is of the practical and the particular, the fine detail, the unique oddities of the people whom I have met face to face or in their writing.

Consequently this chapter is less an argument than a sequence of examples—variations on the theme of personhood; and especially personhood communicated through language, the body, and the social context.

I have ordered my examples roughly according to the relationships in which they occurred, but these are arbitrary divisions, scarcely more significant than to sort the coloured glass of a kaleidoscope into squares or oblongs or triangles.

The essence of our difficulty with personhood in dementia is the scarcity of reports from the inhabitants of that country and hence our reliance on guess-work to reach an empathetic understanding of the experience. I therefore begin with one man's remarkable account of his 'shattered world'.

I continue with other accounts of the relationship of the person with himself as the illness takes hold; I consider personhood in the communication between close family members; then the role of professional carers in sustaining the individuality of the person they care for; and lastly the role of inanimate things.

The man with a shattered world

In 1943 a young soldier in the Russian army endured a shrapnel wound to his head, which destroyed a large part of the temporo-parieto-occipital area of his left cerebral cortex. He came eventually under the care of the celebrated Alexander Romanovich Luria, Professor of Psychology at the University of Moscow, who worked with him for 25 years. Though grievously handicapped in the realms of communication, speech, memory, vision, spatial organization, physical skills, and logical reasoning, Lieutenant Zasetsky painstakingly re-taught himself to write so that he could record the experience of his illness.

The three thousand pages of notes that he wrote over the 25 years were condensed and published by Professor Luria under the title *The Man with a Shattered World* (Luria 1975).

Zasetsky's disabilities derived from a traumatic brain injury rather than from the progressive degeneration of the brain that characterizes the dementias. So his account cannot be taken directly as a description of dementia 'from the inside'; nevertheless he offers us unequalled insights into the phenomena (such as amnesia, word-finding difficulties, visual agnosia) that form part of the outsider's 'objective' description of dementing illnesses.

Zasetsky was so handicapped in communicating that in many settings he was regarded as stupid, illiterate, or confused. How was it possible for him to convey the quality of his experience as precisely and movingly as he does in this short book? He describes the process himself:

> I have to read words one at a time until I get the meaning . . . I also have to stop at the fourth letter of every word, because even though I can see it and know how it is pronounced, I've already forgotten the first three letters . . . At first I had just as much trouble with writing—that is, even after I thought I knew the letters, I couldn't remember how they were formed. But one day a doctor whom I'd come to know well . . . asked me to write automatically, without lifting my hand from the paper, and not letter by letter . . . I hardly knew what I had written since I still had trouble reading. I spent weeks thinking about what I wanted to write and how I would do it, but my sick brain couldn't remember the right expressions . . . (Luria 1975, pp. 67, 69, and 72)

He decided to try and write the story of his illness.

> But when I started, I realised I'd never be able to do that since I didn't have enough of a vocabulary or a mind to write well . . . I'd get an idea of how to describe the moment I was wounded and the period immediately afterwards, when my illness began. So I began to hunt for words to describe it and finally I thought up two. But by the time I got to the third word I was stuck . . . Hold on, I'd think, I've got it. But before I could manage to write it down, it was gone, along with the other two words I'd had such a hard time remembering . . . (Luria 1975, p. 73)

It is agonizing just to read his description of the ceaseless efforts he made to capture his slipping and fragmenting thoughts. But there were powerful reasons for him to continue in the effort:

> By working on that one story of mine every day . . . I hoped I'd be able to tell people about the illness and overcome it . . . This writing is my only way of thinking. If I shut these notebooks, give it up, I'll be right back in the desert, in that 'know nothing' world of emptiness and amnesia . . . (Luria 1975, pp. 77–8)

> Perhaps, I thought, if I describe my illness in more detail and give them an account of what's happened, the doctors will understand me. And once they

understand me and my illness, they'll certainly be able to cure it. After all, when I was in the hospital I wasn't really able to remember and tell them what bothered me, so perhaps they still don't realise I'm suffering, since I can't give them any of the details . . .   (Luria 1975, p. 78)

How much more vividly could one convey the qualities of intelligence, courage, and determination that lived on in this man, behind all the handicaps he struggled with? Yet to others, little of this richness was apparent and even his family found it hard to retain contact with the person he truly was:

My family tries to help me converse by asking me questions, but after a while, when they don't get anywhere, they give up on me. It's as if they said to themselves 'There's no point to it, he'll never remember what he wanted to say'.   (Luria 1975, p. 83)

. . . , even now, no matter what circumstances I'm in (with my friends, family, different groups of people, working or just taking a walk), I'm always aware of these defects in my memory and in my ability to speak or think. I sense just how abnormal I am when I talk to people; I'm aware of that idiotic smile on my face, that silly, nervous laugh I have and my constant habit of saying 'yes, yes' while someone is talking to me.   (Luria 1975, p. 58)

Zasetsky's difficulties in communicating were not confined to language. The damage to his brain also hampered communication with his own body:

Often I fall into a kind of stupor and don't understand what's going on around me; I have no sense of objects. One minute I stand there thinking about something, the next I lapse into forgetfulness. But suddenly I'll come to, look to the right of me, and be horrified to discover half my body is gone . . . Sometimes when I'm sitting down I suddenly feel as though my head is the size of a table—every bit as big—while my hands, feet and torso become very small . . .   (Luria 1975, p. 47)

Or, in the weeks following his injury, when he was in a hospital near Moscow:

During the night I suddenly woke up and felt a kind of pressure in my stomach. Something was stirring in my stomach, but it wasn't that I had to urinate—it was something else. But what? I just couldn't work it out. Meanwhile, the pressure in my stomach was getting stronger every minute. Suddenly I realised I had to go to the toilet but couldn't work out how. I knew what organ got rid of urine, but this pressure was on a different orifice, except that I'd forgotten what it was for.   (Luria 1975, p. 49)

Nor could he reliably use his body to communicate with others:

I was lying in bed and needed the nurse. How was I going to get her to come over? All of a sudden I remembered you can beckon to someone and so I tried to beckon to the nurse—that is, move my left hand lightly back and forth. But she walked right past and paid no attention to my gesturing. I realised then that I'd completely forgotten how to gesture with my hands so that someone could understand what I meant.   (Luria 1975, p. 49)

> When I was finally sent home and saw my family, I immediately recognised
> my mother and sisters. They were overjoyed that I was home, threw their
> arms around me, and kissed me. But I wasn't able to kiss them—I had
> forgotten how.   (Luria 1975, p. 87)

These brief fragments of Zasetsky's story introduce some of the themes that
I seek to pursue in the rest of the chapter:

(1) how completely our brains influence our communication, not only with
   others but with ourselves;

(2) the question that all carers of a person in the end stages of dementia ask
   themselves, 'are they still there, inside that altered brain and body?';

(3) are the 'person in the past' and the 'person now' one and the same?

But there is (at least) one crucial difference between Zasetsky and the people
who suffer from dementia. He lost everything in one traumatic moment, then
spent years painstakingly recovering fragments of his old abilities and learning
new ones. The person with dementia contends with an experience that Zasetsky
never faced: the early recognition that something intangible is going fearfully
wrong and the struggle afterwards to hold on to some portion of normality.

The relationship with one's self

What do we know about the experience of dementia through introspection and the
dialogue with oneself that comes about through trying to record experiences
in written form? One beneficial result of increasing public awareness of
Alzheimer's disease and of professional readiness to share the diagnosis
of dementia with the sufferer is the appearance in print of first-hand accounts
of the illness. The account that I shall often refer to here is that of Robert
Davis, a Presbyterian minister in Miami, in his book *My Journey into
Alzheimer's Disease: Helpful Insights For Family and Friends* (Davis 1989).

Everyday clinical practice in old-age psychiatry brings us into contact with
a range of individual responses to the hard fact of having a dementing illness.
Some people appear to be quite unaware of any important alteration
in themselves, though changes are obvious to their closest companions. To
themselves, they feel like the person they always were.

By contrast, other people become sharply and frighteningly aware of a
change, which—at that stage, anyway—neither family nor 'objective tests' are
able to detect. The sensation of being at home in one's head is so much part of
our daily unexamined security and comfort, that when a person reports that they
feel something going wrong with their minds, it has to be taken very seriously.

But, as far as I can tell, this early awareness of something not being right does
not impinge on the person's sense of themselves: typically people will refer to a
'me' that is under threat, rather than a 'me' that has become a different person.

A patient I knew would say: 'What is happening to me? Am I going mad? I don't seem to want to do the things I used to do before'. Objectively, he had lost his usual motivation and engagement with life. His family tried to encourage him to 'get out of the house, you will feel better'; but for him, something vital had disappeared from his experience, which no willed, self-imposed activity could replace.

Many of the early threats to the sense of personhood in dementia come from changes in social role. Among these, the loss of the right to drive a car is perhaps the commonest and sometimes the most severe. There are many reasons for this phenomenon. The act of controlling a car through a rapidly changing and hazardous environment draws on faculties that are compromised in dementia. At the same time, many of the components of driving require no conscious thought, so the person with dementia may feel secure that those abilities are not impaired at all. The rights of others are involved, because errors made by the driver are likely to harm others more than themselves. And, not least, the ability (and entitlement) to drive form a vital part of many people's sense of their place in society.

One of my patients had been the army driver for one of the great commanders of the Eighth Army in North Africa and he had an impeccable driving record in civilian life thereafter. When he was found to have a dementing illness, the advice that he should no longer drive was perceived by him as a contemptuous attack on the worth and achievements of his whole life. The bitterness that this caused made any adjustment to the later losses in his illness much harder for him to bear.

Robert Davis wrote,

> Certainly one of the very real fears felt by anyone with early Alzheimer's disease is the fear of failure. I live with the imminent dread that one mistake in my daily life will mean another freedom will be taken from me . . . The thought that one moment of inattention will change your life forever! . . . In the old days I could easily have a fender-bender in the Miami traffic and it would be no big deal. It happens all the time. Today if I have a fender-bender, in all likelihood it will be the end of my driving career. Mistakes are not easily forgiven or forgotten. They often produce great loss of freedom and sense of person. I find myself becoming much more careful and timid, not from paranoia alone but as a result of these very real fears of failure.   (Davis 1989, pp. 91–2)

For other sufferers from dementia, it is their role as head of the household and controller of finances that forms part of the core of their identity. For others still, it is their professional persona that counts most. Families and friends often do a great deal to preserve even some symbolic remnant of these social roles for the sake of the person they care for.

> A highly productive person has to wonder why he is still alive and what purpose the Lord has in keeping him on this earth. As I struggle with the indignities that accompany daily living, I am losing my sense of humanity

> and self-worth. Blessed is the person who can take the Alzheimer's patient
> back to that happier time when they were worthwhile and allow them to see
> the situation in which they were of some use.   (Davis 1989, p. 103)

We should also consider the body by which the patient lives and ways in which the bodily 'self' changes in dementia. A person's own characteristic and individual habits, addictions, tastes, skills, graces, energies, and rhythms can all be affected. They can be lost, or unexpectedly retained, in different forms of dementia and in different individuals, for reasons that our understanding of brain function is still too crude to supply. One can try some educated guesses. The brain region responsible for the sense of smell is affected early in Alzheimer's disease—was this why one of my patients lost his interest in food to the point where he would only eat fish and chips, lavishly sprinkled with sugar? This may seem a very trivial aspect of 'personhood', but such things contribute to the sense of alienation, of living with a stranger, which many families experience.

Loss of interest in smoking, or in drinking to excess, is not uncommon. It is an ironic comment on our laudable desire to nourish the autonomy of people with dementia that their friends do not usually fight to preserve this addicted aspect of their personhood. Yet it may be part of one's identity. Another of my patients (with a different illness), who had tried to give up smoking, told me she had changed her mind: 'I've decided that it's me, it's one of the things I do' (and indeed there was not much else that she did to fill her day).

One taste that is most strikingly preserved is the appreciation of music; and music also acts as an important medium of communication in people whose dementia seems otherwise to have cut them off entirely. Music therapists cite many examples. Motor skill may be retained in association with music. I remember a patient who had lost all speech but who played carols on the piano for the ward Christmas party year after year and joined enthusiastically in the slow old-fashioned dancing that followed. Luria referred to the enduring 'kinetic melodies' that enabled Zasetsky to recapture the skill of writing automatically—without conscious thought as to how he managed it.

Older people with dementia are often additionally handicapped by the physical infirmities of old age and with advancing dementia comes the loss of control over movement. Many younger sufferers, however, are terrific walkers: walking may be one of the things they are still experts in. A young patient whose admirable physical skills had been part of his profession lost nearly all his abilities when he became ill, but not his desire and his ability to walk—for miles over the roughest country available; and the vigour and determination expressed in this way encapsulated his identity for those who came to know him in his illness.

Robert Davis casts another light on walking.

> Many people have tried to guess why Alzheimer's disease patients are so
> restless and want to walk around at all hours of the day and night. I believe I
> may have a clue. When the darkness and emptiness fill my mind, it is totally

terrifying. I cannot think my way out of it. It stays there, and sometimes images stay stuck in my mind. Thoughts increasingly haunt me. The only way that I can break this cycle is to move. Vigorous exercise to the point of exhaustion gets my mind out of the black hole . . . When I have had a particularly difficult night and awaken foggy and disoriented, I find that a stretch of vigorous activity helps me to clear my head.   (Davis 1989, p. 96)

He also describes vividly the fatigue of dementia, a common symptom, which relatives find hard to understand—or even to forgive, when they attribute it to lack of interest and self-absorption. It would seem, if we accept his description, that they are mistaken.

I do not know the proper medical description for what occurs, but I do know that the ability to function intellectually rises and falls with the amount of time I have been trying to concentrate and the amount of external stimuli to which I have been exposed. If I do not listen to my body and withdraw from the overstimulation, it takes several days for my intellectual abilities to return. This is very frightening, because I can't help wondering each time this happens if I have pushed myself totally over the line of no return . . . If I want to function at the top of my limited capacity, I must establish a routine and keep to it. I must stay away from crowds, blinking lights, too much emotional or mental stimulation, and must not become physically exhausted . . .   (Davis 1989, pp. 8–8)

. . . If I press myself with greatest concentration to try to keep up, I feel as though something short circuits in my brain. At this point I become disoriented, have difficulty with my balance if I am standing, my speech becomes slow, or I cannot find the right words to express myself . . .   (Davis 1989, p. 86)

There are situations which we know we cannot handle. In spite of all the pushing and urging of friends and family who insist that we will have a wonderful time, the patient senses that it will lead to his mental devastation. There are times when the patient needs to be alone.   (Davis 1989, p. 89)

Relationships with family and friends

You are destined to live only with the memory of who he was . . . How can you say goodnight to your sweetheart and wonder, will this be the night from which reason will never again waken? Will morning find that new person in my bed, the man who will not know who I am or why I am in his bed? . . . (Betty Davis, in Davis 1989, p. 140)

Today we are alive, today we know each other and share simple joys, a walk along the canal . . . our memories, many of which I alone hold the key to unlock now.   (Betty Davis, in Davis 1989, p. 140)

So much of personal identity belongs not to self reflection but to the mutual recognition between two people. The better they know each other, the more secure the foundations of their two identities. When dementia brings loss of language, coordination, and memory, as with a fragmented image, the knowledge preserved in the relationship can allow the gaps to be partly filled in. It is part of loving, to know another so well that their turns of phrase, their responses, their humour can be predicted. It is part of the joy of being loved, to be so predicted. So it jars the relationship badly when you find the person you love (perhaps your wife or your mother) acting in an unfamiliar and unpredictable way and when for their part they see in your response the sudden revelation that you no longer understand them.

The poignancy of such moments is all the greater precisely because it is the families and friends of people with dementia who are the most important safekeepers of their identities, insofar as they hold their histories, understand what was important to them in their former lives, and remember their preferences and habits of thought. And, as the quotation from Robert Davis's wife reminds us, it is relationships between bodies as well as between minds that we are considering. When people continue to look, feel, and smell the same as they used to, some part at least of their personhood is sustained.

I myself remember from childhood the scent of deep red roses that graced a dear relative of mine and from later years I remember my gratitude that the same beautiful smell was with her as she became helplessly dependent on the care of her family. By sad contrast, I remember the shock caused to the wife of a patient when a well-meaning nurse shaved off his beard as he lay unconscious in hospital. His wife had never in her life seen him clean shaven.

When the daughters of a patient living in a nursing home insisted that she should continue to have a weekly hairdo and manicure, because they knew how much their mother used to care about her appearance and enjoy the feeling of being pampered, who is to say whether they were insisting on preserving this aspect of her personhood for their own comfort, or for hers? What did it matter, so long as the happiness of preserving it entered into the relationship between them?

When the effects of the illness make sophisticated communication impossible, bodily communication can still make the link between individuals, though the carer at the time may have no way of knowing this for sure. Robert Davis, by virtue of his lucid times and his persistent efforts (very similar to Zasetsky's, but with a computer to help him) to make a written record of his experience, is able to assure us of the meaningfulness of that bodily link:

> Sometimes these fears come even in daylight as I am gripped in a trancelike state. In such a condition, people can even talk to me and I can grunt a response while those speaking to me have no idea what is happening inside me. (Davis 1989, p. 108)

> . . . There is a way to help in these terror-filled times, but it is definitely not by reasoning with the patient. This is the time for comfort, reassurance, a soft touch, and a gentle voice with soothing words or even songs if you are so gifted. Whatever body language speaks peace in your family can be put to good use in this situation. As soon as my wife is aware that I am in one of these states, she embraces me and strokes me. She asks me to tell her about

what was bothering me. As I talk about it, the panic subsides and I am made aware that I am in touch with reality again and that I am once more saved from the black hole.   (Davis 1989, p. 109)

At the end stages of the illness, when the person is barely able to communicate anything of their inner experience, when there are no clues to go on and one can only guess, families guess very differently.

I think of the husbands of two patients with dementia, whom I knew from their first contact with our service. As far as any outsider could tell, these marriages were alike in the respect, devotion, love, and care that were expressed between the partners when they were still equals and that were shown by the husbands to their wives as the dementia took hold. Both wives came into nursing homes at the end of their lives. One husband continued to cherish the person that his wife had been, acting towards her as though she was still 'there', hidden inside her unresponsive body and brain—as though she might still be reached by his attention, though he could not know it. The other husband had a clear sense that his wife had gone and that her body was empty. Yet his need to grieve then for her passing seemed denied to him and he was angry that the futile nursing care of her body had to continue. We were giving her no treatment, only basic care, but she lived on.

As I understood it, both husbands longed for the death of their wives: one to release her from the imprisonment, the other to end the charade of caring for a person who was no longer there. Can one presume to judge how they 'should' have responded? It would not be true to say that one was caring and the other indifferent; nor that the former was merely sentimental and the other realistic. What can be said is this: I do not believe that either of them ever thought of their wives, even at these last stages, as non-persons.

Relationships between the person with dementia and professional carers

In general, professional carers (whether the staff of nursing homes or home carers visiting intermittently) will take a person entering their care 'as they are': the relationship between them is built mainly on the present behaviour, communication, and emotional responses, with little regard to their past identities. Over time, relatives who hold the history of the patient may try to educate the carers about them. They will interpret current behaviour by reference to the past ('he was a postman, so he was used to getting up early all his life'). Sometimes this process of education is a painful one for relatives, when they feel that the staff are not paying attention to the real identity of the person. Sometimes there is an unspoken rivalry over 'who knows the person best' and whose interpretation of their current behaviour, their personhood at the present time, is to prevail.

Sometimes there are advantages in this difference in perspective. The person entering the nursing home can leave their dysfunctional relationships behind, can lose the unpleasant identity they carried, and can make a fresh start with people who have no presuppositions about their character or moral qualities, but will relate to them simply as a person needing care.

Respecting the previous social role of the person is conceptually easier. Good care homes make sure that relatives write down the life story of a new resident, or create a scrap book, or search out belongings relating to their previous lives, in order to bring the past identity of the person into their new relationships.

What else forms the basis for the relationship between the resident of a nursing home and the paid carers who attend to their needs? What takes place in that relationship that can define and sustain the resident's individuality? Affection or hostility, appreciation of care or resistance to being cared for, humour, patience, enjoyment of life, cantankerousness, inconsolable distress, or inaccessibility—they all influence the quality of the interaction with the carers. Staff experienced in dementia care will generally try to understand any troublesome responses in terms of illness, rather than as a reflection of the resident's personality. They will generally start from the assumption that 'we are there to meet their needs'. The more uncomplicated the needs are to identify and to meet, the easier it is to make the relationship and to accept the resident as a likeable person who requires a lot of care, rather than as a troublesome and unappealing person.

But it is not uncommon for a person with dementia who is entering a specialist nursing home to be very unwilling to accept any care because they do not perceive themselves as a person needing help. Experienced staff are able to construe this rejection of care as a need in itself; in doing so, they are saying something quite complicated about that person. To respect them as their patient means honouring their sense of their own autonomous personhood, while also respecting the needs of their body, which they themselves ignore.

Relationship with inanimate things

For some people, their home performs the same purpose as the family's life history or scrapbook. One of the reasons why psychogeriatric assessments are carried out in patients' homes is because homes communicate so much information. When the person can no longer describe to the visiting psychiatrist who they are or have been, their home—its atmosphere and the objects in it—can help to do so.

Moreover, the home can play a similar communicative role in a person's relationship with themselves. A patient of mine with dementia, who had lost her husband 2 years earlier, was so lonely and frightened that she called the emergency services a dozen times a day. Nevertheless she would not contemplate leaving her home, because she and her husband had struggled and saved for years to buy it (and all the objects in it) and to defend it against encroaching neighbours. To leave her home would have meant finally losing her husband and herself. This was her way of fighting the battle to retain her identity.

The accompanying stubbornness and the deafness to argument were lifetime characteristics, according to her estranged children. Ironically (but mercifully) when she went to a nursing home for convalescence after an emergency admission to hospital, she rediscovered herself, thanks to the new relationships that the head of the home and the staff created for her.

Conclusions

If I were to offer any generalized conclusions of even a semi-philosophical nature from the vantage point of old-age psychiatry, they would be these.

First, we cannot draw a clear boundary between a personality and the interaction of that personality with its surroundings (with people and things). There is a sense in which some parts of the personality *are* this interaction. At the same time, what Zasetsky and Davis both show is that interaction of a superficial kind may cause others to underestimate grossly the complexity of the inner mental life of the patient with dementia.

Nor, second, can we clearly mark a point—short of terminal coma or death—when we can say that the person whom we knew before their dementia has finally ceased to exist.

As a last illustration of the remarkable resilience of 'personhood' and its expression even through a damaged brain, let me quote again from Davis and Zasetsky:

> Not being able to handle the ministerial role did not mean that I immediately became a blithering idiot. Rather, it meant that I am now limited in my activities . . . I am still human. I laugh at the ridiculous disease that steals the most obvious things from my thoughts and leaves me spouting some of the most obscure, irrelevant information when the right button is pushed. I want to participate in life to my utmost limit.   (Davis 1989, p.100)

> The title I decided on for my writing was 'I'll Fight On!' I wanted to describe how this disaster came about, and how it has continued to plague me ever since I was wounded. I haven't given up hope. I'm trying to improve my situation by developing my ability to remember and speak, to think and understand. I'm fighting to recover a life I lost when I was wounded and became ill.   (Luria 1975, p.18)

References

Davis, R. (1989). *My Journey into Alzheimer's Disease: Helpful Insights For Family and Friends*. Wheaton, Illinois: Tyndale House.

Luria, A. R. (1975). *The Man with a Shattered World*. Harmondsworth, Middlesex: Penguin Education. (First published 1972, New York, USA: Basic Books.)

13 Spiritual perspectives on the person with dementia: identity and personhood

F. Brian Allen and Peter G. Coleman

Spirituality and religious faith

In this chapter we consider contributions from spiritual and theological perspectives to the meaning of personal identity in the face of dementia. In contemporary health and social care literature there has been a growing interest in spirituality and stress has been laid on identifying and meeting the spiritual needs of people, particularly those with mental health problems, learning disabilities, and ill health in later life. Definitions of spirituality are elusive as are concepts of mind, meaning, and personhood—not least in the case of people with dementia.

Spirituality is often described both as being about the intangible and immaterial aspects of life as well as being closely associated with a sense of meaning and purpose. It is particular to each person and yet, by virtue of its essential nature to all human beings, is shared with others. Some would say that spirituality is intuitive or even innate and, therefore, not easily susceptible to rational explication. Whilst it is sometimes described as being distinct from religion, arguably spirituality is essential to religion. One definition claims,

> people of all ages share basic human needs that include love (the giving and receiving of affection), faith (someone or something to believe in), hope (something to look forward to), peace (finding a measure of stability and tranquillity) and worship (a sense of awe and the attribution of value or 'worth' to whomever or whatever is deemed to merit it).   (Jewell 1999, p. 10)

Some of the circumstances of older age give a particular focus to these needs and values. Other definitions emphasize connectivity.

> Spirituality is an intra, inter and transpersonal experience that is shaped and directed by the experiences of individuals and the communities within which they live out their lives.   (Swinton 2001, p. 20)

Spirituality could be described as that which is essential to our humanity, embraces the desire for meaning and purpose, and has personal, social, and transcendent dimensions. The word 'spirit' comes from the Latin for breath and its equivalent in Hebrew and Greek, amongst other languages, similarly denotes that which is fundamental to life. To talk of spirituality, then, is to attempt to put into words things intimate and immanent as well as things other and transcendent.

Spending time with people with dementia and their carers inevitably poses some basic questions about ourselves. Who am I and what is to become of me? What is the meaning and purpose of our lives? Such are the existential questions and dilemmas with which we are faced and which are often seen as fundamental to recent spiritual discourse. Historically, this discourse has taken place within the frameworks of faith traditions, where faith is both the means and the end of the spiritual quest. Clearly history bears witness to how religious faith, as the politics of spirituality, has not lived up to the ideals it has promulgated; fundamental concepts have been lost or diluted in practice. In a secular and post-modern environment, such history is often used as reason to cease taking underlying concepts seriously. Furthermore, post-Enlightenment philosophies have often rejected the premises of religious thought. That beliefs about who we are and what is to become of us can no longer be responded to in religious terms with any reasonable legitimacy or integrity is a notion we wish to challenge.

The apparent renewal of interest in spirituality can be seen as indicative of a positive regard for the identity and personhood of people with dementia. We suggest it also reflects a sense of something essential that is missing from current theory and practice, which goes beyond specific considerations about people with dementia. Without understating the effects of dementia on either those diagnosed or their carers, it appears that people with dementia are showing us something of ultimate concern about the nature of personhood and creation. This is, perhaps, reflected in part by the recent focus on the personhood of people with dementia (Kitwood 1997).

The way in which terms such as 'individual' and 'person' have been employed in both philosophical and religious thought over the centuries is being explored today, perhaps not so much to discover what has hitherto remained mysterious or unknown, but more in an attempt to recover that which has been lost in modern and post-modern thought, or indeed not developed adequately to sustain its case in the contemporary world of ideas.

Individuals and persons

So how far can it be said that what might appear to be the disintegrating self is identifiable as a person? We would argue that it is helpful to think of the seemingly unbecoming self as still being the self despite behaviour and com-munication having changed. In his examination of the philosophy of both Locke and Hume in this regard, Brennan concludes that his own inclination is '. . . to note the more modest possibility that personhood itself may be a matter of degree . . .' (Brennan 1990). He argues that Locke's definition of a person places an unsuitably high standard on what it is to be a unitary person. Neo-Lockean theories also impose implausibly high standards, Brennan argues, on personal identity. We would add that Hume's view that a person is no more than the sum of their experiences reduces the notion of personhood to the point beyond which it is irreducible. We seek to show in this chapter the significance of differentiating between 'individual' and 'person' as well as the essentially relational nature of being human.

Consider the extreme example of Peter Singer (Singer 1994) who, with approval, quotes Locke as defining a person as a being with reason and reflection that can 'consider itself, the same thinking thing, in different times and places' (Locke 1690, p. 211). Accordingly a fully functioning chimpanzee has more moral rights, Singer argues, than a cognitively impaired human being. However, elsewhere he admits that his mother is in the advanced stages of Alzheimer's disease (Toolis 1999) and that he pays for her care.

> What am I doing that I should be doing differently in accordance with my philosophy? Am I supposed to be killing her? For one thing, I would end up in jail. She gets some pleasures from life, the pleasure of eating—rather simple pleasures. Why should she not continue to have those? Because it costs money to look after her! Yes, but there are other things. I am not in dire poverty . . . In an ideal world . . . if there was a way, without punishment . . . of painlessly ending my mother's life and then transferring the resources to look after her to people who would otherwise die of malnutrition, of which there are many, I would say, yes, that would be a better thing to do. But that is not the situation either I or my mother are in. (Toolis 1999)

This demonstrates the brittle nature of neo-Lockean philosophy. As Bernard Williams says in the same article (Toolis 1999), 'Most human beings recognise that . . . personal relationships are a dimension of personal morality'. This points to the impossibility of talking about our selves without reference to others. This was familiarly and succinctly summarized by John Donne almost four centuries ago:

> No man is an Iland, intire of it selfe; everyman is a peece of the Continent, a part of the maine; if a clod bee washed away by the Sea, Europe is the lesse, as well as if a Promontorie were, as well as if a Mannor of thy friends, or of thine own were; Any mans death diminishes me, because I am involved in Mankinde; And therefore never send to know for whom the bell tolls; It tolls for thee. (Donne 1987)

So there are dangers inherent in ignoring the moral implications of discussing persons and personhood. Indeed people with disabilities in North America have campaigned using the slogan, 'No one should have to prove their personhood' and have sought to recognize the frailty of human embodiment by suggesting that the so-called able-bodied (and by implication 'able-minded') majority should regard themselves as being 'temporarily able bodied'. Such comments indicate a view that being human is a process involving both becoming and unbecoming, thus emphasizing our interdependence.

What, then, makes us human? Language becomes problematic when it is regarded as the defining human characteristic. In the case of dementia we can find ourselves literally in a situation beyond words. This can arise when either the person with dementia is not able to communicate verbally or the carer finds it impossible to express their understanding of what is happening to the person. What are we to say when we find ourselves here? Wittgenstein would possibly have us remain silent but other traditions would remind us that words are not the only form of communication.[1] We may have experiences that we cannot describe or attribute accurately, but which we nonetheless experience. We may have experiences that evoke emotions, some of which we may not understand, but which affect the way in which we feel and behave. We may well communicate the effect of these experiences non-verbally, or indeed our words, if we utter them, may not communicate our meaning as clearly as might other means of communication.

In Christian theology the *via negativa* is a reminder that language deals with human relationships but does not in itself deal adequately with the divine–human relationship. In the Western tradition it is seen by St Thomas Aquinas as a necessary precursor to the *via positiva*; in the Eastern Orthodox Church the *via negativa* is stressed and known as the apophatic way. Apophatic spirituality can be seen as a mystical meeting point of different faith traditions, which is beyond words. Furthermore the Judaeo-Christian tradition bears witness to the apparent paradox of inanimate creation praising God in the canticle known as the Benedicite (the Prayer of Azariah and the Song of the Three Young Men (*Daniel*, sections inserted between 3:23 and 3:24))[2], as well as the human counterpart whereby 'the Spirit himself intercedes for us with sighs too deep for words' (*Romans* 8:26). So both the limits of language and the possibility of meaning in non-verbal communication are recognized as contributing to our understanding of what it is to be human.

Major changes in personality and behaviour often involve considerable distress, not least at the losses incurred both by persons with dementia and their carers. There are also, of course, difficult questions posed about the continuity of personality and thus aspects of personal identity, the consequences of which can take us to strange places. Consider Beethoven's *Pastoral Symphony*: to what extent could it be said that it exists only when it is being performed or played on a recording? To what extent could it be said to have existed in the mind of the composer or on the first occasion of its performance, let alone on the many occasions on which it has since been performed and the many different interpretations it has been given? What are we to say about its existence between performances? Or consider a riverbed in a country given to dry and rainy seasons. Is it no longer a riverbed at different times of the year? By analogy we can conceive of personhood as a matter of degree or, perhaps, variation; that is, we become persons and things happen to us that may well be unbecoming but at all times we are persons.

Ray Anderson (Anderson 2003) argues vigorously that practical theology has a particular end in view and therefore differs from empirical (social) science; as such, it is pre-theoretical. Similarly we would argue that in a so-called post-modern world some fixed point needs to be established in order to construct an approach. Our fixed point is the assertion that personhood is relational. This is both the means and the end. We are who we are because of others—the Other. There is, of course, nothing new in this assertion. However, the assertion is particularly poignant in the case of people with dementia, who otherwise can all too easily be relegated to a category of being non-persons.

Much of the Western (Christian) tradition shares a view of 'persons' defined by function and rationality and, thus, dysfunction and irrationality are indicators of non- or sub-persons. This appears as a comment on society, which is itself unable to cope with apparent weakness and dependence, seeing it as meaninglessness and failure. Such attitudes, often born out of fear, can achieve moral and political acceptability; hence, it becomes possible to dispose of those whose brains do not function well. An extreme example of the consequences of this way of regarding persons is the murder of thousands of people in mental hospitals carried out in Nazi Germany by doctors. The Nazis invented a term to apply to such people—*Ballast-Existenzen*—people you could dispose of without losing anything essential. People of many faiths regard this as blasphemy against the Creator. For all people are inseparably connected to others through that creation that gives those others well-functioning brains. A Christian theology of creation embraces the concept of purposeful creativity, lovingly wrought, which includes deviation as a natural part of the process. Here the Creator is involved within creation and shares risk and self-exposure to ambiguities and 'failures'.

Person-centred care

The theory underpinning the new culture of dementia care as expounded by the late Tom Kitwood (Kitwood 1997) owes much to the Jewish writer Martin Buber (Buber 1958) and the way in which dialogical personalism has been interpreted in practice. This requires much of the carer, who must maintain a positive regard for the person with dementia *as a person*. Both are themselves in relation to the other. Recently Faith Gibson has questioned the demands made upon carers by the high standards set by Buber's concept of 'dialogical living' (Gibson 1999) as interpreted and applied by Kitwood and others. Her conclusion is, however, that we can do nothing less; for to ignore one person's diminishment would be to diminish us all. We would add that people with dementia demand much of others but also show others much about the range of human communication and, therefore, much about what it is to be human. And Buber himself claims, 'The primary word I-Thou can only be spoken with the whole being' (Buber 1958, p. 11). Thus if we are to understand the human experience of dementia it is essential to see personhood in relational terms.

Tom Kitwood's work focused on confronting what he termed the 'malignant social psychology', which operates to the detriment of people with dementia—so much so that they are regarded as less than persons. Martin Buber's classic *I and Thou* influences much of Kitwood's promotion of the new culture of dementia care, which sees people with dementia as primarily persons and persons in relationship. Characteristically Hebraic, and part of the Judaeo-Christian tradition, Buber—in a similar way to another Jewish thinker, Levinas (1998)—describes life as dialogue: in the beginning is relationship. Buber points to the irreducibility of the personal and of the communion between persons, suggesting that the locus of meaning is in the encounter, the communication of the one with the other/Other.

> In the beginning and in the end is relationship, which can never be tran-scended or absorbed—even in God. There is the closest possible mystical unity between I and Thou, but always it is a mysticism of love, which insists upon and respects the non-identity of the other.   (Robinson 1979, p. 9)

With Buber very much as his starting point John Robinson, in this discus-sion about the significance of dialogue, seeks to show how the apparent opposites contained within Christian and Hindu belief systems belong together (almost as if they are on a Möbius strip, that is, where a single-sided surface is formed by joining a long rectangle after twisting one end through 180°). Robinson makes the point that this argument could be pursued by an examina-tion of other religious traditions and their relationship one with another, not so much to demonstrate that this is the case, but rather to show the centrality of dialogue and therefore relationship to life, including perspectives afforded by the study of religions. We seek to exemplify this later with reference to one particular tradition within Christianity.

The I–Thou relationship is the one of subject to subject, of self-disclosure and intimacy; but this can fall away into subject–object, I–It, that is, coolness and detachment. So Kitwood says, realistically, 'daring to relate to the other as Thou may involve anxiety and suffering but Buber sees it as the path to fulfil-ment and joy' (Kitwood 1997, p.10). Stephen Post explores this theme further in his discussion about solicitude or care:

> As Soble (1990) puts it, this view of care, which is consistent with the Jewish *chesed* and the Christian *agape*, denies the need to be grounded 'in Y's attractive properties S or in X's belief or perception that Y has S' [Soble op. cit., p. 5]. Such solicitude is not based on property or capacity, nor is it explic-able or easily comprehensible. Such solicitude is a matter of bestowal rather than appraisal, it is unconditional rather than based on certain properties in its object, and it is therefore never extinguished. This solicitude 'is its own reason and love is taken as a metaphysical primitive. Such is the structure of agapic personal love' [Soble op. cit., p. 6].   (Post 2000, p. 25)

If personhood is essentially relational then becoming a person is at once both simple and immensely complex. We become a person by being born of human parents and by the many layers of internal and external influences we experience (Habgood 1998). And so we may also experience a stripping away of these layers in unbecoming circumstances, such as dementia. Diminishment and passivity are regarded negatively in the world of activity or agency and the age of information or cognition. At times, however, it is more possible to be known than to know and to have one's desires interpreted by another when one can be said no longer to know them oneself. Finding meaning not only in the activities of life but also in the passivities is something Teilhard de Chardin addresses in his devotional classic *Le Milieu Divin* (de Chardin 1960), with its world view that makes room for the 'divinisation of our passivities' and the negativities of life, including death. 'Death is the sum and consummation of all our diminishments' (de Chardin 1960, p. 61). Thus he describes the ultimate encounter with the Other, the ultimate Thou.

Meaning in pastoral encounters

Consider the encounter between a chaplain and the husband of a resident in a nursing home whilst he helps his wife with her lunch. The husband says he is there because he loves his wife and, having coped with her dementia for too many years on his own, wants to be with her in the extreme stages of her illness whilst she is cared for by others. The relatives of another resident who has died recently join them briefly and express the hope that his wife will soon be better. The husband replies that this is not possible. The chaplain, recognizing that as both a false hope to the husband but a necessary hope for the visitors, offers no comment at the time. Later the bereaved relatives and chaplain talk about how death can bring necessary healing both to those who have died as well as to the bereaved (Allen 2004).

Consider also the case of a woman at the threshold of the severe stages of dementia, a lifelong practising Roman Catholic, with a past and future, but where meaning is found in the encounter in the present moment. While she could still express herself verbally but was no longer able to receive the sacrament of Holy Communion as had been her custom, she offered a prayer of her own. Her words are recorded:

> Dear God
> You are all that matters
> Help us to be happy
> Helps us to be welcoming
> We need each other.[3]

How are we to interpret this? There is indeed much to understand about the 'ecology of the mind' (Brennan 1990) and the limits to philosophy and psychology's potential to recover the concept of the person. However, the hermeneutic perspective to which Widdershoven and Berghmans refer (see Chapter 11) is helpful here. It provides a philosophical reinforcement to some of the more recent psychological approaches to dementia care. Cheston and Bender (1999), for instance, employ the analogy of attempting to focus a camera to describe the psychological strategies people with dementia might use to understand (and therefore give meaning to) what is happening to them. Words show something beyond themselves; we need to reflect on more than just the text to understand what is being said, in a way similar to Anton Boisen's concept of 'living human documents' (Foskett 1996, p. 58). Perhaps if we regard persons as living documents we need to read between the lines to reach the meaning and thereby develop (what we might call) an interlinear interpretation of, or approach to, understanding personhood. We recall that Heidegger's theological training concerned ancient texts, out of which grew his interest in the interpretation of the being or the person who interprets the texts.

So we could offer an interpretation of the prayer offered by the woman in the midst of her experience of dementia. We could say that she addresses the Other, the ground of our Being, the 'I am that I am' about the importance of our shared moods and feelings as well as recognizing our essential interdependence. Such an insight comes out of the furnace of her experience of increasing diminishment and articulates the divinization of her passivities (de Chardin 1960).

Members of Christian churches share responsibility for the churches' mission to sustain people with mental as well as physical infirmities and those caring for them. The last decade or so has seen several pieces of work in the UK dedicated to responding to these needs, by groups such as the Christian Council on Ageing's Dementia Group, the Leveson Centre for the Study of Ageing, Spirituality and Social Policy, and the MHA Care Group.[4] Although the major tasks involved are person centred and practical, it is important to cultivate and promote a theology of dementia that can underpin pastoral work. Otherwise the thinking of even the best intentioned caregiver is liable to be affected by the negative, perhaps soul-destroying, perspectives on dementia current in modern society.

There is undoubtedly much to be learned from what various religious and spiritual traditions have to say about dementia. As a result of immigration and the greater intermingling of religions within their major cities, British and other Western societies now have a multi-faith character. This provides a valuable opportunity to listen to what these diverse traditions have to say about caring for disabled people, including those with dementia. The Eastern Orthodox Christian tradition is one with which we have become acquainted as a result of the diaspora of Eastern Christians, especially from Greek and Russian cultures, in the course of the twentieth century. Before that, Eastern Christianity was largely hidden by the great schism that separated the Western and Eastern churches already in the eleventh century. We realize that this is only one possible view on the person with dementia, even among Christian perspectives, let alone other world faiths. But we consider it more useful, for appreciating theology's potential contribution to understanding dementia, to concentrate on one tradition rather than trying to amalgamate different religious perspectives in a short space, which might be blander.

The Eastern Orthodox perspective on the person and the person with dementia

As other contributors to this collection have made clear, we operate with different concepts of identity and the self. In Britain we have been particularly influenced by the debate on the nature of personal identity begun by Locke and Hume. But the concept of the person has a much longer and even more complex history. In Western culture it began with the ancient Greek concept of 'persona', meaning 'mask'. This term was given quite a different usage by the early fathers of the Christian church as they reflected on the centrality for their faith of the person of Christ. Whereas the classical world did not have a concept of 'person' as distinct from an 'individual', early Christianity used the term person to refer to the individual in relationship. It is interesting that this sense of personhood is largely lost today, with the result that the words 'person' and 'individual' have become interchangeable in most contexts of use. Post-modern thought has in turn recovered the notion of 'mask' in the image(s) of the self that we present to the world around us.

The loss of the concept of the person in relationship and the increased importance given to the individual in isolation coincides with the growing emphasis on reason and reflection as a mark of moral status in discussions of human value and rights. The views of Peter Singer (Singer 1994) and others in this regard can be interpreted as following in the line of the Western philosophical tradition. However, we need to acknowledge that we no longer live in a culture with homogeneous values and that the minimum requirement on all of us is to understand the basis of our differing views. The Judaeo-Christian concept of the person, although a basic root of Western culture, has been neglected and requires restatement.

Central to Christianity is the concept of the Trinity of God—Father, Son, and Holy Spirit—and its reflection in the human person. The Trinity is a doctrine about the identity of God, but by implication it is also about the identity of the human person. Because the aim of human life in Christian understanding is to share in God's life, this means sharing in the life of the Trinity. Just as God is not an isolated person but is considered always in relationship, Father to Son to Spirit, so a human person is never to be considered in isolation from the rest of humanity.

The doctrine of the Trinity grew out of the early Christians' reflection on the Christian message. It was not an easy doctrine to formulate and, for a people with strongly monotheistic roots in Judaism who wanted to remain monotheistic, it involved much intellectual and moral struggle. Considering the effort that went into its formulation, it is surprising that the Trinity is now taken so much for granted that its important implications are poorly realized. The failure to have communicated its message adequately lies at the basis of the claim (often made) that Christianity has hardly begun to influence human society (Roberts and Shukman 1996).

Christianity has constantly struggled to realize its original vision. The difficulties of communicating a religion of love and interrelationship were compounded by the growing splits within Christianity, which began in its early history and have continued to the present day. Of these, the most significant is the split generally known as the Great Schism, which separated Western from Eastern Christianity. Although the split is dated to the mutual ex-communications delivered between Rome and Constantinople in 1054, marked divergences of attitude had been present for a long time. The events of the Crusades formalized a state of hostility, which has only recently been constructively addressed.

One of the most considerable intellectual contributions of Western Christianity to modern culture, but also at the same time one of its limiting features, is its considerable emphasis on rationality: man's power of reason as the distinguishing mark of humanity. This line of thought was developed strongly in the scholastic tradition of which Aquinas was the prime exemplifier. Most of the attitudes adopted by Western Christianity are shaped by considerations of man defined in the terms of rational faculty. Eastern Christianity, despite its many faults, does not have this inheritance and has remained truer to the original, more social understanding of human nature created in the image of the Trinity. Traces of this thinking can also be found in the West too. For example, Richard of St Victor (died 1173), a native of Scotland, wrote an engaging presentation on the inner meaning of the doctrine of the Trinity in his book entitled *De Trinitate*.

The following is taken from Kallistos Ware's account of Richard's teaching (Ware 1986). Richard starts from the central revelation of Jesus Christ that God is love. Because love is the perfection of human nature, the highest reality within our personal experience, it is also the quality within our experience that brings us closest to God. Love expresses, better than anything else that we know, the perfection of the divine nature. But self-love is not true love. Love is a gift and exchange and so, to be present in its fullness, it needs to be mutual. It requires a 'Thou' as well as an 'I' and can truly exist only where there is a plurality of persons: 'The perfection of one person requires fellowship with another' (Ware 1986, p. 9)[5]. This is the case not only with humans but also with God: divine love, as well as human, is characterized by sharing and communion. In God's case, as also that of humans, writes Richard, 'nothing is more glorious . . . than to wish to have nothing that you do not wish to share' (Ware 1986).

He then goes on to argue that the sharing of love cannot exist among any less than three persons. 'Perfect love casts out fear' (*I John* 4:18). Love in its perfection is unselfish, without jealousy, without fear of a rival. Where love is perfect, then, the lover not only loves the beloved as a second self, but also wishes the beloved to have the further joy of loving a third, jointly with the lover, and of being jointly loved by that third. So God is seen by Richard in terms of interpersonal community, although this is, as he recognizes too, no more than an analogy.

Richard was later criticized by Aquinas and others for this analogy and its implications that God needs love, as love must be a striving to gain what one does not yet possess. But it is inconceivable that God should be lacking in anything, so applying the analogy of humans sharing love is not applicable to God.[6] In formulating this argument Aquinas places himself within the tradition of thinking about love as a deficiency. Plato's argument in the *Symposium* that eros is the offspring of poverty is probably the most well-known example (Plato 1961). But it is possible to argue that Richard's dynamic view of God as exchange, giving and taking, is closer to the spirit of the Christian revelation than is the scholastic idea of a self-sufficient God in 'splendid isolation'.

What are the implications for our understanding of dementia? In the Judaeo-Christian-Muslim view of a fallen world we are tormented by evils. Dementia is one of these torments. But perhaps we focus too much on the debilitating effect of brain damage on the mind, rather than on its social consequences. Isolation is one of the greatest evils we know. This takes various forms in our experience of each other—lack of connection, opaqueness, deception, failure of communication. Dementia intensifies many of these socially based problems (Kitwood and Bredin 1992), although it can lighten others as some people appear to lose inhibitions and (re)gain trust as their mental faculties wane.

Christians are presented with the Trinitarian image of God—whose being is perfect relationship—as a model for their lives. The central notion employed by the early patristic writers in referring to this aspect of God is, in Greek, *perichoresis*, usually translated as 'coinherence' or 'mutual indwelling'. But the connotations are broader than this. *Choros* is the word for dance. *Perichoresis*, therefore, is 'round dance'. In the Trinity each person contains the other two and moves within them in an unceasing movement of mutual love. Andrei Rublev's fifteenth-century icon (in the Tretyakov Gallery, Moscow) of the three angels who visited Abraham and Sarah in the Old Testament passage is often taken to be the closest and most beautiful representation of this sense of the Trinity as timeless intercommunion, of prayer in community, not only of persons praying but being prayed in.

This image can be employed by those seeking a Christian perspective on understanding our life with people suffering from dementia. We need to soften the Western mind's concern with the isolated reasoning individual. For example, much Christian writing on suffering emphasizes intellectual awareness as being integral to man's dignity. As a consequence, pastoral writings are often silent on dementia and mental illness. One of the most troubling fears about dementia concerns how a person can retain their identity if they cannot remember who they have been. It has to be admitted that memory is also a very important aspect of the Judaeo-Christian tradition, which is built upon faith in historical events and in particular the recollection of God's saving acts in history. In their central act of worship, the Eucharist, Christians are urged to 'do this in remembrance of me'. Remembering becomes increasingly difficult for people with dementia. But the importance of the Trinitarian concept of the person is that we are not alone. Others can and do remember for us and in the last analysis we are remembered by God, who is not bound by our limitations, however great they become.

We suggest that recovering the distinction between 'individual' and 'person' is very important to future developments in Christian thinking on dementia. 'Individuality' refers to our fragmentation, in that we are separated from one another and broken up within ourselves. This broken aspect is also emphasized in the writings of Kitwood and his colleagues (Kitwood and Bredin 1992). 'Personhood' refers to our deepest essence, which is distinct from that of others, but through which we are called into relationship with man and God. Anthony Bloom notes how St Paul captures in his epistles both notions of relationship and fragmentation in referring to how 'we carry things holy in broken vessels' (Bloom 1997, p. 7). Our brokenness and our need for relationship go together. The belief that we must have in one another rests in Jewish, Christian, Muslim, and much other religious thought on God's belief in humankind, in each one of us, individually, but most importantly in our relationship with one another and with Him (Coleman and Mills 2001).

Missing dimensions and lost icons

We have argued that personal identity is inextricably bound up with the dialogical nature of being human and that this is no less the case for persons with dementia than anyone else. Furthermore it is possible that the narratives, or texts, of the lives of persons with dementia are indicating to us the significance of the loss of a meta-narrative. According to Philip Sheldrake (Sheldrake 2001), the French philosopher Paul Ricoeur has influenced modern theological thought through his stress on the importance of narrative to human identity and thus for the possibility of reconstructing a viable 'historical consciousness'. As with post-modernist thinking Ricoeur rejects the idea of using history 'to decipher the supreme plot' (Ricoeur 1988, p. 103). However, he 'recognizes that humans cannot live without narratives of meaning' lest we risk undermining 'human solidarity (we bond together by sharing stories)' and risk being 'trapped by the immediacy of the present' (Sheldrake 2001, p. 19). So it is by means of narrative that the particularity of time and place is related to the universal. In the case of people with dementia the moral dilemma often centres on whether their narratives are being told at all.[7]

It was observed more than half a century ago that,

> [We] have lost those cultural formations which once served to provide fundamental values; which once provided life-plans, identities and visions; which once determined a sense of worthwhile duty.   (Eliot 1939, p. 21)

More recently Rowan Williams has reflected on cultural bereavement:

> what is lost is what I want to call the soul . . . not the soul of early modern philosophy, an immaterial individual substance, but something more complex—a whole way of speaking, of presenting and 'uttering' the self, that presupposes *relation* as the ground that gives the self room to exist, a relation developing in time, a relation with an agency which addresses or summons the self, but is in no way part of the system of interacting and negotiating speakers in the world. In religious terms, this agency has been seen as the source of the self's life in such a way as to establish that any self's existence is a simple, unnecessary and gratuitous act on the part of the source. The self *is*, not because of need but because of gift.   (Williams 2000, p. 160)

Where memory is problematic, not least for guaranteeing continuity, being remembered by God (Goldsmith 1999, p. 131) 'in the land of forgetfulness' (*Psalm* 88:12) is a statement not only of faith, but also one which opens up the possibilities for the location of memory. Rather than limited by definition, as a function of the individual, it is seen as that which resides in community, tradition, and place and so is not entirely dependent on any one individual's level of cognitive function. Clearly the practice of communities observing ritual and a special sense of place, or sacred space, as a way of 're-membering' is not the monopoly of any one tradition. Sheldrake's 'fundamental contention is that there can be no sense of place without narrative' because 'the hermeneutic of place progressively reveals new meanings in a kind of conversation between topography, memory and the presence of particular people at any given moment' (Sheldrake 2001, p. 17). Concerning Heidegger's concept of a person as *Dasein*, he says, 'in other words to be a person is literally "to be there", to be in a particular place' (Sheldrake 2001, p. 7). Eileen Shamy, who pioneered a Christian ministry in New Zealand specifically with and for people with dementia and their carers, has commented that to ask of a Maori person what had happened to their memory was to make a category mistake, for their memory was understood to reside in the community and the place and not to be the possession of the individual.[8] Similarly, it is not the case that relatedness as an essential attribute of personhood, or indeed nationhood, is unique to certain religious or cultural traditions, as an examination of the African concept of *Ubuntu* would demonstrate.

The essential nature of human relatedness is seen in Christianity as God given and thus a reflection of the nature of God in humankind. It has been claimed recently (Habgood 1998) that the development of the word 'person' in Christian thinking has not contributed much to our understanding of the nature of human relatedness and the way in which—in the light of some current ethical dilemmas—it is essential to being a person. This warns against making an appeal to the Christian doctrine of the Trinity too quickly as the model for our essential relatedness. On the other hand, a contemporary re-examination of the doctrine of the Trinity can be shown to inform discussions of ethical and political relations: 'It is in dialogue . . . that one can be a person in the true sense and it is therefore persons-in-dialogue who are in the image of God' (McFadyen 1990, p. 44).

The divine economy of the Holy Trinity, which is the perfect relationship exisiting between God as Father, Son, and Holy Spirit, is the icon of perfect loving and community. It was this understanding that inspired Basil the Great in the fourth century to found one of the first hospitals in Caeserea where he was bishop. It grew in significance so much that a new town grew up with it at the centre. As well as founding the Eastern Monastic tradition, he was one of the great teachers in early Christendom. The Cappadocian Fathers were used to both political and theological dispute as, amongst other topics, the early church sought to understand and explain the person of Christ in relation to the Godhead. Some of his most important teaching was on the distinction between *ousia* and *hypostasis*, intricate and complex terms with various philosophical and metaphysical meanings in different contexts. Broadly speaking they are used by Basil to

> explain how one substance can be simultaneously present in three persons . . . [by appealing] . . . to the analogy of a universal and its particulars . . . [thus] the universal . . . essence and the particularizing characteristic or identifying peculiarity . . . are differentiated.   (Kelly 1968, p. 265)

However, it is important to note that this was not an abstract theoretical notion (in the pejorative sense that the term 'theology' is often used today in political debate). This is, rather, an example of practical theology founded upon the ethic of relatedness as both God given and personally fulfilling. In his research on ageing in the early Christian church, Rob Merchant has drawn attention to the considerable emphasis on social welfare reflected in the sermons, writings, and actions of church leaders such as Basil and John Chrysostom. Their commitment to vulnerable older people was evident in the design of homes for the aged whose direction was a major responsibility of the local bishop (Merchant 2003).

We have attempted to show the centrality of relationship to spiritual perspectives on the person with dementia. This calls for a re-examination of the contribution of some aspects of Christian teaching, as in the example we have given from the Eastern tradition, along with continuing careful listening to the voices and stories of people with dementia and their carers. The ethical implications of such spiritual dimensions are demonstrable and transcend rationalist arguments, represented by Singer (1994). The elusive nature of definitions of spirituality, personhood, and identity is by no means particular to the case of people with dementia. However, what we do discover by examining their situation and experience is that they contribute much to the exploration of what it is be fully human.

Endnotes

1 This sentence refers, of course, to the famous last sentence of Wittgenstein's *Tractatus Logico-Philosophicus*: 'Whereof one cannot speak, thereof one must be silent' (Wittgenstein 1922, Section 7). Of course, the use of Wittgenstein in this way is ironic. There is nothing to suggest in his writings that he was unaware of the possibility of non-verbal communication! Indeed, one interpretation of the *Tractatus* is to say that he wished to demonstrate what had to be shown rather than said.

2 References to the Bible in this chapter are to the Revised Standard Version (1965)—details in bibliography (*The Holy Bible* 1965). References are cited thus: *Book* Chapter:verse(s).

3 See Christian Council on Ageing (1997). The story of 'Ellen's Prayer' is also told by Audrey Ball, in Dinning (2005) and reproduced in Hughes (2005).

4 The Leveson Centre for the Study of Ageing, Spirituality and Social Policy (Temple Balsall, Knowle, Solihull, West Midlands B93 0AN) has published, with the MHA Care Group (which is made up of the charity Methodist Homes for the Aged and its sister registered housing association), a useful directory and their website includes a link to the Christian Council on Ageing and its Dementia Group: www.levesoncentre.org.uk. The Leveson Centre explores multi-cultural aspects of ageing and welcomes people of all faiths and none.

5 Ware is quoting directly here from Richard of St Victor's *De Trinitate*, III, 6.

6 A fuller account of Aquinas's thought on this matter will be found in Davies (1992), pp. 190–1.

7 The relevance of Ricoeur and the importance of narrative are explored further in Chapter 5 of this book by Radden and Fordyce.

8 See Shamy (2003), but these comments mainly come from an unpublished contribution to a Christian Council on Ageing Conference in York, England, in 1992 at which FBA was present.

References

Allen, F. B. (2004). Review. *Leveson Centre Newsletter*, **11**: 18–19.

Anderson, R. (2003). *Spiritual Caregiving as Secular Sacrament*. London: Jessica Kingsley.

Bloom, A. (1997). The whole human person: body, spirit and soul. In: *To Be What We Are: The Orthodox Understanding of the Person* (ed. B. Osborne), pp. 5–14. London: Russian Orthodox Diocese of Sourozh.

Brennan, A. (1990). Fragmented selves and the problem of ownership. *Proceedings of the Aristotelian Society*, **90**: 143–58.

Buber, M. (1958). *I and Thou*, 3rd edn. Edinburgh: Clark.

Cheston, R., Bender, M. (1999). *Understanding Dementia—The Man with the Worried Eyes*. London: Jessica Kingsley.

Christian Council on Ageing (1997). *Is Anyone There?* Newcastle upon Tyne: Christian Council on Ageing Dementia Project. (Video.)

Coleman, P. G., Mills, M. A. (2001). Philosophical and spiritual perspectives on dementia. In: *A Handbook of Dementia Care* (ed. C. Cantley), pp. 62–76. Buckingham: Open University Press.

Davies, B. (1992). *The Thought of Thomas Aquinas*. Oxford: Clarendon Press.

de Chardin, T. (1960). *Le Milieu Divin*. London: Collins.

Dinning, L (2005). The spiritual care of people with severe dementia. *Nursing and Residential Care*, **7**: 36–9.

Donne, J. (1987). Seventeenth meditation. In: *Devotions upon Emergent Occasions* (ed. A. Raspa), p. 87. New York: Oxford University Press.

Eliot, T. S. (1939). *The Idea of a Christian Society*. London: Faber and Faber.

Foskett, J. (1996). Christianity and psychiatry. In: *Psychiatry and Religion* (ed. D. Bhugra), pp. 52–64. London: Routledge.

Gibson, F. (1999). Can we risk person-centred communication? *Journal of Dementia Care*, **7**: 20–4.

Goldsmith, M. (1999). Dementia. A challenge to Christian theology and pastoral care. In: *Spirituality and Ageing* (ed. A. Jewell), pp. 125–35. London: Jessica Kingsley.

Habgood, J. (1998). *Being a Person*. London: Hodder and Stoughton.

Hughes, J. (ed.) (2005). *Palliative Care in Severe Dementia*. London: Quay Books.

Jewell, A. (ed.) (1999). *Spirituality and Ageing*. London: Jessica Kingsley.

Kelly, J. N. D. (1968). *Early Christian Doctrines*, 4th edn. London: Adam and Charles Black.

Kitwood, T. (1997). *Dementia Reconsidered*. Buckingham: Open University Press.

Kitwood, T., Bredin, K. (1992). Towards a theory of dementia care: personhood and well being. *Ageing and Society*, **12**: 269–87.

Levinas, E. (1998). *On Thinking-of-the-Other: Entre-Nous*. London: Athlone.

Locke, J. (1690). [1964] *An Essay Concerning Human Understanding* (ed. A. D. Woozley). Glasgow: William Collins/Fount.

McFadyen, A. (1990). *The Call to Personhood*. Cambridge: Cambridge University Press.

Merchant, R. (2003). *Pioneering the Third Age. The Church in an Ageing Population*. Carlisle: Paternoster Press.

Plato (1961). *Collected Dialogues* (ed. E. Hamilton and H. H. Cairns). Princeton: Princeton University Press.

Post, S. (2000). *The Moral Challenge of Alzheimer Disease*, 2nd edn. Baltimore and London: Johns Hopkins University Press.

Ricoeur, P. (1988). *Time and Narrative, Volume 3*. Chicago: University of Chicago Press.

Roberts, E., Shukman, A. (ed.) (1996). *Christianity for the Twenty-First Century: The Life and Work of Alexander Men*. London: SCM Press.

Robinson, J. A. T. (1979). *Truth is Two-eyed*. London: SCM Press.

Shamy, E. (2003). *Guide to the Spiritual Dimension of Care for People with Alzheimer's Disease and Related Dementia* (ed. A. Jewell). London: Jessica Kingsley.

Sheldrake, P. (2001). *Spaces for the Sacred Place, Memory and Identity*. London: SCM Press.

Singer, P. (1994). *Rethinking Life and Death*. Oxford: Oxford University Press.

Soble, A. (1990). *The Structure of Love*. New Haven: Yale University Press.

Swinton, J. (2001). *Spirituality and Mental Health Care*. London: Jessica Kingsley.

The Holy Bible (1965). London: Thomas Nelson (Revised Standard Version, Old and New Testaments together with the Apocrypha of the Old Testament.)

Toolis, K. (1999). The most dangerous man in the world. *The Guardian Weekend*, **6th November**: 52–6.

Ware, K. (1986). The human person as an icon of the Trinity. Revised text of a university sermon preached in Great St Mary's Cambridge (13 October 1985). *Sobernost*, **2**: 6–23.

Williams, R. (2000). *Lost Icons*. Edinburgh: T. and T. Clark.

Wittgenstein, L. (1922). *Tractatus Logico-Philosophicus* (trans. C. K. Ogden). London: Routledge and Keegan Paul.

14 *Respectare:* moral respect for the lives of the deeply forgetful

Stephen G. Post

Introduction

'Respect' derives from the Latin word *respectare*, which means 'look' (*spectare*) 'again' (*re*). This chapter sets out the reasons why we should look again and more carefully at the experience of persons with dementia, rather than dismiss them after a first superficial glance. The more we can appreciate the continuities between their experience and our own, the less likely we are to cast aside the deeply forgetful as 'life unworthy of life'—that is, as life unworthy of equal consideration in the forms of respect and care. What I hope to indicate is that while persons with dementia suffer many losses in function and capacity, they do not lose their essential humanity. And it is the sharing of a common humanity that ensures their moral status. Hypercognitive snobbery is moral blindness.

Memory is, of course, a wonderful evolutionary gift and we rightly treasure it. The greatest Western writer on memory was of course St Augustine. In the Tenth Book of his *Confessions*, Augustine wrote these elegant words about the majesty of memory—lines that would echo over the centuries in Western thought:

> All this goes on inside me, in the vast cloisters of my memory. In it are the sky, the earth, and the sea, ready at my summons, together with everything that I have ever perceived in them by my senses, except the things which I have forgotten. In it I meet myself as well. I remember myself and what I have done, when and where I did it, and the state of my mind at the time. In my memory, too, are all the events that I remember, whether they are things that have happened to me or things that I have heard from others . . . (Augustine *Confessions*, x, 8)

Memory, which remains in many ways mysterious, is one of the miracles of neurological evolution and the source of all the connections between past and present experience that allow us to have self-identity and autobiography. Note that for Augustine it is the temporal glue between past and present that allows us to 'meet myself as well'. People with progressive dementia feel the immensity of their decline and if there is any 'kind' point in this progression, it must be when affected individuals forget that they forget, losing insight into this decline.

Inclusion and a common humanity

An adequate ethical theory or moral life requires us to include everyone within the moral domain of care and respect. This universalism pertains to the scope of moral concerns, asserting that all human lives count equally. There is a troubling tendency, however, to exclude certain human beings from moral concern. This occurs most frequently when we differentiate 'them' from 'us', depersonalizing and dehumanizing the other for reasons of race, class, gender, age, sexual orientation, religion, culture, or cognitive abilities including forgetfulness. There is a proneness toward elitisms of various sorts, all of which assert that some people are worthy of our moral concern and some are not, or are much less so. Under such circumstances of exclusion, we easily set aside the principle of the inviolability of the other and we ignore the requirement of meeting their basic human needs. *The core concern of ethics, then, is the deep affirmation of a common humanity and there is no reason to exclude anyone from that affirmation based on the mere fact that they have become more deeply forgetful than the rest of us.* In this sense, the moral quality of a civilization depends in part on how it treats those who struggle with diminished memory and other cognitive capacities.

We sometimes want to exclude the deeply forgetful because we know how important good memory is to our full functioning and power and thus the very last thing we want is to suffer through the diminution of what is a nearly sacred human capacity. Memory is so crucial to our experience and we are all subtly anxious about losing it. We easily demean those whose memory has dissipated by treating them with indifference or even with cruelty. This indifference is seen when we approach a person with dementia and neglect to speak with them directly, or to make eye contact with them, or to call them by their name expecting a response. Whether the waiter in a restaurant or the doctor in the clinic, there is a tendency to speak about or around someone with dementia, rather than with them. Outright cruelty is seen in programmes like T-4, in 1939, when persons with dementia were taken out of German mental asylums and left to freeze in the cold overnight air in the early hypothermia experiments (Muller-Hill 1988). Because memory is a form of power, we can sometimes find in those who have lost such power the opportunity to mock and ignore, sending the message that their very existence rests on a mistake (Post 2000). Power is the ability to punish and we do punish people for being forgetful. How often a spouse will use the memory lapse of a husband or wife as an opportunity to make a humiliating comment. We see this 'power to humiliate' quite vividly in those (hopefully rare) cases of a family caregiver who now finds opportunity to assert a new-found dominance.

It is a morally useful exercise to consider the fact that we are all a little forgetful. We take memory for granted until it begins to wane, as it does, actually, by the fourth decade of life. Most of us eventually become more noticeably forgetful in later years and this normal loss is troubling enough. Yet we are still functional and lucid of mind. As the saying goes, 'It is all right to forget where you parked your car, but not that you have a car that is parked.' With a diagnosis of dementia we enter the domain of the deeply forgetful and slowly but intractably we experience in grief the erosion of the temporal glue. Past, present, and future begin to disconnect. We begin to lose the stories of our lives. Yet the differences between 'them' with dementia, and 'us' without it are a matter of degree more than of kind.

How should we think about the deeply forgetful? What value do they have that requires us to treat them with equal regard? Does deep forgetfulness imply a diminution of the moral obligation to regard well-being highly? What moral status do the deeply forgetful retain? These are the questions to which we will return throughout this chapter.

It is remarkable that despite the advance of dementia, people seem to want to do the best they can for the deeply forgetful. We like to think that the quality of a civilization is measured in part by our compassionate love for those whose minds are in the grip of dementia. The ordinary response in families and in society is not that of the occasional philosopher who asserts on paper that those who have lost temporal glue, who are more or less consigned to the pure present, no longer have moral status and therefore should be painlessly eliminated. Even the eminent preference utilitarian Peter Singer (Singer 1993, p. 97), who has long defended senicide, when confronted with the diagnosis of probable Alzheimer's disease in his mother, became in practice a dutiful, caregiving son. So what is at work when we affirm the continuing moral status of the deeply forgetful? Perhaps a brief case will help clarify the fact that we do consider their ill treatment unacceptable.

Ms H and the arrogance of exclusion

In the summer of 2004 I was asked to provide a court deposition on behalf of the Muslim son of a woman who had been raped in a nursing home. Ms H had been faithfully married for many years before her husband died. Following the dictates of Islam and of her local Imman, Ms H had neither dated nor been sexually intimate for 10 years after her spouse's passing. Then came her diagnosis of probable Alzheimer's disease and her eventual placement in a nursing home. Ms H was a wanderer and one night she ambled down the hall into the bedroom of a somewhat younger resident with mild learning difficulties and a history of sexual aggression. An evening nurse, who made 15-minute checks on Ms H, discovered the two naked and in the bed. Ms H was weeping. Several days later, Ms H was able to mention this incident to her Muslim daughter-in-law, but was fearful of bringing it directly to the attention of her son, who also practised Islam, for there was family dishonour associated with being raped. The son brought a legal suit against the nursing home for negligence and I was asked to give a deposition.

The attorney defending the nursing home argued that in fact, even though Ms H was apparently briefly upset about the violation of her long-established religious values and about this assault itself, she soon forgot about the incident. Therefore, the defence attorney argued, she had not experienced significant 'lasting' harm and thus the case was frivolous—if indeed she did actually express her grief and agitation to her daughter-in-law over having been sexually intimate and if indeed she really could have authentic religious commitments at her stage of dementia.

In a 4-hour long deposition, I argued that significant harm was done. First, Ms H was harmed with respect to remaining self-identity, for she was a deeply committed Muslim throughout her life and still found meaning in her faith as evidenced by occasional moments of prayer and a protective attitude toward sacred objects in her room. While she had lost a significant portion of her memory, there were episodes of insight into her past and her meaning system. Thus, it was wrong to assert that the sporadic nature of her insights made the violation of her self-identity unimportant. Instead of dismissing her past as irrelevant, we should work to create an environment in which her connections with the past are cultivated in order to enhance her sense of security and well-being. Second, Ms H was harmed emotionally, even if she recovered from her agitation quickly, because she could not retain vivid memories of what had occurred after several days had passed. The emotional life of Ms H is an aspect of her experience that should be especially respected as the source of her well-being and quality of life. Yet at every turn, the defending lawyer had his intense counterarguments, most of which amounted to the assertion that someone who is demented cannot experience harm with regard to self-identity or affect, at least not in any significant 'lasting' manner. And in response, I asserted that the cognitive, autobiographical, emotional, relational, and sentient aspects of the deeply forgetful should be respected just as they are in humans whose memories have not faded so deeply. Concern with confidentiality precludes me from writing more. Suffice it to conclude that the reader will find such callousness appalling.

In sharp contrast to the lawyer's attitude regarding the experience of Ms H, the respect for the deeply forgetful that ought to be espoused is evident in the following e-mail written by a daughter soon after her father passed away:

Hello Dear Friends:

As many of you know, my father has been suffering from Alzheimer's disease for the past 4.5 years. It has been a long and often very hard road for him, for my mom, and for me too. However, as of 7 p.m. last night, my father no longer has to struggle with the disease that robbed him of every part of his being, except one. He never once stopped recognizing my mom and never, ever stopped reaching out to her and wanting to give her a kiss. No matter how many parts of his personality were lost, no matter how many hospital visits full of needles and catheters, no matter how many diapers, he always retained his kind, gentle sweetness and his European manners as a gentleman.

> In the end, things went very quickly for him. He simply closed his eyes and closed his mouth, indicating no more food or water.

The man described above was in the advanced and therefore terminal stage of dementia, marked by some combination of the inabilities to communicate by speech, to recognize loved ones, to maintain bowel and/or bladder control, to ambulate without assistance, and to swallow without assistance. Yet throughout he seems to have benefited greatly from the giving and receiving of love, consistent with the relational context found meaningful over the course of his life. There was no assertion of a radical disconnection between the 'then' intact self and the 'now' demented self—rather, the subtle expressions of continuity in subjective experience and lingering self-identity were honoured.

With these contrasting vignettes of exclusion and inclusion as background, I wish to ask what it is in the deeply forgetful that compels us to continue to count them among the morally considerable, rather than as a person who is brain dead or in the persistent vegetative state where all higher brain function has died out?

Respect for residual self-identity: the example of religious commitment

I reject all attempts to pick out one property as the basis for moral consideration, for this monism is inevitably arbitrary and invites exclusion. Some philosophers pick the property of rationality as that one property and they generally define rationality procedurally as an ability to do certain things, such as to act consistently based on clear thinking, to arrive at decisions by deliberation, to envisage a future for oneself, and so forth. But in fact rather few of us go through life with consistent rationality (Zagzebski 2001). We act on emotion, on intuition, on impulse, and the like. We go through periods of considerable irrationality because of variation in mood. Young children have limited reasoning capacities, but we do not devalue them as a result of this. Moreover, what is morally important is not rationality as a decisional capacity, but rather as a source of self-identity—of 'who' we are rather than of 'how' we proceed.

Because it is rarely addressed in the discussion of ethics and dementia care—in contrast to the hospice literature—initial attention regarding self-identity will be directed to religion in the lives of persons with dementia. For example, in the case of Ms H, her self-identity was deeply rooted in her Islamic commitments. Indeed, serving as an expert witness in her case prompted me to consider religious belief and self-identity more than might otherwise have been the case.

Metaphysics aside, the simple uncontroversial point is that people with a diagnosis of dementia and their caregivers have to cope with very difficult circumstances. Their lives are disrupted and they tend to turn toward whatever it is in the universe that they believe can offer solace and meaning. Pastoral care, even for those who are quite demented, is meaningful as a way of manipulating symbols through ritual in order to create a greater sense of security and connectedness despite fragmentation and loss. An interdisciplinary team model of dementia care that includes pastoral care, following the hospice model, is appropriate. Chaplains should have a significant role in the disclosure of a diagnosis as serious as dementia. They must be able to encourage hope despite the perils of forgetfulness. Hope is a multi-dimensional, dynamic attribute of an individual that concerns dimensions of possibility and confidence in future outcome. Hope can address secular matters such as future plans and relationships, or religious matters of ultimate destiny. Hope is an aspect of 'religious' well-being.

One autobiographical account of religious self-identity and coping with dementia is Reverend Robert Davis's *My Journey into Alzheimer's Disease: Helpful Insights for Family and Friends* (Davis 1989). As Davis 'mourned the loss of old abilities', he nevertheless could draw on his faith: 'I choose to take things moment by moment, thankful for everything that I have, instead of raging wildly at the things that I have lost' (p. 57). Even as he struggled to find a degree of peace through his faith, he was also keenly aware of people who 'simply cannot handle being around someone who is mentally and emotionally impaired' (p. 115). Such a faith-based coping with this serious diagnosis is rather widespread.

People with a diagnosis of dementia often pray, for they are thrown back onto whatever faith they have in the meaningful and beneficent purposes underlying the universe. The person with a diagnosis of dementia will often desire to pray with family members, to pray in religious communities, and to pray alone. The word prayer comes from the Latin *precari*, 'to entreat', or ask earnestly. It comes from the same root as the word precarious and it is in the precariousness of emerging forgetfulness that often the person with dementia is driven to prayer. Prayer is one way of enhancing hope in the future despite dementia. Chaplains and clinicians can encourage this propensity to gain strength through prayer in the midst of cognitive decline.

Even in the more advanced stages of dementia, the symbolic self will persist to degrees. One man with dementia clutched his cowboy hat whenever he went to bed, as though he knew that his self-identity was somehow connected with this symbol. It turns out that he had worn country and western garb as a steel worker for many years. He continued to clutch his hat until the day he died. Pastoral caregivers, then, may be able to reach the person with dementia at some deeper symbolic level of the self, although more needs to be learned about the best forms of pastoral care in the most deeply forgetful.

Caregivers often pray for loved ones with dementia. In a study of religious variables in relation to perceived caregiver rewards, African–American women caring for elderly persons with major deficits in activities of daily living perceived greater benefits through caring based on a spiritual–religious reframing of their situation. Religiosity indicators (that is, 'prayer, comfort from religion, self-rated religiosity, attendance at religious services') are especially significant as coping resources in African–American women caregivers (Picot *et al.* 1997). Spirituality is a clear stress deterrent and therefore also impacts on depression rates, which are extraordinarily high in dementia caregivers. These authors suggest that,

> if religiosity indicators are shown to enhance a caregiver's perceived rewards, health care professionals could encourage caregivers to use their religiosity to reduce the negative consequences and increase the rewards of caregiving. (Picot *et al.* 1997)

This seems self-evident.

Other studies indicate that spirituality is an important factor in coping with the sometimes ruthless stress induced by caring for someone with dementia (Murphey 1988). Spirituality among dementia caregivers is a central means of coping (Whitlatch *et al.* 1992). In an important study, 32 family caregivers of persons with dementia and 30 caregivers of persons with cancer were compared cross-sectionally to determine whether the type of illness cared for affected the emotional state of the caregiver and to identity correlates of both undesirable and desirable emotional outcomes (Rabins *et al.* 1990). While no prominent differences in negative or positive states were found between the two groups, correlates of negative and positive emotional status were identified. These included caregiver personality variables, number of social supports, and the feeling that one is supported by one's religious faith. Specifically, 'emotional distress was predicted by self-reported low or absent religious faith' (Rabins *et al.* 1990). Moreover, spirituality predicted positive emotional states in caregiving. Interestingly, the study suggests that it was 'belief, rather than social contact, that was important'.

Self-identity will diminish, but there is no justification for asserting that it is ever entirely gone. Such an assertion would only apply to people in the persistent vegetative state, or who are brain dead. John Locke wrote of the person as a being able to 'consider itself, the same thinking being, in different times and places'.[1] Self-identity is preserved in memory, which provides continuity over time. In this sense, Locke is consistent with Augustine. The Augustinian–Lockean position formulates the idea of a person as a 'who' rather than as a 'what.'

Our task as moral agents is to remind persons with dementia of their continuing self-identity. We must serve as prostheses, filling in the gaps and expecting that now and again the cues we provide will connect with the person and perhaps even elicit a surprising verbal or affective response. In other words, our task is to preserve identity and it is for this reason that many nursing homes will post biographical sketches on the doors of residents' rooms, or family members will remind a loved one of those events and people who have been meaningful along life's journey. We must see the glass of self-identity as half full rather than as half empty and understand that metaphors such as 'gone' or 'husk' are dehumanizing and empirically suspect.

Even when a person has lost connection with many aspects of their self-identity and perhaps on any given moment feels autobiographically lost, there is nevertheless a remaining self-consciousness. 'I' can be anxiously aware of my disorientation to time, place, and past, and yet still be conscious of myself as a self. Such periods of confusion over the past in relation to the present are frightening, but even in such periods we can perceive this loss of groundedness in a past and ask 'Who am I?' In other words, even when self-identity has waned deeply—although there are always faint glimmers of identity—the self is still aware of itself in its confusion. Self-consciousness and self-identity are not neatly divided and it is probably the case that self-consciousness correlates with self-identity in its weakest form.

Sometimes, in such states of confusion, people with moderate and advanced dementia will go back in their autobiographical journey to a period earlier in life where they find security. They have lost much of their sense of identity in the present and seek it in their earlier life. For example, I met a man with advanced dementia who handed me a twig while displaying a huge smile. The nurse told me that when he was a boy, his father gave him the daily chore of bringing kindling in for the fireplace. Now, he was reliving that boyhood doing something he associated with fatherly love. A person may not be projecting plans into the future, or acting autonomously, or able to explain their behaviour, or even abiding in the present. But they can reside in the past, wherever retained deep memories allow.

It is residual self-consciousness, rather than the rational capacity to set ends, that we must respect and, when possible, through relational stimulation, enhance. This is why, for example, it is important to address every person with dementia, no matter how advanced, by name. Bend down, make eye contact, and call the person by name expecting an answer, even if one does not come. This action is more than symbolic—it is a way of affirming residual self-consciousness and this affirmation is morally crucial.

There is nothing morally relevant about the ability to project rational purposes into the future. What is morally relevant is the experience of subjectivity, of myself as a subject in the sense of being conscious of self as self. And as for the ability to communicate by speech, this too is not morally relevant. Indeed, subjectivity exists in the absence of speech. Alasdair MacIntyre, in his work entitled *Dependent Rational Animals: Why Human Beings Need the Virtues* (MacIntyre 1999), a revision of his 1997 Carus Lectures, has said nothing that those involved in the world of cognitive disabilities would not readily affirm: human beings are vulnerable, mutually dependent, as well as often imperiled by the fact that we overestimate the moral significance of the capacity for speech. We assume that those who cannot communicate are of lesser value and this pertains even to advanced non-human species. MacIntyre is most concerned with the virtue of 'just generosity' toward those who are disabled, especially with regard to independence and practical reasoning.

Many utilitarians make the error of combining the principle of the greatest happiness of the greatest number (that is, a tyranny of the majority unhampered by constitutional rights) with a narrow 'hypercognitive' definition of personhood. Peter Singer (Singer 1993), Dan W. Brock (Brock 1988), and others, who indicate that persons of moral status must have desires for the future, exclude those without ample temporal glue. The most deeply forgetful must then ultimately be devalued. I coined the term 'hypercognitive' in 1995 to underscore a persistent bias against the deeply forgetful that is especially pronounced in modern philosophical accounts of the 'person' (Post 1995). I did not anticipate that the term would catch on so widely in the literature. Only 'persons' narrowly defined, it is often argued, have moral standing. Human beings with significant cognitive disabilities would have little or no moral status under such a system. The philosophers of hypercognitive personhood seem to state that if we do not wear the personae dictated by their intellectualist leanings, we count less or not at all under the protective principles of non-maleficence and beneficence.

Ethics requires us to afford moral status to those who are no longer autonomous, rational decision makers—if indeed any of us ever really are autonomous—through an appreciation of self-identity and self-consciousness. Rationality is too severe a ground for moral standing, allowing (if not requiring) the disregard of many individuals who share our common humanity from the edges of decline. Incidentally, there are countless family members who will base respect for the deeply forgetful on the religious assertions of a non-material soul that still exists intact underneath all the neurological losses of dementia. Such a view has its defenders among the contemporary philosophers of the 'mind–body' problem, such as Sir John Eccles.[2] Family members and also those affected with dementia may take solace in the presence of a non-material soul, lying fully intact beneath the surface of radical communicative breakdown. I do not take such a view, but appreciate it as a way of asserting the moral intuition concerning the inviolability of the deeply forgetful, as well as some degree of continuity of self.

The radical differentiation between the formerly intact or 'then' self and the currently demented or 'now' self, as put forward by some commentators, is simply a misrepresentation of the facts. The reality is that until the very advanced and even terminal stage of dementia, the person with dementia will usually have sporadically articulated memories of deeply meaningful events and relationships ensconced in long-term memory. It is nonsense to bifurcate in any strong sense the self into 'then' and 'now,' as if continuities are not occasionally quite manifest. This is why it is essential that professional caregivers be aware of the person's life story, making up for losses by providing cues toward continuity in self-consciousness. Even in the advanced stage of dementia, as in the case presented at the outset of this section, one finds varying degrees of emotional and relational expression, remnants of personality, and even meaningful non-verbal communication (as in the reaching out for a hug).

Respect for residual emotional and relational capacities

In his book entitled *Dementia Reconsidered: The Person Comes First*, Tom Kitwood's definition of love within the context of dementia care includes comfort in the original sense of tenderness, closeness, the calming of anxiety, and bonding (Kitwood 1997). Kitwood and Kathleen Bredin developed a description of the 'culture of dementia' that is useful in appreciating emotional and relational aspects of quality of life. They provide indicators of well-being in people with severe dementia: the assertion of will or desire, usually in the form of dissent despite various coaxings; the ability to express a range of emotions; initiation of social contact (for instance, a person with dementia has a small toy dog that he treasures and places it before another person with dementia to attract attention); affectional warmth (for instance, a woman wanders back and forth in the facility without much socializing, but when people say hello to her she gives them a kiss on the cheek and continues her wandering) (Kitwood and Bredin 1992).

There is an emotional and relational reality in the lives of the deeply forgetful. The first principle of care for such persons is to reveal to them their value by providing attention and tenderness in love. As a culture of care we must set aside the distorted position that a person's worth, dignity, and status as a human being under the principles of non-maleficence and beneficence depend entirely on their cognitive capacities. I prefer an 'I-Thou' view of personhood, which takes into account the emotional and relational capacities of the person (Rudman 1997). Insofar as we live in a culture that is dominated by heightened expectations of rationalism and economic productivity, clarity of mind and productivity inevitably influence our sense of the worth of a human life. But on the emotional level, there is no difference between 'them' and 'us.'

Persons with cognitive disabilities need the emotional sense of safety and joy, *and seem to reveal in the clearest way our universal human needs*. The first principle of care for such persons is to reveal to them their value by providing attention and tenderness in love. Kitwood defined the main psychological needs of persons with dementia in terms of care or love. He drew on the narratives of caregivers to assert that persons with dementia want love, 'a generous, forgiving and unconditional acceptance, a wholehearted emotional giving, without any expectation of direct reward' (Kitwood 1997, p. 81). The first component of love is comfort, which includes tenderness, calming of anxiety, and feelings of security based on affective closeness. It is especially important for the person with dementia who retains a sense of their lost capacities. Attachment, the second component of love, includes the formation of specific bonds that enhance a feeling of security. Other components of love are inclusion in social experiences, genuine occupation that draws on a person's abilities and powers, and, finally, acknowledgement of identity.

The person with dementia, then, is part of our common humanity as an emotional and relational being and therefore must be treated with care and respect.

Only a view of humanity that excludes emotion and relationality would ignore this and such a view would be both callous and inhumane.

Reflections

This chapter began with the notion of respect as 're-looking.' If we pass by the person with dementia just once and reach superficial conclusions, we fail morally. When we pass by a second time and begin to observe the complexity of a life lived in deep forgetfulness, respect becomes possible. The more we re-examine these lives, the more we come to honour them.

The fitting response to the increasing prevalence of dementia in our ageing society is to enlarge our sense of human worth to counter an exclusionary emphasis on rationality, efficient use of time and energy, ability to control distracting impulses, thrift, economic success, self-reliance, 'language advantage', and the like. We make too much of these things. Here I would distinguish the heritage of Stoic rationalism from Judaism and Christianity. The great Stoic philosophers achieved much for universal human moral standing by emphasizing the spark of reason (*logos*) in us all. Yet this is clearly an arrogant view in the sense that it makes the worth of a human being entirely dependent on rationality and then gives too much power to the reasonable. Reinhold Niebuhr concluded that,

> since the divine principle is reason, the logic of Stoicism tends to include only the intelligent in the divine community. An aristocratic condescension, therefore, corrupts Stoic universalism. (Niebuhr 1956, p. 53)

Jewish and Christian ethics, however, are able to include even those with cognitive disabilities under the protective umbrella of beneficence. Equal regard based on the cognitive, emotional, relational, and symbolic–expressive aspects of persons with dementia (including advanced dementia) lead me to reject the notion 'I think, therefore I am' and replace it with the less arrogant notion 'I feel and relate, and therefore, I am'.

Endnotes

1 For further consideration of this view, see Matthews's discussion in Chapter 10 of this book and see Hughes (2001).
2 For further background discussion of the mind-body or mind-brain problem, see Chapter 1 of this book, pp. 7–20.

References

Augustine, St. *Confessions*. (Numerous editions available, for example, 1961 (trans. R. S. Pine-Coffin). Harmondsworth: Penguin.)

Brock, D. W. (1988). Justice and the severely demented elderly. *Journal of Medicine and Philosophy*, **13**: 73–9.

Davis, R. (with help from his wife Betty) (1989). *My Journey into Alzheimer's Disease: Helpful Insights for Family and Friends*. Wheaton, Illinois: Tyndale House.

Hughes, J. C. (2001). Views of the person with dementia. *Journal of Medical Ethics*, **27**: 86–91.

Kitwood, T. (1997). *Dementia Reconsidered: The Person Comes First*. Philadelphia: Open University Press.

Kitwood, T., Bredin, K. (1992). Towards a theory of dementia care: personhood and well-being. *Ageing and Society*, **12**: 269–97.

MacIntyre, A. (1999). *Dependent Rational Animals: Why Human Beings Need the Virtues*. Chicago: Open Court.

Muller-Hill, B. (1988). *Murderous Science: Elimination by Scientific Selection of Jews, Gypsies, and Others: Germany 1933–1945*. New York: Oxford University Press.

Murphey, C. (1988). *Day To Day: Spiritual Help When Someone You Love Has Alzheimer's*. Philadelphia: Westminster Press.

Niebuhr, R. (1956). *An Interpretation of Christian Ethics*. New York: Meridian.

Picot, S. J., Debanne, S. M., Namazi, K. H., Wykle, M. L. (1997). Religiosity and perceived rewards of black and white caregivers. *Gerontologist*, **37**: 89–101.

Post, S. G. (1995). *The Moral Challenge of Alzheimer Disease*, 1st edn. Baltimore and London: Johns Hopkins University Press.

Post, S. G. (2000). *The Moral Challenge of Alzheimer Disease: Ethical Issues from Diagnosis to Dying*, 2nd edn. Baltimore and London: Johns Hopkins University Press.

Rabins, P. V., Fitting, M. D., Eastham, J., Fetting, J. (1990). The emotional impact of caring for the chronically ill. *Psychosomatics*, **31**: 331–6.

Rudman, S. (1997). *Concepts of Person and Christian Ethics*. Cambridge, UK: Cambridge University Press.

Singer, P. (1993). *Practical Ethics*. Cambridge, UK: Cambridge University Press.

Whitlatch, A. M., Meddaugh, D. I., Langhout, K. J. (1992). Religiosity among Alzheimer's disease caregivers. *American Journal of Alzheimer's Disease and Related Disorders and Research*, **12**: 11–20.

Zagzebski, L. (2001). The uniqueness of persons. *Journal of Religious Ethics*, **29**: 401–23.

15 Understandings of dementia: explanatory models and their implications for the person with dementia and therapeutic effort

Murna Downs, Linda Clare, and Jenny Mackenzie

Introduction

There are many different ways of understanding the experience of living with dementia. These understandings can be thought of as explanatory models. None of them reflects, or indeed is capable of reflecting, the one and only truth. Rather, they represent the attributions we make for why people behave as they do. By inference, they provide us with guidance as to the most appropriate and helpful response.

Individuals, families, professionals, and communities all have belief systems about what causes dementia. The explanatory models of dementia, which we as individuals and societies adopt, will affect both the experience of living with dementia and how we support people and their families living with these conditions (Cassell 1976). Explanatory models are ways of conceptualizing how illness is recognized, understood, and interpreted, from popular, folk, and professional perspectives (Kleinman 1981).

The purpose of this chapter is to describe four explanatory models of dementia and to examine their implications for a person with dementia and the nature of the therapeutic effort required to provide support. The models are not intended to be exhaustive. For example, psychoanalytic explanatory models are omitted. The models included are dementia as normal ageing; dementia as a spiritual experience; dementia as a neuropsychiatric condition; and dementia as a dialectical process involving an interplay between biological, psychological, and social components. While these are presented as discrete models, we recognize that in real life they rarely appear in a pure form. Rather, as individuals and societies, we adopt an eclectic approach to explaining dementia. Our separation of the models into discrete categories is only for purposes of discussion.

We shall demonstrate that, in general terms, different explanatory models dominate at different time periods, and, within the same time period, between and within ethnic groups. We shall describe how some explanatory models place more or less emphasis on the therapeutic effort required to ensure quality of life and on the form such therapeutic effort may take. We shall conclude by stressing the ethical imperative to promote understandings that both emphasize the essential humanity of the person with dementia and maximize quality of life for people with dementia and their families.

Dementia as normal ageing

Many people and peoples consider the memory difficulties and behavioural changes associated with dementia to be the result of normal ageing. In this explanatory model, changes in cognitive functioning and behaviour are caused by age-associated physiological changes or by social circumstances that exacerbate these naturally occurring effects, such as bereavement or migration (Braun and Browne 1998; Elliott *et al.* 1996).

This view of the inevitability of impaired mental functioning with age was the dominant view in Western cultures until the 1970s. It continues to be a contemporary view within some Western societies (Pollitt 1996), Chinese Americans (Elliott *et al.* 1996), and some Asian and Pacific Islander Americans living in Hawaii (Braun and Browne 1998). Gubrium (1986) in his book *Oldtimers and Alzheimer's: The Descriptive Organization of Senility* discussed the difficulty of distinguishing between normal ageing and dementia at a neurobiological level. He argued that attempting to do so was a social construction on the part of the cognitively intact, aimed at creating order from the disorder manifested by people with dementia. Research reviewed by Huppert (1994) suggests that the difference between dementia and age-associated changes in cognitive functioning is more quantitative than qualitative, one of degree rather than of kind.

Implications for people with dementia and their families

The implications for the person with dementia of their experience being attributed to changes associated with normal ageing are that they maintain whatever their status was prior to the development of these changes. In cultures where to be old is to be revered, older people with dementia are also revered. In cultures rife with ageism (Byetheway 1994), older people with dementia experience this ageism. Arguably people with dementia are at increased risk from the negative effects of ageism given their reduced capacity for coping.

Implications for therapeutic effort

Where dementia is viewed as an inevitable part of ageing, there is no justification for offering additional health and social service resources over and above those already provided for older people—which of course may in any case already be inadequate. No specialist therapeutic effort is expected or expended. No specialist skills are considered to be required. This can result in a failure of care to meet the individual needs of people with dementia adequately, as documented in the article from the UK's *Independent* newspaper in October 2002 (Fig. 15.1).

Woman, 71, died of thirst because carer couldn't spell 'Alzheimer's'

BY JEREMY LAURANCE
Health Editor

A WOMAN died of thirst in an old people's home after the deputy manager failed to record that she was suffering from Alzheimer's disease because she could not spell it.

A pathologist told an inquest into the death of Edith Pyett, 71, that it was the worst case of dehydration she had seen. Mrs Pyett had been in the Belmont Care Centre in Eastbourne for a week. Annette Ducille-Horton, the home's deputy manager, admitted failing to enter Mrs Pyett's Alzheimer's disease – which left her unable to eat or drink without assistance – in her care plan. She told the jury at the inquest in Eastbourne: "The reason I did not put Alzheimer's in the care plan was because I couldn't spell it. I was going to do it later but I didn't. I had not come across it before. I thought it was Old Timers' disease."

The omission meant staff did not realise the severity of Mrs Pyett's problems or understand her needs. She was not assigned a named carer and, despite the concerns of several care assistants that she was not drinking, a fluid monitoring chart to record what she drank was not set up

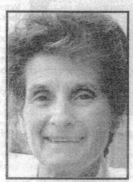

Edith Pyett: Staff didn't know she needed help

for her, as it was for others.

James Pyett, 77, a retired hospital porter, had cared for his wife full-time since she developed the disease in 1995 but had placed her in the home while he visited his daughter in Surrey for a short break.

When he returned after a week he told the jury he was shocked at the state she was in. "I hardly recognised her. She was unkempt. Her head and eyes were rolling all over the place. I thought she was very ill," he said.

He gave her juice, which she "gulped down", and although staff knew she was incontinent and she was wearing an incon-

tinence pad he found her trousers were saturated and her buttocks were "red-raw".

Her condition deteriorated and she was admitted to hospital, where she died of renal failure on 7 March this year.

Mr Pyett said he had told staff at the home when his wife was admitted that she could not give herself food or drink, although she had a good appetite and liked to drink. "I spent an hour telling staff her needs. She liked a cup of tea but she could not indicate that she was thirsty. I told them she needed help with her food and drink."

The care assistant Caroline Carpenter said there was no record of her having Alzheimer's or dementia. She said: "There was nothing in Mrs Pyett's notes to explain her constant smiling. I looked in there to check on general health information but there was nothing to suggest she suffered from dementia."

Dr Jane Mercer, who performed the post-mortem examination, said Mrs Pyett's kidneys had failed due to dehydration. "It was extremely severe. I have not seen worse results."

The jury returned a verdict of death from dehydration, aggravated by neglect.

Fig. 15.1 Article from the UK's *Independent* newspaper in October 2002. Reproduced with kind permission from Independent Newspapers Ltd.

Spiritual explanations of dementia

Some cultures have placed more emphasis on spiritual explanations of dementia, where dementia is viewed, for example, as the result of forces of good or, more commonly, of evil. In non-Western and minority ethnic communities within the West, spiritual forces are often presented as the reason for changes in an older person's behaviour and functioning. This belief in a spiritual power is often more acceptable than the concept of a mental illness as an explanation for changes in behaviour (Hussain 2001). Witchcraft, or *nazar* in the Islamic world, is frequently associated with signs of mental illness. It is common in Muslim communities to believe in possession by ubiquitous semi-human spirits (jinn or ginn) that can cause ill-health in the person so possessed.

Similarly, Elliott *et al.* (1996) found that Chinese living in the USA may recognize dementia as an illness, but attribute it to spiritual forces making retribution for family wrong doing or the sins of ancestors, an imbalance of yin and yang, misalignment of property, or possession by evil spirits or fate. A further example of a belief in sorcery commonly held in South Asian culture concerns a belief in *ayn nazar* (the evil eye) seen as a negative force or spell cast on a person to cause them illness.

These types of belief structure are not confined to South Asian culture. Helman (2000) traces the concept of the evil eye through a series of anthropological studies conducted throughout Europe, the Middle East, and North Africa. In each presentation the person possessing the evil eye is usually unaware of their power and causes harm unintentionally rather than deliberately. Citing Underwood and Underwood (1981), Helman (2000), describes the characteristics of someone possessing the evil eye as 'a stranger or local person whose social activity, appearance, attitudes or behaviour is to some degree unorthodox or different, especially a person who stares rather than speaks' (Helman 2000, p. 94). It is easy to see parallels in this descriptor with some presentations of dementia.

Uwakwe's interviews with 10 religious leaders in Nigeria suggest dementia results when: ' ... an evil spirit through demonic attack possesses the brain leading to loss of memory, bad dreams, hallucinations, irrational talk etc.' (Uwakwe 2000, p. 1152). In some languages no word exists to describe dementia. For example, in Urdu, the closest term for dementia means 'crazy' or 'insane' (Forbat 2002). Pollitt (1997) discusses the lack of an equivalent term for dementia in Aboriginal and Torres Strait Islander communities. Similarly in many Asian languages there is no word for 'care' (Gunaratman 1997). Ineichen (1998) explains that families in the Middle East tended to attribute declining memory and cognitive abilities to normal ageing.

Implications for people with dementia and their families

As possession is generally considered to be inversely proportionate to religious conviction, a person showing signs of mental illness or dementia easily becomes stigmatized and outcast. Belief in the evil eye means that the person with dementia risks being seen as the possessor of the evil eye and thus becomes feared, avoided, and isolated by the community (Mackenzie in press). On the other hand, a person with dementia may be revered, be seen as having been specially chosen by God or especially spiritually rich, or be considered to be in close communion with the spiritual side of life (see for example, Henderson 2002). More commonly, however, they may be stigmatized by being seen as possessed by evil spirits through lack of faith, paying the price for wrong doing.

An overriding factor in the process of stigmatization, which arises from all spiritual explanations for the presence of dementia-type symptoms, is the effect on the family and also on subsequent generations. Immediate family members are implicated in having contributed to their relative's condition by their lack of faith. A family shamed by the presence of mental illness or dementia-like symptoms attributed to spiritual forces could not hope to secure good marriages for their younger members; neither could they expect to retain *izzat* (an honourable reputation) in their local communities (Mackenzie in press). As a result, families may resort to hiding the older person away to protect the wider family from stigma and shame (Forbat 2003).

Implications for therapeutic effort

When dementia is viewed as a result of the spiritual side of life, prayer is seen to provide the necessary salvation (Rassool 2000). In this sense, within Muslim tradition when an illness such as dementia is believed to be written in a person's destiny—*naseeb* (fate or fortune)—older people and their family carers tend to seek spiritual treatment from a *Molvi* (priest) as a folk healer who would provide holy water to drink and/or a *taweez* (amulet) to wear around the neck. In cases where dementia is viewed as being the result of jinn, its successful defeat depends on strength of faith and the power of prayer.

Belief in the evil eye leads towards reliance on folk healing (Mackenzie in press). Uwakwe (2000) provides us with a range of interventions that may be used when someone is seen to have dementia resulting from spiritual forces: fasting, special prayers, counting the rosary, penance, reading the Bible, home visits, chastisement (beating), material and financial assistance, exorcism, crusade, night vigil, testimonies, and music and dancing (Uwakwe 2000, p. 1152). As a result of these beliefs, Forbat (2003) describes a 'clash in discourses, terminology and interests' between 'service users' and professionals in the UK.

Dementia as a neuropsychiatric condition

In Western cultures, a neuropsychiatric model of dementia predominated throughout most of the twentieth century and continues to exert a powerful influence. An explanatory model of dementia as a neuropsychiatric condition views the experience as being the result of underlying progressive brain disease, most commonly reflecting the neuropathological changes associated with Alzheimer's disease or vascular dementia, or both. Viewed as a psychiatric disorder, the cognitive and behavioural changes are described as 'symptoms' (which the patient complains of) and 'signs' (which the doctor notices).

This explanatory model proposes a kind of biological determinism where cognitive symptoms (deficits in memory, thinking, orientation, comprehension, calculation, learning capacity, language, and judgement), behavioural signs (including wandering and repetitive questioning), and psychotic symptoms and signs (hallucinations and delusions) are attributed directly to neurological impairment (Coffey and Cummings 1994, 2000). Thus, in this explanatory model, living with dementia entails living with both cognitive and non-cognitive symptoms or signs, the non-cognitive features being frequently referred to as 'behavioural and psychological signs of dementia' or 'challenging behaviour'. As illustrated in the textbook cover shown in Fig. 15.2, these symptoms are associated with 'suffering' and require management[1].

This explanatory model, which continues to dominate among professional understandings of dementia, has been criticized for neglecting the social and psychological factors involved in the expression and experience of the illness (Cotrell and Schulz 1993; Kitwood 1987; Lyman 1989; Snowdon 1997). Snowdon's nun study demonstrated the lack of a direct correlation between brain disease and symptomatology. Rather, he argued, the expression of neuropathology can be mediated by prior levels of education and by the current environment (Snowdon 1997).

Implications for people with dementia and their families

As this explanatory model views the person as having a brain disease, it therefore naturally positions the person as a patient. The person is viewed as a passive victim of a condition over which they have no control, thus inevitably as a 'sufferer'. An explanatory model of dementia which attributes the person's experience entirely to a neuropsychiatric illness means that the person experiences the stigmatizing and depersonalizing effects commonly experienced by older people with mental disorders (Graham et al. 2003). Some argue that the effect of a psychiatric label is as disabling as the condition to which the label was assigned.

Furthermore, a process of diagnostic overshadowing can result where all actions and expressions are attributed to the labelled condition. This was famously described by Rosenhan (1973). The person with dementia experiences the same disenfranchisement as others with a psychiatric condition. Sayce (1999) challenges us as a society to reinstate psychiatric patients as citizens, a call echoing Kitwood's plea that we should see the person first and foremost as a person, rather than just in terms of a brain disease (Kitwood 1993).

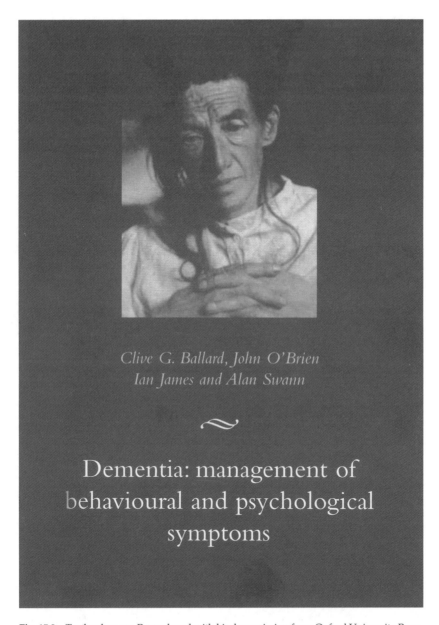

Clive G. Ballard, John O'Brien
Ian James and Alan Swann

Dementia: management of
behavioural and psychological
symptoms

Fig. 15.2 Textbook cover. Reproduced with kind permission from Oxford University Press.

For people with dementia, this disenfranchisement is even more severe. Just as notions of brain and mind and person tend to be viewed as interrelated (if not identical) concepts, progressive brain diseases tend to be viewed as inevitably leading to the loss of self (Cohen and Eisdorfer 1986). As can be seen in the

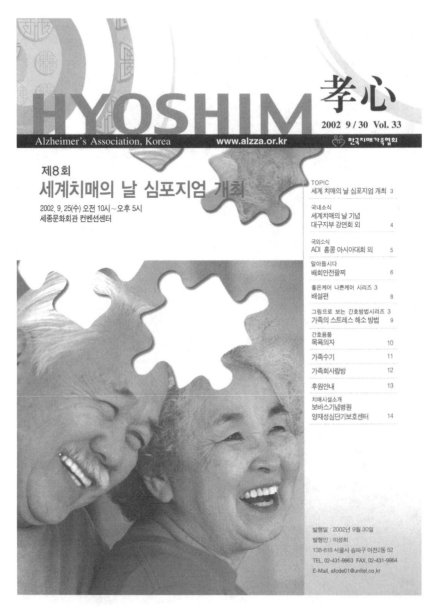

Fig. 15.3 Korean Alzhiemer's Association leaflet. Reproduced with kind permission from the Alzheimer's Association, Korea.

Korean Alzhiemer's Association leaflet (Fig. 15.3), this interest in brain disease can prevent us from seeing the person as whole.

This explanatory model positions family carers as inevitably burdened, leading them to be patients in their own right. Twigg and Atkin (1994) argue that the same process that turns older people into patients turns families into carers facing inevitable 'burdens' of care. In this explanatory framework, carers themselves become patients whose psychological and physical morbidity needs to be treated. A chapter in a key textbook of old age psychiatry uses the language of 'prescribing' to describe the provision of services for carers of people with dementia (Brodaty and Green 2000). Indeed since the 1980s families have been viewed as 'hidden victims' because the need for such support and services was ignored (Brodaty and Green 2000; Zarit *et al.* 1985).

Caring for a relative with dementia puts demands on families. Many feel poorly informed for, and poorly supported in, this role. In response to a health care system better suited to meeting the needs of acute conditions, carers have formed mutual aid societies, which have resulted in today's Alzheimer's societies operating locally, regionally, nationally, and internationally (Fox 2000). It can be asked to what extent the burden associated with caring for a relative with dementia can be attributed to their relative's neuropsychiatric condition or to a fragmented and inadequate health and social care response (Audit Commission 2000).

Implications for therapeutic effort

Viewing the mental frailty of old age as a psychiatric condition caused by brain disease implies the need and moral obligation for specialist intervention (Shenk 2002), particularly from old age (O'Brien *et al.* 2000) and geriatric (Coffey and Cummings 2000) neuropsychiatry. Psychiatric input involves three main areas: the diagnosis of dementia, the prescription of cognitive enhancers, and the management of behavioural symptoms (Bullock 2002).

The diagnosis of dementia is a key service provided by psychiatry. In particular, specialist input into differential diagnosis is essential for appropriate drug prescription of both cognitive enhancers and psychotropic medication (Burns and McKeith 2002). Support for coming to terms with the diagnosis and adjusting to life with a progressive condition is less well developed. In the UK the prescription of cognitive enhancing medication is restricted to old age psychiatry. The growth in these treatment options has changed the status of old age psychiatry from being a poorly resourced service to one with recognized therapeutic potential (Burns and McKeith 2002). Despite the hope these drugs offer professionals and patients alike, their efficacy is time limited.

The role of medication in the management of behavioural symptoms is perhaps the most controversial of roles played by old age psychiatry. Many psychiatrists on the ground describe their reluctance to prescribe psychoactive medication for behavioural aspects of dementia, preferring instead to seek psychosocial solutions (Bird 2000). It is recognized that the emphasis on drug treatments for the management of behavioural symptoms may be misguided or harmful (Ballard and O'Brien 1999). Brodaty *et al.* (2003) provide a useful typology of behavioural symptoms, suggesting that as few as 10% require specialist psychiatric input, the remaining 90% requiring specialist psychosocial approaches. Nevertheless an explanatory model that views behaviour as symptoms of an underlying brain disease leads, by deduction, to a treatment modality that relies on psychoactive medication.

While there is a recognition that adequate support requires the involvement of specialist mental health services that are comprehensive, accessible, responsive, individualized, multi-disciplinary, accountable, and systematic (Audit Commission 2002; Burns *et al.* 2001), it is also recognized that such services are not the norm (Audit Commission 2000). In England, the National Service Framework for Older People has few resources devoted to it, unlike a similar government initiative—the National Service Framework for Mental Health. In the UK the majority of people in care homes have dementia (Macdonald and Dening 2002) and thus require specialist dementia care, yet in many cases the 'quiet' people with dementia are not recognized as having dementia and thus do not receive any specialist care (Macdonald and Dening 2002).

A dialectical process explanatory model of dementia

In the West, the neuropsychiatric explanatory model of dementia was considered by some to be too reductionist in its biological determinism and thus unable to account for several facts about dementia (Gubrium 1986; Kitwood 1987; Lyman 1989). Histopathological evidence suggested that there was not a one-to-one correlation between brain disease and clinical expression (Snowdon 1997). Rather, Snowdon (1997) documented cases of people who were relatively cognitively intact who, on post-mortem, showed the characteristic plaques and tangles of Alzheimer's disease. He concluded that there were protective factors that could resist and delay the expression of brain disease. Brody (1971) pointed to the deleterious effects of environment on brain disease leading to what she coined as 'excess disability' in many people with dementia; that is, disability which is in excess of what one might expect from brain disease alone. This suggests that at least some aspects of an individual's decline in functioning might be reversible or might have the potential to be postponed for longer.

In the UK, Kitwood (1990) proposed that dementia could best be understood as a dialectical process. Such an explanatory model sees the experience of living with dementia to be the result of a dialectical interplay between neurological impairment (or brain disease) and psychosocial factors—health, individual psychology, and the environment, with particular emphasis on the social context. This model has much in common with the biopsychosocial model of illness promoted by the World Health Organization (2002) and the social or disability model described by Gwilliam and Gilleard (1996) and Downs (2002). Post (2000) lends support to the mediating effects of non-biological variables on the experience of living with dementia by arguing that the cultural context in which one lives will affect the experience of dementia. He refers to our 'hypercognitive' culture in the West, where intellect and reasoning are valued above relational and aesthetic aspects. Thus, the cultural significance of intellectual impairment will further jeopardize people with dementia living in the West. What Kitwood's dialectical process model of dementia provides above and beyond a biopsychosocial model is that it allows for the environment to have as much effect on the brain as the brain has on the person's abilities. In this way the model has much in common with the research on enriched environments published by Diamond (1993, 2001). Following this line of argument, people with a brain disease such as dementia will be adversely affected at a neurological level by an impoverished environment and enhanced by an enriched environment. For Kitwood and Bredin (1992) the most disabling effects of brain disease are to be found, not in functional impairment, but in threats to one's sense of self and one's personhood. For Kitwood and Bredin (1992), personhood is dependent on other people. Kitwood and Bredin (1992) and Sabat (1994) describe a malignant social psychology, which depersonalizes the individual.

Nevertheless, viewing dementia as the result of interacting influences positions the person with dementia at the centre of those influences. The development of a person-centred approach in dementia care is based on the argument that people with dementia, far from being passive victims, are active agents in their lives, actively seeking meaning, responding, and attempting to act on their world (Sabat and Harré 1994; Sabat 2001).

Viewed from within this explanatory framework, 'challenging behaviour' is seen as an attempt to express or meet psychological or physical needs, or to express will (Kitwood 1997a; Stokes 2001). Recent empirical research (Cohen-Mansfield 2000; Beattie et al. 2004) and clinical experience (Stokes 2001) testify that much of what is labelled as challenging behaviour can be explained as a person's attempt to meet their needs or to communicate needs to others, be they for physical comfort, stimulation, or emotional belonging. It is perhaps not surprising that much of the documented literature on challenging behaviour is conducted in nursing home settings, which are notorious for failing to meet people's needs for occupation or engagement (Nolan et al. 1995).

Furthermore it is recognized that the meaning of much behaviour can be fully understood only within the context of the person's life history. In this explanatory model, biography and life history are seen as mediators in the expression of dementia. Stokes (2001) describes how many actions made by people with dementia have meaning when viewed within the context of their life story. For example, someone who finds it difficult to sleep at night and wants to walk around while others are sleeping may have been a night watchman.

This dialectical model makes it possible to account for both the weak correlations between symptoms and pathology and the heterogeneity of clinical presentation observed with similar pathology. The manifestation of dementia in any one individual, therefore, can be understood only by considering the interplay of neurological impairment, physical health (including sensory acuity), personality and agency, biography and past experience, social psychology, and social resources.

Such a model addresses some of the shortcomings of the neuropsychiatric model where a form of biological determinism was assumed. It provides a theoretical basis for Snowdon's findings of the lack of correlation between brain disease and manifest symptoms (Snowdon 1997) and for the phenomenon of 'excess disability' first described by Brody (1971).

Implications for people with dementia and their families

The central implication of the person-centred approach is that the person with dementia has the same value as any other person, a similar broad range of needs, and the same rights as a citizen, which must be safeguarded. The person-centred approach to dementia emphasizes the importance of understanding the person's experience of living with the condition (Kitwood 1997b; Harris 2002), rather than solely making assumptions about what this is like and, therefore, what is required. In this explanatory model there is recognition that people with dementia have a unique expertise without which we shall neither fully understand the condition, nor provide effective support strategies (Cotrell and Schulz 1993; Harris 2002).

It is increasingly accepted that people with dementia can express views, needs, and concerns, even in the later stages and that the challenge is to find effective ways of communicating (Goldsmith 1996; Killick and Allan 2001). A number of personal accounts directly describe the experience of early-stage dementia (for example, McGowin 1994; Simpson and Simpson 1999; Lee 2003; Snyder 1999). Researchers have interviewed people with dementia and worked with them to develop an understanding of their experience and derive theoretical models that reflect this experience (Keady and Nolan 1995a,b; Clare 2002, 2003; Phinney 2002; Harris 2002; Sabat 2001). Approaches are being developed to explore the experiential world of people with more advanced dementia (Killick and Allan 2001; Normann et al. 2002). Most importantly, people with dementia are finding a voice through self-help groups (see, for example, www.dasni.org) and are increasing their profile in advocacy and representation.

The person-centred approach also has significant implications for carers and family members of people with dementia. Rather than assuming a loss of self, the model implies an on-going, evolving relationship. It is recognized that this can present significant challenges and difficulties for carers. Carers, like their relatives with dementia, will need support. From this perspective, carers are not inevitably victims, but with adequate support and appropriate information will have the opportunity to renegotiate their relationship and become enriched. The carer's challenge is to escape the medical confines of the disease and to assemble a new humanity in the loss (Shenk 2002, p. 93). This humanity that comes from being with a person with dementia is illustrated in Fig. 15.4.

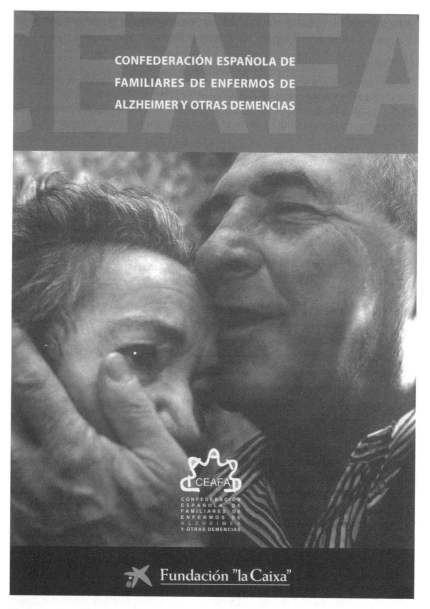

Fig. 15.4 Leaflet from Spanish carers' organization. Photograph reproduced with kind permission of Diego Alquerache. Leaflet reproduced with kind permission of Confederación Espanola de Familiares de Enfermos de Alzheimer y Otras Demencias (CEAFA).

Implications for therapeutic effort

The central aim of dementia care within Kitwood's dialectical model is the preservation and enhancement of the personhood of the individual with dementia. In this respect the model is firmly rooted within a philosophical tradition that argues that self is not reliant on cognition. The implication here is that while the self, or at any rate its coherent expression, may be under threat with neurological disease, it is the moral duty of those around the person to support and enhance its expression. As Kitwood writes, 'personhood is bestowed ... by others' (Kitwood 1997a, p.8). Thus the central goal of care within this tradition is to become attuned to, and to support, the experience and perspective of the person with dementia, previously a neglected aspect of dementia research and care (Cotrell and Schulz 1993). Services are more likely to be effective and appropriate if people with dementia have been able to contribute their perspective when service developments are discussed (Clare and Cox 2003; Cox et al. 1998).

Viewing dementia as a dialectical interplay between biology, psychology, and the environment, particularly the social environment, implies a compelling argument for therapeutic effort. While relatively little can be done to arrest the underlying brain disease, much can be done to promote health and well-being. It prompts the development of supports and services that address the many facets of a person's life that might hasten or delay the onset, or ameliorate or exacerbate the effects, of neurological disease. These include health promotion, self-management, support groups, and other ways of addressing social, emotional, and spiritual needs. Similarly, behaviours that have been explained by the neuropsychiatric paradigm as 'symptomatic' of the underlying disease and therefore either meaningless, irrational, or problematic are viewed within the biopsychosocial model as an active agent's attempt to communicate feelings and needs, or as an expression of will (Cohen-Mansfield 2000; Rader et al. 1985; Stokes 2001). Bird (2000) argues for the need for a comprehensive approach to understanding behaviour and criticizes the neuropsychiatric model as inappropriate and inadequate in its reductionism.

A biopsychosocial approach emphasizes maintaining and enhancing quality of life over and above simply controlling or managing symptoms (Lawton and Rubinstein 2000). This focus on factors that can be manipulated to ameliorate or exacerbate the effects of neurological impairment has been described as a cultural revolution (Morton 1999) and as providing the foundation for a 'new culture' in dementia care (Kitwood and Benson 1995).

The implications for therapeutic effort can be described under three main domains: (1) supports for active coping; (2) the provision of enriched social environments; and (3) the promotion of rehabilitative approaches.

Supports for active coping

The dialectical model emphasizes the dynamic interplay between neurology and social context. This interplay is mediated in part through individual psychology in terms of the way in which the individual adapts to the onset and progression of dementia. The importance of the psychological impact of dementia on the self is implicit within the dialectical model. A compensatory approach that considers how the individual copes with the changes resulting from dementia is integral to a psychological understanding of dementia (Woods and Britton 1985). Here the individual is viewed as an agent who actively seeks to bring to bear whatever resources are available in order to adapt and cope (Cotrell and Schulz 1993; Droes 1997; Hagberg 1997). Recent work has explored aspects of the active coping engaged in by people with dementia and couples where one partner has dementia (for example, Clare 2003; Clare and Shakespeare 2004; Keady and Nolan 2003).

One implication for intervention is that it is important to support the maintenance of selfhood and identity so as to optimize the personal resources available for on-going coping and adjustment. This can be done in a number of ways. Interventions may aim to address some of the factors influencing individual psychological reactions, or to change the psychological reactions themselves, or to adapt the resulting coping behaviour. For example, cognitive rehabilitation supports practical coping and adjustment (Clare 2003), while self-maintenance therapy (Romero and Wenz, 2001) focuses directly on the need to support and strengthen the sense of self. Kitwood (1997*a*) categorizes care approaches as 'positive person work' when they serve to enhance personhood; examples include validation, holding, and affirmation.

While emphasizing the perspective of the person with dementia and the role of individual psychology, it is also important to consider the wider systemic context that surrounds the person. The concept of self in this model refers to a socially-constructed sense of identity that is embodied and rooted in a temporal and environmental context. Thus, the context may also become a focus for intervention, both at the immediate level and also in terms of reducing stigma and negative perceptions at a socio-cultural level.

> Our goal . . . is to try to help these people live a quality life, to help them gain some coping mechanisms for their deficits, and to help them feel better as human beings. (Support group for people with dementia worker interviewed by Shenk (Shenk 2002))

> While scientists did battle with this disease, victims and their families had the opposite task: to make a certain peace with it, to struggle to understand the loss, come to terms with it, create meaning out of it. (Shenk 2002, p. 32)

As yet relatively little is known about the possibilities that Kitwood's dialectical model might hold for primary prevention of dementia, although findings such as those from the nun study (Snowdon 1997) support the view that this area is worth investigating further. The model does, however, have important implications for prevention or reduction of excess disability, in terms of offering avenues for maintaining well-being and optimizing coping and everyday functioning within the constraints imposed by dementia.

Providing an enriched social environment

Sabat (2001) argues that having dementia affects the possibilities available for the social presentation of self in the context of relationships. Lyman (1998) suggests that the social consequences of cognitive impairment are the most difficult for people with dementia. Where the social context is 'malignant', Kitwood (1997a) argues, the result is a vicious circle of deterioration. Where the social psychology is benign, neurological impairment can be mitigated by positive interactions, so that the person is able to function as effectively as possible and retain a sense of well-being and personhood. A malignant social context might contribute to structural changes in the brain while a benign social context coupled with an enriched environment might even facilitate some regeneration (Karlsson et al., 1988).

The most central implication of Kitwood's model is the need for high-quality interpersonal care that affirms personhood—that is, person-centred care. A useful contemporary overview of person-centred care (Brooker 2004) suggests that four key components are integral to this approach: valuing people with dementia and those who care for them, treating people as individuals, looking at the world from the perspective of the person with dementia, and providing a positive social environment in which the person living with dementia can experience relative well-being. Each of these four elements emphasizes the importance of relationships and interactions in dementia care. Traditionally, the perspectives of caregivers and of people with dementia were considered separately and little consideration was given to the complex interactional relationship between the person with dementia and the carer. Recent work building on the dialectical model places a focus on the relationship between the person with dementia, the family member or other supporter, and the health care provider. For example, there is a developing focus on the experience and interactions of couples (for example, Lyons et al., 2002; Clare and Shakespeare 2004; Robinson et al., in press) and Nolan et al. (2004) have applied the term 'relationship-centred' to optimal dementia care.

Alongside this, there is a developing focus on the interactions among 'health care triads' (Fortinsky 2001) and on the ways in which physical surroundings can support self and relationship (Marshall 2000; Teresi et al. 2000). Imagery used by *Alzhiemer's Disease International* reflects this belief in the importance of interactions for people with dementia (see Fig. 15.5).

Rehabilitative approaches

The influential World Health Organization model of disability (World Health Organization 1980) highlighted the important distinction between impairment, disability, and handicap and the potential of rehabilitation as a means of addressing the effects of disability. Rehabilitation can help to optimize well-being in the context of progressive disorders, even though the underlying

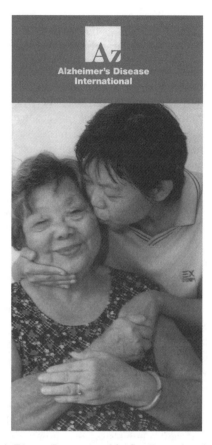

Fig. 15.5 Alzheimer's Disease International leaflet. Reproduced with kind permission from *Alzheimer's Disease International*. Photograph copyright of *The Star*, Malaysia.

impairment cannot be cured or reduced. The relevance of a rehabilitation model for dementia care was noted by Cohen and Eisdorfer (1986) and recent years have seen the development of rehabilitation approaches (Marshall 2004) aimed at addressing particular areas of disability, such as cognitive rehabilitation (Clare 2003; Clare and Woods 2001). People with a diagnosis of dementia have themselves begun to advocate for a rehabilitation-oriented approach (Friedell 2002).

Conclusion

We began by saying that there are many different ways of understanding what dementia is and what it is like to live with dementia. These understandings can be thought of as explanatory models. We have described four influential explanatory models and have attempted to demonstrate how they underpin different kinds of attributions about the features shown by people who have what we describe as dementia. In each case, we have considered what guidance the models offer as to the most appropriate and helpful response.

While the four models have been presented in this chapter in discrete sections, in actuality any one person or society can hold one or more of these at the same time, or can fluctuate between one model and the next. The emphasis in the chapter has been on presenting these models as discrete explanatory frameworks and examining the extent to which, as explanatory frameworks, they assist us in accounting for why people behave as they do.

Certainly different understandings lead to different emphases. Viewing dementia as a normal part of ageing leaves the older person needing as much help and support as any other older person, without any requirement for specialist input. Viewing dementia as a result of spiritual intervention puts the older person in the potentially stigmatized position of having attracted negative attention owing to moral shortcomings, which in turn brings shame to the family. This stigmatized state requires that the family keep the situation secret, hide the person away, and care as best they can alone, without any outside help. The only role for the broader society is in the use of traditional healing approaches.

Viewing dementia as a neuropsychiatric disease places the older person in the sick role. The psychiatrically labelled older person experiences a loss in social worth. As with labelling effects in general, most of the person's behaviour is attributed to the disease process. As such, the person is viewed predominantly in terms of deficits. This model places the family in the caring role, with an assumption that they will experience psychological and physical morbidity as a result of their relative's disease. It puts psychiatry in the relatively powerful expert position where symptom management—primarily of a pharmacological nature—is the goal. It confers a moral obligation on part of the medical community to intervene and suggests that care for people with dementia is specialist care.

Viewing dementia from the perspective of the person-centred approach where the expression of the disease and its experience are viewed as the result of a dialectical process between neurological impairment, individual psychology, physical and mental health, and the social and physical environment keeps the person at the centre of all our efforts to help. It focuses on the person's abilities and strengths and suggests a citizenship model of inclusion. It views a person's experience as a valuable source of information that contributes to understanding what constitutes effective support.

Such a model offers the most comprehensive approach to understanding and supporting the person's experience. It recognizes the need for a multi-disciplinary approach and the many aspects of a person's life that can be enhanced. Its theoretical framework provides professionals and practitioners with the basis for addressing all aspects of the person's life rather than restricting the focus to brain disease. It argues for the need for multi-disciplinary assessment and support, along with an integrated health and social service.

Endnote

1 The use of this particular book is solely for its cover. Ironically its content provides a useful overview of all that can be done to prevent distress and promote quality of life.

References

Audit Commission (2000). *Forget Me Not: Mental Health Services for Older People.* (Available at www.audit-commission.gov.uk.)

Audit Commission (2002). *Forget Me Not 2002: Developing Mental Health Services For Older People In England.* (Available at www.audit-commission.gov.uk.)

Ballard, C., O'Brien, J. (1999). Treating behavioural and psychological signs in Alzheimer's disease: the evidence for current pharmacological treatment is not strong. *British Medical Journal*, **319**: 138–9.

Beattie, E. R. A., Algase, D. L., Song, J. (2004). Behavioural symptoms of dementia: their measurement and intervention. *Ageing and Mental Health*, **8**: 109–16.

Bird, M. (2000). Psychosocial management of behaviour problems in dementia. In: *Dementia* (ed. J. O'Brien, D. Ames, and A. Burns), pp. 603–14. London: Hodder Arnold.

Braun, K. L., Browne, C. V. (1998). Perceptions of dementia, caregiving, and help seeking among Asian and Pacific Islander Americans. *Health and Social Work*, **23**: 262–74.

Brodaty, H., Green, A. (2000). Family carers for people with dementia. In: *Dementia* (ed. J. O'Brien, D. Ames, and A. Burns), pp. 193–205. London: Hodder Arnold.

Brodaty, H., Draper, B., Low, L. F. (2003). Behavioural and psychological symptoms of dementia: a seven tiered model of service delivery. *Medical Journal of Australia*, **178**: 231–4.

Brody, E. (1971). Excess disabilities of mentally impaired aged: impact of individualised treatment. *Gerontologist*, **25**: 124–33.

Brooker, D. (2004). What is person centred care for people with dementia? *Reviews in Clinical Gerontology*, **13**: 215–22.

Bullock, R. (2002). New drugs for Alzheimer's disease and other dementias. *British Journal of Psychiatry*, **180**: 135–9.

Burns, A., McKeith, I. G. (2002). Old age psychiatry. *British Journal of Psychiatry*, **180**: 97–8.

Burns, A., Dening, T., Baldwin, R. (2001). Care of older people: mental health problems. *British Medical Journal*, **322**: 789–91.

Byetheway, B. (1994). *Ageism.* Buckingham: Open University Press.

Cassell, E. J. (1976). Disease as an 'it': concepts of disease revealed by patient's presentation of symptoms. *Social Science and Medicine*, **10**: 143–6.

Clare, L. (2002). We'll fight it as long as we can: coping with the onset of Alzheimer's disease. *Aging and Mental Health*, **6**: 139–48.

Clare, L. (2003). Managing threats to self: awareness in early-stage Alzheimer's disease. *Social Science and Medicine*, **57**: 1017–29.

Clare, L., Cox, S. M. (2003). Improving service approaches and outcomes for people with complex needs through consultation and involvement. *Disability and Society*, **18**: 935–53.

Clare, L., Shakespeare, P. (2004). Negotiating the impact of forgetting: dimensions of resistance in task-oriented conversations between people with early-stage dementia and their partners. *Dementia*, **3**: 211–32.

Clare, L., Woods, R. T. (eds.) (2001). *Cognitive Rehabilitation In Dementia: A Special Issue of Neuropsychological Rehabilitation*. Hove: Psychology Press.

Coffey, C. E., Cummings, J. L. (eds.) (1994). *The Textbook of Geriatric Neuropsychiatry*. Arlington: American Psychiatric Publishing.

Coffey, C. E., Cummings, J. L. (eds.) (2000). *The American Psychiatric Textbook of Geriatric Neuropsychiatry*. Arlington: American Psychiatric Publishing.

Cohen, D., Eisdorfer, C. (1986). *The Loss of Self: A Family Resource for the Care of Alzheimer's Disease and Related Disorders*. New York: W. W. Norton.

Cohen-Mansfield, J. (2000). Approaches to the management of disruptive behaviours. In: *Interventions in Dementia Care: Toward Improving Quality of Life* (ed. M. Powell Lawton and R. L. Rubinstein), pp. 39–64. London: Springer.

Cotrell, V., Schulz, R. (1993). The perspective of the patient with Alzheimer's disease: a neglected dimension of dementia research. *Gerontologist*, **33**: 205–11.

Cox, S., Anderson, I., Dick, S., Elgar, J. (1998). *The Person, the Community and Dementia*. Stirling: Dementia Services Development Centre, University of Stirling.

Diamond, M. C. (1993). An optimistic view of aging. *Generations*, **17**: 31–3. (Special issue on mental health.)

Diamond, M. C. (2001). Enrichment, response of the brain. In: *Encyclopedia of Neuroscience*, 3rd edn (ed. G. Adelman), pp. 396–7. Amsterdam: Elsevier Science.

Downs, M. (2002). Dementia as disability: Implications for practice. In: *Dementia Topics for the Millennium and Beyond* (ed. S. Benson), pp. 4–7. London: Hawker Publications.

Droes, R. M. (1997). Psychomotor group therapy for demented patients in the nursing home. In: *Care-Giving in Dementia: Research and Applications, Volume 2* (ed. B. M. L. Miesen and G. M. M. Jones), pp. 95–118. London: Routledge.

Elliott, K. S., Di Minno, M., Lam, D., Mei Tu, A. (1996). Working with Chinese families in the context of dementia. In: *Ethnicity and the Dementias* (ed. G. Yeo and D. Gallagher-Thompson), pp. 89–108. Washington DC: Taylor and Francis.

Forbat, L. (2002). There is no word for dementia in Urdu: researching minority ethnic family carers and dementia. (Paper presented at the International Alzheimer's Congress, Barcelona, September 2002.)

Forbat, L. (2003). Concepts and understandings of dementia by 'gatekeepers' and minority ethnic 'service users'. *Journal of Health Psychology*, **8**: 645–55.

Fortinsky, R. (2001). Health care triads and dementia care: integrative framework and future directions. *Aging and Mental Health*, **5 (Suppl. 1)**: S35–48.

Fox, P. (2000). The role of the concept of Alzheimer disease in the development of the Alzheimer's Association in the United States. In: *Concepts of Alzhiemer's Disease:*

Biological, Clinical and Cultural Perspectives (ed. P. J. Whitehouse, K. Maurer, and J. F. Ballenger). London: Johns Hopkins University Press.

Friedell, M. (2002). Awareness: a personal memoir on the changing quality of life in Alzheimer's. *Dementia: The International Journal of Social Research and Practice*, **1**: 359–66.

Goldsmith, M. (1996). *Hearing the Voice of People with Dementia: Opportunities and Obstacles*. London: Jessica Kingsley.

Graham, N., Lindesay, J., Katona, C., Bertolote, J., Camus, V., Copeland, J. K. *et al.* (2003). Reducing stigma and discrimination against older people with mental disorders: a technical consensus statement. *International Journal of Geriatric Psychiatry*, **18**: 670–8.

Gubrium, J. F. (1986). *Oldtimers and Alzheimer's: The Descriptive Organization of Senility*. Greenwich, Connecticut: JAI Press.

Gunaratman, Y. (1997). Breaking the silence: Black and ethnic minority carers and service provision. In: *Community Care: A Reader* (ed. J. Bornat, J. Johnson, C. Pereira, D. Pilgrim, and F. Williams), pp. 114–23. London: MacMillan.

Gwilliam, C., Gilliard, J. (1996). Dementia and the social model of disability. *Journal of Dementia Care*, **4**: 14–15.

Hagberg, B. (1997). The dementias in a psychodynamic perspective. In: *Care-Giving in Dementia: Research and Applications, Volume 2* (ed. B. M. L. Miesen and G. M. M. Jones), pp. 14–35. London: Routledge.

Harris, P. B. (ed.) (2002). *Pathways to the Person: The Subjective Experience of Alzheimer's Disease*. Baltimore: Johns Hopkins University Press.

Helman, C. G. (2000). *Culture, Health and Illness*, 4th edn. London: Hodder Arnold.

Henderson, J. N. (2002). The experience and interpretation of dementia: cross-cultural perspectives. *Journal of Cross Cultural Gerontology*, **17**: 195–6.

Huppert, F. A. (1994). Memory function in dementia and normal aging—dimension or dichotomy? In: *Dementia and Normal Aging* (ed. F. A. Huppert, C. Brayne, and D. W. O'Connor), pp. 291–330. Cambridge: Cambridge University Press.

Hussain, A. (2001). Islamic beliefs and mental health. *Mental Health Nursing*, **21**: 2 and 6–9.

Ineichen, B. (1998). The geography of dementia: an approach through epidemiology. *Health and Place*, **4**: 383–94.

Karlsson, I., Brane, G., Melin, E., Nyth, A. L., Rybo, E. (1988). Effects of environmental stimulation on biochemical and psychological variables in dementia. *Acta Psychiatrica Scandinavica*, **77**: 207–13.

Keady, J., Nolan, M. (1995*a*). IMMEL 2: working to augment coping responses in early dementia. *British Journal of Nursing*, **4**: 377–80.

Keady, J., Nolan, M. (1995*b*). IMMEL: assessing coping responses in the early stages of dementia. *British Journal of Nursing*, **4**: 309–14.

Keady, J., Nolan, M. (2003). The dynamics of dementia: working together, working separately, or working alone? In: *Partnerships in Family Care* (ed. M. Nolan, U. Lundh, G. Grant, and J. Keady), pp. 15–32. Buckingham: Open University Press.

Killick, J., Allan, K. (2001). *Communication and the Care of People with Dementia*. Buckingham: Open University Press.

Kitwood, T. (1987). Explaining senile dementia: the limits of neuropathological research. *Free Associations*, **10**: 117–40.

Kitwood, T. (1990). The dialectics of dementia: With particular reference to Alzheimer's disease. *Ageing and Society*, **10:** 177–96.

Kitwood, T. (1993). Discover the person not the disease. *Journal of Dementia Care*, **1**: 16–17.

Kitwood, T. (1997*a*). *Dementia Reconsidered: The Person Comes First*. Buckingham: Open University Press.

Kitwood, T. (1997*b*). The experience of dementia. *Ageing and Mental Health*, **1**: 13–22.

Kitwood, T., Benson, S. (1995). *The New Culture of Dementia Care*. London: Hawker Publications.

Kitwood, T., Bredin, K. (1992). Towards a theory of dementia care: personhood and well-being. *Ageing and Society*, **12**: 269–87.

Kleinman, A. (1981). *Patients and Healers in the Context of Culture: An Exploration of the Borderland Between Anthropology, Medicine and Psychiatry*. Berkeley: University of California Press.

Lawton, M. P., Rubinstein, R. L. (2000). *Interventions in Dementia Care: Towards Improving Quality of Life*. New York: Springer.

Lee, J. L. (2003). *Just Love Me: My Life Turned Upside-Down by Alzheimer's*. West Lafayette, Indiana: Purdue University Press.

Leighton, A. H., Lambo, T. A., Hughes, C. C. (1963). *Psychiatric Disorder among the Yoruba*. Ithaca: Cornell University Press.

Lyman, K. (1989). Bringing the social back in: A critique of the biomedicalisation of dementia. *Gerontologist*, **29**: 597–605.

Lyman, K. (1998). Living with Alzheimer's disease: the creation of meaning among persons with dementia. *Journal of Clinical Ethics*, **9**: 49–57.

Lyons, K. S., Zarit, S. H., Sayer, A. G., Whitlatch, C. J. (2002). Caregiving as a dyadic process: perspectives from caregiver and receiver. *Journal of Gerontology: Psychological Sciences*, **57B**: 195–204.

Macdonald, A., Dening, T. (2002). Dementia is being avoided in NHS and social care. *British Medical Journal*, **324**: 548.

Mackenzie, J. (in press). Stigma and dementia: South Asian and Eastern European family carers negotiating stigma in two cultures. *Dementia: The International Journal of Social Research and Practice*.

Marshall, M. (2000). Homely: the guiding principle of design for dementia. In: *Dementia*, 2nd edn (ed. J. O'Brien, D. Ames, and A. Burns A), pp. 233–40. London: Arnold.

Marshall, M. (ed.) (2004). *Perspectives on Rehabilitation and Dementia*. London: Jessica Kingsley.

McGowin, D. F. (1994). *Living in the Labyrinth: A Personal Journey through the Maze of Alzheimer's*. Cambridge: Mainsail Press.

Morton, I. (1999). *Person-centred Approaches to Dementia Care*. Bicester: Winslow.

Nolan, M., Grant, G., Nolan, J. (1995). Busy doing nothing: activity and interaction levels amongst differing populations of elderly patients. *Journal of Advanced Nursing*, **22**: 528–38.

Nolan, M. R., Davies, S., Brown, J., Keady, J., Nolan, M. (2004). Beyond 'person-centred' care: a new vision for gerontological nursing. *International Journal of Older People Nursing*, **13**: 45–53.

Normann, H. K., Norberg, A., Asplund, K. (2002). Confirmation and lucidity during conversations with a woman with severe dementia. *Journal of Advanced Nursing*, **39**: 370–6.

O'Brien, J., Ames, D., Burns, A. (eds.) (2000). *Dementia*. London: Hodder Arnold.

Perrin, T. (1997). Occupational need in severe dementia : a descriptive study. *Journal of Advanced Nursing*, **22**: 528–38.

Phinney, A. (2002). Fluctuating awareness and the breakdown of the illness narrative in dementia. *Dementia: The International Journal of Social Research and Practice*, **1**: 329–44.

Pollitt, P. A. (1996). Dementia in old age: an anthropological perspective. *Psychological Medicine*, **26**: 1061–74.

Pollitt, P. A. (1997). The problem of dementia in Australian Aboriginal and Torres Strait Islander communities: an overview. *International Journal of Geriatric Psychiatry*, **12**: 155–63.

Post, S. (2000). *The Moral Challenge of Alzheimer's Disease: Ethical Issues from Diagnosis to Dying*. London: John Hopkins.

Rader, J., Doan, J., Schwab, M. (1985). How to decrease wandering, a form of agenda behaviour. *Geriatric Nursing*, **6**: 196–9.

Rassool, G. H. (2000). The crescent and Islam: healing, nursing and the spiritual dimension. Some considerations towards an understanding of the Islamic perspectives on caring. *Journal of Advanced Nursing*, **32**: 1476–84.

Robinson, L., Clare, L., Evans, K. (in press). Making sense of dementia and adjusting to loss; psychological reactions to a diagnosis of dementia in couples. *Aging and Mental Health*.

Romero, B., Wenz, M. (2001). Self-maintenance therapy in Alzheimer's disease. *Neuropsychological Rehabilitation*, **11**: 333–55.

Rosenhan, D. (1973). On being sane in insane places. *Science*, **179**: 250–8.

Sabat, S. R. (1994). Excess disability and malignant social psychology: a case study of Alzheimer's disease. *Journal of Community and Applied Social Psychology*, **4**: 157–66.

Sabat, S. R. (2001). *The Experience of Alzheimer's Disease: Life Through a Tangled Veil*. Oxford: Blackwell.

Sabat, S. R., Harré, R. (1994). The Alzheimer's disease sufferer as a semiotic subject. *Philosophy, Psychiatry, & Psychology*, **1**: 145–60.

Sayce, L. (1999). *From Psychiatric Patient to Citizen: Overcoming Discrimination and Stigma*. London: Palgrave Macmillan.

Shenk, D. (2002). *The Forgetting. Understanding Alzheimer's: A Biography of a Disease*. London: Harper Collins.

Simpson, R., Simpson, A. (1999). *Through the Wilderness of Alzheimer's: A Guide in Two Voices*. Minneapolis: Augsburg.

Snowdon, D. (1997). Ageing and Alzheimer's disease: lessons from the nun study. *Gerontologist*, **37**: 150–6.

Snyder, L. (1999). *Speaking our Minds: Personal Reflections from Individuals with Alzheimer's*. New York: W. H. Freeman.

Stokes, G. (2001). *Challenging Behaviour in Dementia: A Person-Centred Approach*. Bicester: Speechmark.

Teresi, J. A., Holmes, D., Ory, M. G. (2000). The therapeutic design of environments for people with dementia: further reflections and recent findings from the National Institute on Aging collaborative studies of dementia special care units. *Gerontologist*, **40**: 417–21.

Twigg, J., Atkin, K. (1994). *Carers Perceived: Policy and Practice in Informal Care*. Milton Keynes: Open University Press.

Underwood, P., Underwood, Z. (1981). New spells for old: expectations and realities of Western medicine in a remote tribal society in Yemen, Arabia. In: *Changing Disease Patterns and Human Behaviour* (ed. N. F. Stanley and R. A. Joshe), pp. 271–97. London: Academic Press.

Uwakwe, R. (2000). Knowledge of religious organizations about dementia and their role in care. *International Journal of Geriatric Psychiatry*, **15**: 1152–3.

Woods, R. T., Britton, P. G. (1985). *Clinical Psychology with the Elderly*. London: Croom Helm.

World Health Organization (1980). *International Classification of Impairments, Disabilities, and Handicaps*. Geneva: World Health Organization.

World Health Organization (2002). *Towards a Common Language for Functioning, Disability and Health*. Geneva: World Health Organization.

Zarit, S. H., Orr, N. K., Zarit, J. M. (1985). *The Hidden Victims of Alzheimer's disease: Families Under Stress*. New York: New York University Press.

16 Personhood and interpersonal communication in dementia

Lisa Snyder

Overview

In the safety afforded by a group of his peers, a man diagnosed with Alzheimer's disease describes a dream he had the previous night. He was trying to get to a gathering of some kind but when he finally arrived, 'the door was locked.' After knocking repeatedly, someone finally answered the door, but did not understand him when he tried to speak. 'I'm standing there and wondering why I can't get in and they don't understand.'

The need to communicate and to be understood is fundamental to the human experience. We live amidst swiftly flowing currents of verbal and non-verbal exchanges that transmit messages for our interpretation and response. We connect, we interrelate, we belong when we are afforded the opportunity to engage in these currents—to define our*selves* and express that selfhood in the act of being acknowledged and 'understood' by another. In this light, interpersonal communication is a mutual, co-constructed process in which each person offers definitions of self and of what is real for others to interpret, affirm, or challenge. Although these definitions and interpretations are subjective, they often shape the contours of dialogue. Communication builds upon the interlocutors' previously assembled definitions of selfhood as well as the schemas previously used to interpret verbal and non-verbal cues. Relationships are formed around attachments to certain supportive, destructive, or relatively neutral communication exchanges that evolve from these constructs. The experience of dementia, however, often threatens previously recognized co-constructions of self and reality resulting in progressively alienating communication between those who have symptoms of the disease and those who do not. Misunderstandings abound and it is not uncommon for persons with the disease to feel shut out.

In his seminal work, *I and Thou*, philosopher Martin Buber writes, 'All real living is meeting' (Buber 1958, p. 11). Beyond the confines of language, communication is also—in a pure form—an act of being with another: not only is a space created where messages are given and received, but also connections occur in mutual acknowledgment of the uniqueness of the other. Buber perceives open and honest communication as a true encounter between equals and termed such rare meetings 'dialogical' moments. For each person's humanity to be most fully realized they must 'imagine the real': imagine as clearly as possible what another person is wishing, feeling, perceiving, and thinking. This chapter introduces a context (namely support groups) as a means to imagine the real, to facilitate dialogical encounters, and to affirm selfhood in people with dementia. Throughout the chapter, statements from individuals with dementia guide and shape the discussion.

Effects of dementia on communication

The neuropsychological effects of dementia on language functions are well documented in the scientific literature. Test batteries reveal progressive deficits in verbal fluency, naming, and recognition. Words such as aphasia, anomia, agnosia, and apraxia alliterate definitions of the unfortunate outcomes of degenerative disease on the person's ability to interpret and express language. These objective measures provide a superficial basis, however, for understanding the more complex dynamics of interpersonal communication.

Sabat (2001) underscores the limitations of neuropsychological testing in evaluating the dynamic nature of language. Although such tests attempt to evaluate distinct cognitive domains relative to language,

> in the course of daily social experience and interaction, a whole panoply of cognitive functions is called upon more or less simultaneously, each 'separate' elementary function thus interacting with others.   (Sabat 2001, p. 11)

Just as one cannot fully understand communication abilities solely in terms of isolated neuropsychological tests, neither can one fully appreciate the capacity for communication apart from social context and the spontaneous interplay of human rapport. In their case study of an aphasic woman with Alzheimer's in an adult day centre, Sabat and Cagigas (1997) note that evaluation in a more natural social setting can reveal many intact communication strengths and abilities not otherwise observed in objective neuropsychological testing. Extralinguistic communication via body language, voice tone, facial gestures, and mime may be used despite moderate to severe language problems. Emotional expressions of anger, joy, and empathy can communicate affect and responses to interpersonal interactions. Through her experience of working with people with dementia in an adult day centre, Seman (2002) confirms that communication with participants is best understood as a complex set of interactions that exist in the context of environment and affective relationships. She notes the wise comment made by a day centre participant with dementia to staff: 'listen with the ears of your heart' (Seman 2002, p. 139).

Indeed, the most compelling insights into issues of communication and dementia come directly from the testimony of those experiencing its often exasperating and demoralizing trickery. When given the opportunity, people with dementia can often communicate very effectively about their communication 'deficits'. In her qualitative analysis of interviews with five people with dementia, Phinney (1998) discerns a theme of conversation breakdown. Those interviewed revealed how they were less comfortable speaking with others. They found they had trouble staying on track in a discussion and were less confident they could find the right words to convey their thoughts. Many others with dementia reiterate these concerns.

Bill, a retired editor, describes word-finding difficulty since the onset of his dementia. He states,

> For a while, I'll search for a word and I can see it walking away from me. It gets littler and littler. It always comes back, but at the wrong time. You can't be spontaneous. (Snyder *et al.* 1995, p. 98)

In his book *Partial View—an Alzheimer's Journal*, Cary Henderson, diagnosed with Alzheimer's disease writes,

> I really can't converse very well at all. So that's very limiting. I can't think of things to say before somebody's already said it and they've superseded what I have to say. The words get tangled very easily and I get frustrated when I can't think of a word. Every time I converse with somebody, there's always some word I can't remember. I really cuss when I can't remember a word. (Henderson 1998, p. 18)

Such exasperation with basic communication tools can result in feelings of increased isolation and devaluation. Holst and Hallberg (2003) explored the meaning of everyday life as expressed by 11 people with dementia. One theme that emerged in dialogue was 'losing the ability to reach out to others'. Participants felt they were no longer being acknowledged as persons, which itself restricted their communication. They discussed feelings of anger, shame, and sadness about their impaired ability to speak. Some felt insulted when others misunderstood or ignored them, or expressed feeling 'sad about losing their ability to enter into a relationship in which they could share experiences with others' (Holst and Hallberg 2003, p. 363). This series of progressively more alienating events was articulated by a woman who confided to friends in an early-stage dementia social club:

> I'm aware that I'm losing larger and larger chunks of memory . . . I lose one word and then I can't come up with the rest of the sentence. I just stop talking and people think something is really wrong with me. (Trabert 1997)

Some people with dementia are able to describe the conscious use of creative social skills to compensate for their embarrassing communication. A retired social worker said,

> I think I've learned to slow down and pay better attention. I don't want to get involved in a conversation and take a leap from here to there without being clear about that intermediate step. I want to make sure I know what I'm talking about.

> My caution does, in some instances, slow my response because when I'm spontaneous, I have to be sure that I don't put my foot in my mouth. I might say something to person A that really was meant for person B. And that's not necessarily a good thing! You commit a few more faux pas than you do ordinarily. So sometimes you have to cover up. I will find something to praise in someone as a means of disarming them about mistakes that I might make. It somehow makes them less upset if I lose track. I've discovered that this is very helpful. It's amazing what you can do to protect yourself! (Snyder 2000, pp. 121–2)

This need to protect oneself from the real or felt stigma of dementia can result in withdrawal from interpersonal communication and feelings of diminished value and belonging. One woman described the feeling that her personhood was under threat:

> I still would like to be treated like a person, you know, because I'm still a person whether I do it wrong or right . . . I want to feel like somebody because a lot of times with this—already with what I have . . . I really don't belong anyplace. (Alzheimer's Association 1994)

The emergence of support groups for persons with dementia

Subjective accounts describing the effects of dementia on selfhood, interpersonal relationships, and communication have been a catalyst for a worldwide burgeoning movement of support groups for people with dementia. Support group facilitators report on the decreased sense of isolation expressed by participants, as well as the significant level of self-disclosure, empathy, altruism, and cohesion observed early on among group participants (Caron 1997; Snyder *et al.* 1995; Yale 1995). Case examples and participant quotes reveal positive outcomes in effective peer group problem solving, the alleviation of depression, increased acceptance of the diagnosis, and increased communication between group participants and between group participants and their care partners (Hawkins and Eagger 1999; Morhardt and Johnson 1998; Yeh *et al.* 2001). Common topics for discussion in support groups include receiving the diagnosis, disclosing the diagnosis to others, developing coping strategies for cognitive and functional loss, finding meaningful activity, reconciling losses and existential issues of identity and mortality, and struggling with role changes and autonomy. Beyond specific content discussed within support groups, the interpersonal communication dynamics allow affirming, engaged discourse that is rarely afforded to people with dementia as they attempt to navigate mainstream life. These dynamics allow understanding and validation. A participant of a support group for younger persons with dementia in Scotland said,

> Having this illness is a lonely experience, even when you have a close family who gives you a lot of love. There is a part of me that they can't reach or

understand, but when I'm with my buddies I don't have that lonely feeling because they can understand me.   (Duff 1998)

Participants of other groups also report a sense of safety; they self-disclose because they do not face the same risks of judgement or misunderstanding encountered elsewhere. One man stated, 'You're in a secure place with bastions all around shielding you from outer forces who wish to do you in.'

Members of a different group had the following conversation when reflecting on their experience together.

I: All of us are all together. We're one. It's amazing to talk to people differently. This is like a sanctuary for me, it's safe. I was scared that this was going to be gone. It all goes together. These are my friends. I feel we should be able to stay here until we want to die.

M: It's wonderful and I look forward to it every week. It's nice meeting each week and you get more and more attached. I get tips on how to keep your brain from letting you down. I love it here. We improve with this kind of meeting.

C: It is good to know other people are experiencing what you are experiencing. This is a support group. We will never forget each other in this group. Never. The bond is that strong.

L: We need each other and it is a valuable, valuable thing. I wouldn't have survived this without the group. I was suicidal. I transformed from that. The group keeps me on my toes and makes me think of the experiences I've had. It's not as bad as I thought it was. You can improve.

G: It's comfortable. I'm a private person, but I feel easy and free to talk about what is going on because you all are going through it. Other people put you down for being incompetent.

C: Sharing our experiences gives us greater insight into ourselves as well.

R: I can't remember names, but I can remember thank you in seven languages. It's comforting to be here.

This sense of commonality, trust, and feeling of being understood affords a degree of security and protection that often prompts participants to refer to their group as a safe haven or to invoke a metaphor referring to survival. One man stated, 'This group is my lifeline' (Yeh *et al.* 2001). In another group a participant reflects on communication among group members and says,

It's a different kind of communication in the sense that you're not taking any chances here whereas in other situations you're taking a chance that whatever they hear or whatever they perceive is not registering the way we would like to see it registering. That doesn't happen here. We're all in the same lifeboat (ibid).

The feelings of vulnerability and the risk of misinterpretation or judgement by others is fundamental to many communication challenges for people with dementia. However, the capacity to 'register' what someone else says often has as much to do with the capabilities of the listener as it does with those of the speaker. At the root of these interchanges lies an entangled relationship between the personal and social constructions of reality and communication and the maintenance of selfhood.

The philosophy of 'as if'

In his discussion of fictionalism, Vaihinger argued that in order to make sense of our world, we construct systems of thought or 'fictions' (Vaihinger 1925). These individual or socially constructed fictions are conscious or unconscious ideas, not based in objective reality, but which enable us to deal more effectively with reality than we would do otherwise. Unlike a hypothesis, which is offered up for testing and verification, fictions are subjective constructs that we assemble and then live with 'as if' they are true regardless of their factual accuracy (Ansbacher and Ansbacher 1956, p. 77). These fictions are malleable; although we employ them with some degree of certainty, they can also be discarded or revised as needed or as dictated by changing circumstances. In a support group meeting where the theme of increased dependency and reliance on others was being discussed, one participant stated,

> All my life I've lived with certain clichés—"I'm an independent person". "I can do what I want". The idea of independence is a cliché. That's what I was brought up to think I could do.

This man's example of a 'cliché' exemplifies what Vaihinger calls a fiction: an idea that is constructed to facilitate effective or meaningful living when lived 'as if' it were true.

Our personal and collective fictions about dementia can have a significant impact on our communication with affected persons. If we consider a prevailing fiction, 'people with dementia have difficulty communicating', the reality of this statement is based on the scientific or social fictions we have constructed that define effective, legitimate, meaningful communication. The fiction may do little, however, to help us register comments from a speaker with dementia if we believe the fiction is absolute truth and then listen 'as if' the comments no longer have full legitimacy. One man described the resulting communication chasm:

> It seems my main trouble is with communication. Sometimes, I'm about to say something that is very important to me and it's nearly impossible to transmit the information because everyone listening has the presumption that what I'm about to say is unscrewed. There's essentially no way for me to convince anybody that although I'm affected by Alzheimer's in many ways, there's still a lot that's up there in my mind that has reason to be communicated. (Barlow and Snyder 1997, p. 6)

In contrast, if we harbour this same fiction but we listen to people with dementia 'as if' what they say has meaning despite their communication difficulties, the outcome of conversations may be quite different and the fiction may begin to change. Philosopher Daniel Dennett discussed adopting an intentional stance (Dennett 1987). The listener who invokes the intentional stance assumes that when a person speaks, they are intending to communicate something with thought and feeling. When pre-verbal children speak their first words, we listen 'as if' they are learning language and forming thoughts. A few simple words engender our rapt attention. When people with dementia speak with a similar functional capacity, we hear their messages 'as if' they have been reduced to the un-understandable, their sparse words a reflection of the degenerative loss of meaningful communication. Many will have witnessed dialogue between two residents of a nursing home, however, in which the communication is animated, gestured, verbal and reciprocal, yet quite incomprehensible to the 'normal' listener. These persons, severely affected by dementia, do not appear to operate under the fiction that their communication is less effective. By invoking an intentional stance towards one another, by listening 'as if' there is a message to receive, they engage in moments of mutual communication and connection.

Vaihinger's theory of 'as if' applies not only to how we listen to people with dementia, but also to how their communications align with our fictions about truth. Nietzsche wrote,

> The erroneousness of a concept does not for me constitute an objection to it; the question is—to what extent is it advantageous to life? (Ansbacher and Ansbacher 1956, p. 86)

Because most constructions of reality are fictional, it is more important to ask how a particular construction serves us. To invoke the intentional stance and to listen 'as if' the communication of the person with dementia has meaning is to acknowledge that personal fictions are less important in their absolute truth than in their subjective truth and personal significance. For example, a person with dementia may develop the fiction, 'someone is stealing from me'. This individual begins to hide precious objects or become vigilant about possessions. Perhaps no one is literally stealing objects from the person and missing items are recovered upon diligent hunting by the carer. As a result, professionals and the carers respond 'as if' the disease is now talking and the person is no longer in touch with reality. The affected person's fiction is labelled 'delusional', or 'suspicious and paranoid', or 'confabulation'. Medication may be prescribed. The person with dementia, however, continues to live 'as if' the fiction were true. A communication barrier forms when the fiction of the carer is affirmed, whilst the fiction of the person with dementia is discounted.

If, on the other hand, we listen to the message of the person with dementia 'as if' it had subjective reality and was not simply a figment of disease, we might gain deeper insight into the meaning and purpose of that fiction. In reflecting on his long period of paranoia about his finances and reasons why people with dementia may hoard or guard their possessions, Robert Davis, diagnosed with Alzheimer's disease, wrote,

> The loss of self, which I was experiencing, the helplessness to control this insidious thief who was little by little taking away my most valued possession, my mind, had made me especially wary of the rest of my possessions in an unreasonable way. (Davis 1989, p. 91)

Davis's fiction served the purpose of projecting his intolerable, internal fears onto the world of external tangible objects where he felt he could exert more control. Henderson (1998) confesses apologetically to feelings of suspiciousness and paranoia towards family:

> ... The feeling of being put on and the feeling nobody loves us, I think those are perfectly normal feelings ... I think for a lot of us the feeling of being cheated, or the feeling of being belittled and somehow made jokes of, I think that's one of the worst things about Alzheimer's.   (Henderson 1998, p. 37)

> ... We miss a lot of things and there are times when I feel people are plotting against me, mainly because I don't hear anything from them, I don't hear good words from them all the time.   (Henderson 1998, p. 81)

Whether his reflections about his 'paranoia' are based on fact is of less importance than the expression of devaluation and isolation inherent in his message. Although the listener's receptivity to the speaker's reality does not necessarily alter the fiction, there is a greater likelihood of understanding its purpose or meaning for the speaker and on that basis, the potential for empathic communication is enhanced.

These feelings of inferiority and devaluation, common to people with dementia, are in contrast to the experiences of participants in support groups, where both facilitators and participants commonly invoke the intentional stance. While carers or professionals may strive to maintain positions grounded in 'reality', or their own personal fictions, support group members often respond to one another's fictions 'as if' they are real and therefore meaningful. Astute facilitators are often themselves guided into this process and mentored by the non-judgemental responses of the participants. Facilitators Goldsilver and Grunier (2001) reported,

> At the first meeting of a newly formed group, two members recognized each other from elementary school. They delighted in their rediscovery of each other, and at each of the following seven sessions they 'rediscovered' each other as if for the first time. As group facilitators, we were prepared to intervene each time they replayed their recognition. However, we took our cues from the other group members, who accepted their behavior without stigma and, in fact, seemed to derive a sense of satisfaction and joy from their interplay.   (Goldsilver and Grunier 2001, p. 112)

Contrast the pleasant result of the group's ability to support each discovery 'as if for the first time' with the demoralizing feelings that might well have occurred were the pair informed each week of the 'reality' of their obvious forgetfulness. As one man said appreciatively about his support group, 'No one ever says, "You already told us that."'

Respect for personal fictions does not, however, preclude honest discourse. To listen to another 'as if' their comment has meaning also implies that one needs to try to ascertain, to the extent possible, the true meaning and not engage in artificial or patronizing expressions of understanding as a means of avoiding conflict. Whilst discussing the topic of communication, an exchange in one support group meeting revealed this dynamic.

> L: Once you have that label [Alzheimer's], it changes the way people communicate with you. Everyone treats you with . . . uh . . . you know, they don't want to . . .
>
> K: Upset you.
>
> L: Yeah, upset you or anything like that. You're just treated differently.
>
> FACILITATOR 1: And I suspect that then translates into being communicated with differently?
>
> L: Yeah, and I'm sure that they may not be even totally aware of it.
>
> FACILITATOR 1: Is it less authentic then?
>
> L: Yes, it is less authentic or at least that's the way I feel.
>
> FACILITATOR 2: More deferential—deferring to you?
>
> L: No, not really deferring . . . ordering! . . . It's like 'you need help' is the attitude. I think that's just . . . they just feel that way.

A sense of diminished authenticity in communication can result in people with dementia experiencing a diminished sense of self. Communication is not only built on constructions and interpretations of reality, but also on fundamental perceptions of the self as a unique and autonomous being. The onset of dementia poses threats to the expression of self and results in further challenges to communication. An examination of the social and relational constructions of self reveals how support groups sustain expressions of selfhood.

The social construction of communication and selfhood

Social Constructionism has its basis in the work of the twentieth-century philosopher Ludwig Wittgenstein (Wittgenstein 1958). While Realism holds that an objective external world exists independently of our representations, Social Constructionists argue that such objectivity is impossible to have: all reality has both subjective and relative aspects. There is no objective knowledge; rather, knowledge is formed from the views and meanings that people, situated in their own history and context, ascribe to a particular experience (Shotter and Gergen 1989). Language is a primary means of constructing meaning and is more than what is expressed or performed between speaker and hearer; it emerges from the cultural practices that shape human interaction. Words do not have meaning in themselves; rather they derive their meaning from their contexts. Within language, thoughts, feelings, and behaviours are expressed; but because it is a historical language and cultural context such expression cannot be taken as absolute 'truth' (Gergen 2001).

Thus, our understanding of health and illness are mediated through language. People learn what it is to be an 'Alzheimer's patient' based on the messages used to convey or conceal the diagnosis, the medical ascription of neurological, cognitive, and functional deficits and the manner in which families and society interact with them. A focus on the tragic effects of dementia has prompted socially constructed fictions such as 'the loss of self', 'empty shell', and the prospect of 'a long goodbye'. Once a diagnosis is made, these fictions affect communication in both subtle and dramatic ways. If we communicate with people with dementia 'as if' their self is diminished, we are less able to hear the intact messages that are expressions of personal identity. However, if we communicate 'as if' there is still a self trying to be recognized, we may open the door for dialogue or greater understanding. Indeed, case studies illuminate the intact social and cognitive abilities in persons with dementia despite cognitive impairment. Individuals can still display the ability to attend, to initiate social contact, and to exhibit self-respect, social sensitivity, creativity, helpfulness, and politeness (Sabat and Collins 1999; Temple *et al.* 1999). These abilities thrive in the support group environment. One member helps another take off their coat; another member offers to make a cup of coffee for a participant who can no longer accomplish this task. Participants take turns in dialogue without interrupting one another; one member offers a handkerchief when another begins to cry.

In their discussion of the application of Social Constructionist theory to selfhood, Sabat and Harré (1992) wrote that selfhood is socially expressed through language—through discursive practices between people that reveal autobiographical stories and attributes, feelings and opinions, and socially constructed personae. One's identity or personhood is developed, sustained, and transformed in and through communicative relationships, both immediate and within society at large. Sabat's three distinct expressions of selfhood—Self 1, 2, and 3 (for a description of which see Chapter 9, p. 146 in this book)—are readily heard throughout support group dialogue and reveal the capacities of persons with dementia to communicate their selves to others.

This retention of selfhood in dementia is often heard well into the disease process and is encouraged in the support group setting. Indeed the facilitation of I-messages, which demonstrate Self 1, is fundamental to group processes. For example, one man discusses the challenge of losing his train of thought to peers in his support group: 'I think that when I start to say these things that are important to me, I blank out. It's very discouraging to me (Snyder *et al.* 1995, p. 98). This man articulates awareness of a self through references to 'I' and 'me' and reveals feelings and experiences that *he* (that is, his Self 1) claims.

The mental and physical attributes of Self 2 are a significant part of identity. Support group participants have an opportunity to reveal and communicate these attributes to one another in an affirming environment. One participant who spends considerable time volunteering in his community remarked, 'I'm a person that likes to help people and that is part of my life. That's me.' In a weekly support group there are opportunities for the uniqueness of each Self 2 to be revealed and acknowledged. In one support group meeting when the facilitator asked V about her response to the topic of discussion, the following spontaneous interchange occurred:

FACILITATOR: You're smiling V. Is this resonating with you or not?

J: She's always smiling. You've got the nicest smile I've ever seen!

V: Oh, aren't you nice! Thank you very much. I really appreciate it.

J: You really do.

These acknowledgements of Self 2 can be tinged with camaraderie and humour, which convey the trust and familiarity inherent to authentic relationship. One group member playfully banters with another:

D: I have a daughter who is very argumentative.

J: The apple doesn't fall far from the tree!

Another exchange reveals the way in which group members acknowledge the value of the group and their positive feelings for one another in affirming personal attributes:

K: [referring to the support group] 'It's so helpful—in what stage and how we're handling it. It gives a sense of bravery in self that is so wonderful.'

R: That's very nice that you think that way—we all think that way on that count.

L: We're all such nice people.

R: We're great people!

Self 3, the socially presented self or persona, can have many facets and is best fostered within the context of an interaction where presentations of self are honoured and valued. For Self 3 to be honoured in a person with dementia requires that others uphold this existence of selfhood in the face of the threatening symptoms of disease. During a group discussion of the growing news coverage about advances in dementia research, one group member turns to another who is a retired physician and asks, 'What does our resident doctor hear from the mail—the reams of things you get—What do you hear about Alzheimer's?' The question afforded the opportunity to have the person's Self 3 as physician and authority on health matters acknowledged and he was able to respond as a person held in esteem by the peers in his group. Another member of the group was a poet who provided a rich closing ritual to each group meeting by reading one of his poems. When profound aphasia began to limit his ability to recite his poems, he continued the ritual by picking a poem at the end of each session and giving it to the facilitator to read. One day this participant came to the group distressed about his failing ability to maintain the tradition of writing a poem for his wife on the occasion of their anniversary.

He had brought with him a game comprising over one hundred words, each singularly printed on small magnetic squares. Largely through mime, he gathered the group around the table and one by one pointed to the words he wanted to use in a poem. Through the support and encouragement of his peers, he then arranged these words in a poem for his wife. The following prose was then typed up by the facilitator and presented by this participant to his wife on their anniversary:

> My love
>
> You are gorgeous.
>
> There is so much beauty in my life with you.
>
> I have visions of
>
> flowers
>
> forests
>
> earth
>
> petals
>
> gardens
>
> trees
>
> and the sun.
>
> I treasure you.
>
> I feel so much pleasure in my life with you.

Thus, in the face of significant cognitive and functional disability, the expression of his verse, as well as his treasured Self 3 persona as gifted poet and loving husband, was co-constructed and maintained by the group.

The power of group affirmation for Self 3 can also inspire confidence in participants to maintain their social personae in ways that support their engagement in, and communication with, the community. One woman, a lifelong health care advocate, joined a support group following her diagnosis. Within the group she shared stories and experiences and recognized remaining strengths and abilities. In a television interview, she convincingly acknowledged firmly held beliefs,

> People with Alzheimer's don't need to be pushed into a corner and forgotten—left to rot essentially. I'm looking after my own needs and being sort of pushy in making sure others understand those needs and I see myself as an advocate for people with Alzheimer's disease. (WGN TV News, Chicago 2003)

By not acquiescing to the dominant fictions about people with dementia and by readily speaking to the media, she was a powerful voice against stigma. With the help of others (support group, family, and health professionals) who validate her social persona and help to co-construct this self, she is not diminished in the face of a degenerative illness, but strengthened. She is creating her own reality and living 'as if' she is a person of worth and influence despite her diagnosis.

Marginalization and malignant social positioning

Stigmatizing negative images of dementia have often resulted in a dismissal of the discourse of persons with the disease and an invalidation of Self 3 expression. In their study of 17 individuals with mild dementia, Harris and Sterin (1999) examined social psychological interactions that either affirmed or devalued the sense of self. They described one man who was well aware of the labelling process that occurred when he was diagnosed with Alzheimer's. This resulted in him feeling 'pushed off to the side and no longer a part of society' (Harris and Sterin 1999, p. 254). Participants of one support group described a process of 'marginalization', which occurred outside their group whereby they felt on the 'margin' of relationships, often 'ignored, demeaned and minimized' (Group Members 2003). They expressed an on-going sense of devaluation within a variety of social, medical, and media contexts and felt that the support group was a 'sanctuary', where they could feel accepted, understood, and valued. Drawing from the concept of Kitwood's malignant social psychology (Kitwood 1997), Sabat (2001) describes this process of marginalization as 'malignant positioning' whereby the primary social personae of persons with dementia that is acknowledged by others is that of 'patient'. Persons are positioned 'as if' they are in an inferior status and their ability to express themselves in relationship is diminished. Pre-existing Self 3 personae that require the cooperation of others for affirmation is extinguished. In his communication with persons with dementia, Killick (1999) quotes one man who is aware of his suspicious feelings and tendency to isolate himself from others owing to perceived malignant positioning:

> I was the most happy-go-lucky fellow. I used to go down to the club and the pub and drink whisky. Now I don't want to go out. And I don't want anyone coming in here. I weigh people up. I'm watching them. In my position, the way that I feel, I don't have trust. And I never was like that. (Killick 1999 p. 160)

At the root of much malignant positioning or marginalization is an erosion of mutual communication and a depersonalization of relationship. A person with dementia risks being experienced as 'less than' by others and this can unintentionally result in objectification. In his discussion of types of relationships, Buber describes distinctions between 'I–Thou' relationships, which are engaged with 'the whole being' as distinct from 'I–It' relationships, which are more bounded and objectified. I–It relationships involve treating others impersonally, like objects. At this level, a person may hardly acknowledge the existence of another. A woman with Alzheimer's disease described the demeaning experience of being ignored:

> Some people when my husband and I are together, they refer to me as her, not us or them or you two. It's like I'm there but they can't see me . . . And it's so aggravating—I want to stick my tongue out and say, 'I have Alzheimer's but I can still comprehend and speak for myself most of the time'. (Alzheimer's Association 1994)

In contrast, I–Thou relationships involve engaging another as a unique, fully human individual. This is the highest, most complex form of communication that Buber calls 'being'. In his writings on client-centred therapy, Carl Rogers states,

> In those rare moments when a deep realness in one meets a deep realness in the other, a memorable 'I–Thou relationship' as Martin Buber would call it, occurs. Such a deep and mutual encounter does not happen often, but I am convinced that unless it happens occasionally, we are not living as human beings. (Rogers 1980, p. 19)

Discussing the importance of the quality of attention the listener gives a person with dementia, Killick quotes the gratitude expressed by one woman when she stated,

> I want to thank you for listening. You see, you are words. Words can make or break you. Sometimes people don't listen, they give you words back, and they're all broken, patched up. But you will permit me to say that you have the stillness of silence, that listens and lasts. (Killick 1999 p. 154)

In a compelling essay on his experience of living with Alzheimer's and his fears about being relegated to I–It relationships, Professor Richard Taylor (unpublished communication) writes,

> Twenty-five years ago Theologian Martin Buber was concerned that our society was moving from I–Thou relationships to I–It relationships. We were treating each other as if we were objects rather than human beings. This dynamic occurs in the relationship between caregivers and Alzheimer's patients. It is happening to me. As the weave of the lace curtain becomes thicker, as the wind blows away even the most recent of memories, people do not have time to explain to me over and over again, things that I don't understand. They tire of telling me the same things over and over. They cannot depend on me to remember the simplest of instructions. My conversations are punctuated with 'I forgot' and a long pause while I search for the right words. The trust relationship between husband and wife, father and son, grandfather and grandchild is breaking. Not because we do not love each other as much as in the past, in fact now it is even more. It is strained to the point of breaking by the symptoms of Alzheimer's disease.
>
> So, how do you relate to a Thou who does not act or think like Thou? Inevitably, I will become an It. I will look, smell, and walk like a Thou, but I will not think and act like a Thou. It's no one's fault this happens. It just does.

The Thous start lying to the It because they are tired of arguing with It. 'The car has been sold', when in reality it's in the garage and we just don't trust It to drive. 'The accountant is writing our checks' when in reality we just do not want to argue over the fact It cannot manage the family money. We still love Thou, but for its own safety and our own peace of mind we treat Thou as an It.

I don't have a solution. I don't want it to happen to me. I don't know how to avoid it.

Healing through meeting

If one examines the experiences of marginalization and malignant positioning in light of interpersonally and socially constructed I–It relationships, real confirmation of the humanity of persons with dementia requires change at both individual and collective levels. Through their interpersonal communication in support groups, participants affirm one another through their deep empathy and their capacity to enter one another's reality. Through valued I–Thou relationships they experience trust and interdependence; they communicate concern for, and reliance on, one another. In contrast to dominant social constructs whereby people with dementia are at risk of diminishment, each person is a member of equal standing in the support group setting. One may question whether these qualities are not functions of therapeutic groups in general and why this should be a distinguishing factor of dementia support groups. Although groups formed around other concerns or interests may establish norms of respectful dialogue, it is the very fact that this opportunity for human discourse is dramatically reduced in the lives of people with dementia that renders the group a place of refuge.

Support groups for people with dementia are not artificial utopias; they are environments where communication can occur in the context of authentic relationships that involve disagreement and honest rapport, where the self and the other are affirmed not only by the acknowledgment of common ground but also by the courage and safety afforded to express differences. 'Hypercognitive' (Post 1995) rapid-paced Western culture is replaced by a group culture co-constructed by the members—an environment that facilitates the opportunity to listen and to be listened to 'as if' there is nothing more important to do for that time. Comparing the culture within his support group to the dominant one outside the group, one man stated,

> Here we can go slow enough to honour each other's words and so I think that we may be the healthy ones in this manner and the other people are sick!

In forming his theory of 'individual psychology' at the turn of the twentieth century, German psychiatrist Alfred Adler was influenced by Vaihinger's philosophy of 'as if' and asserted that human development and personality are based in part on the meanings and fictions we create to shape and interpret the events of our lives. (For a general overview of Adler's work, see Ansbacher and Ansbacher (1956) and Mosak and Maniacci (1999).) Adler argued against the role of unconscious sexual and aggressive drives in favour of the significant influence social constructs play in psychological well-being. Individuals cannot be considered apart from their social environment. All important problems become social problems; all values are social values. Because we are embedded in social situations, the experiences of social interest and belonging are essential to well-being. Psychotherapist and Buber scholar Friedman (1985) concurs,

> No amount of therapy can be of decisive help if a person is too enmeshed in a family, community, or culture in which the seedlings of healing are constantly choked off and the attempts to restore personal wholeness are thwarted by the destructive elements of the system. (Friedman 1985, p. 3)

In his transcribed statements on finding meaning in his experience of Alzheimer's, psychologist Victor DiMeo spoke eloquently about the paradigm shift needed to facilitate respectful communication and meaning-making for people with dementia.

> Some people with Alzheimer's are happy because they have something good going on with them inside or with their family. A lot of them keep busy and that's important, but what I don't like is that we're getting more isolated from what people are doing and what they're like. A lot of people are being left like they are unknown. I'd like to help people find meaning instead of just sitting home and disappearing. I would like to be part of something where I belong and it has meaning to me. Margaret Mead told about somewhere where the culture celebrates people who have problems and gives them a feeling of expertise and knowledge and health whereas we in our society, we make them sick. If you're different and unusual, you're made to feel like there is something wrong with you. So I feel we're on the wrong track. We don't have to live with that. We should help people to feel good about who they are. Why don't we create a society in which these people are given some meaning in who they are? Let's not abandon them. So we have to change that to where people with Alzheimer's feel part of something regardless of whether they remember a name of something. (DiMeo 2003, pp.1–2)

For persons with dementia to find meaning and feel a part of something requires that we deconstruct the barriers we individually and collectively erect that separate our common humanity. If we are to imagine the real, if we are to honour the enduring selfhood of each person with dementia, we must humble ourselves as we confront the alienating influences of our own fictions. We must position people with dementia as our teachers and we must listen to them as if the well-being of humanity depended on our understanding.

Acknowledgement

This work was supported by the National Institute on Aging grant P50AG05131. Grateful acknowledgement is due to Darby Morhardt MSW, for her generous clinical and theoretical contributions to the essence of this chapter.

References

Alzheimer's Association (1994). *Alzheimer's Disease Inside Looking Out*. (Video produced by the Cleveland Area Chapter of the Alzheimer's Association, USA, by Post Production Classic Video Incorporated.)

Ansbacher, H. L., Ansbacher, R. R. (eds.) (1956). *The Individual Psychology of Alfred Adler*. New York: Harper Torchbooks.

Barlow, D., Snyder, L. (1997). A communication barrier. *Perspectives—A Newsletter for Individuals with Alzheimer's Disease*, **3**: 6.

Buber, M. (1958). *I and Thou*. New York: Charles Scribner.

Caron, W. (1997). Finding the person in dementia: experiences in a group for persons with Alzheimer's disease. In: *The Shared Experience of Illness—Stories of Patients, Families and their Therapists* (ed. S. McDaniel, J. Hepworth, W. Doherty), pp. 313–23. New York: Basic Books.

Davis, R. (1989). *My Journey into Alzheimer's Disease*. Wheaton, Illinois: Tyndale House.

Dennett, D. C. (1987). *The Intentional Stance*. Cambridge, MA: Bradford Books/ MIT Press.

DiMeo, V. (2003). Finding meaning in Alzheimer's. *Perspectives—A Newsletter for Individuals with Alzheimer's or a Related Disorder*, **9**: 1–2.

Duff, S. (1998). Alzheimer Scotland—action on dementia: younger person's group in Grampian, north east Scotland. *Early Alzheimer's*, **1**: 4–5.

Friedman, M. (1985). *The Healing Dialogue in Psychotherapy*. New York: Jason Aronson.

Gergen, K. J. (2001). *Social Construction in Context*. Newbury Park: Sage.

Goldsilver, P. M., Grunier, M. R. B. (2001). Early stage dementia group: An innovative model of support for individuals in the early stages of dementia. *American Journal of Alzheimer's Disease and Other Dementias*, **16**: 109–14.

Group Members (2003). Reflections of an early-stage memory loss support group for persons with Alzheimer's and their family members. *Alzheimer's Care Quarterly*, **4**: 185–8.

Harris, P. B., Sterin, G. J. (1999). Insider's perspective: defining and preserving the self of dementia. *Journal of Mental Health and Aging*, **5**: 241–56.

Hawkins, D., Eagger, S. (1999). Group therapy: sharing the pain of diagnosis. *Journal of Dementia Care*, **7**: 12–14.

Henderson, C. (1998). *Partial View—an Alzheimer's Journal*. Dallas: Southern Methodist University.

Holst, G., Hallberg, I. (2003). Exploring the meaning of everyday life for those suffering from dementia. *American Journal of Alzheimer's Disease and Other Dementias*, **18**: 359–65.

Killick, J. (1999). Dark head amongst the grey—experiencing the worlds of younger persons with dementia. In: *Younger People with Dementia—Planning, Practice and Development* (ed. S. Cox and J. Keady). London: Jessica Kingsley.

Kitwood, T. (1997). *Dementia Reconsidered*. Buckingham: Open University Press.

Morhardt, D., Johnson, N. (1998). Effects of memory loss support groups for persons with early stage dementia and their families. (Paper presented at Gerontological Society of America Annual Meeting.)

Mosak, H., Maniacci, M. (1999). *Primer of Adlerian Psychology—The Analytic, Behavioral, Cognitive Psychology of Alfred Adler*. Philadelphia: Taylor and Francis.

Phinney, A. (1998). Living with dementia from the patient's perspective. *Journal of Gerontological Nursing*, **24**: 8–15.

Post, S. (1995). *The Moral Challenge of Alzheimer's Disease*. Baltimore: Johns Hopkins University.

Rogers, C. (1980). *A Way of Being*. Boston: Houghton Mifflin.

Sabat, S. (2001). *The Experience of Alzheimer's Disease — Life through a Tangled Veil*. Oxford: Blackwell.

Sabat, S., Cagigas, X. (1997). Extralinguistic communication compensates for the loss of verbal fluency: a case study of Alzheimer's disease. *Language and Communication*, **17**: 341–51.

Sabat, S., Collins, M. (1999). Intact social, cognitive ability, and selfhood: a case study of Alzheimer's disease. *American Journal of Alzheimer's Disease*, **14**: 1–19.

Sabat, S., Harré, R. (1992). The construction and deconstruction of self in Alzheimer's disease. *Ageing and Society*, **12**: 443–61.

Seman, D. (2002). Meaningful communication throughout the journey—clinical observations. In: *The Person with Alzheimer's Disease—Pathways to Understanding the Experience* (ed. P Harris), pp. 134–49. Baltimore: Johns Hopkins.

Shotter, J., Gergen, K. J. (1989). *Texts of Identity*. London: Sage.

Snyder, L. (2000). *Speaking our Minds—Personal Reflections from Individuals with Alzheimer's*. New York: W. H. Freeman.

Snyder, L., Quayhaygen, M. P., Shepherd, S., Bower, D. (1995). Supportive seminar groups: An intervention for early stage dementia patients. *Gerontologist*, **35**: 691–5.

Temple, V., Sabat, S., Kroger, R. (1999). Intact use of politeness in the discourse of Alzheimer's sufferers. *Language and Communication*, **19**: 163–80.

Trabert, M. (1997). The DRC Club. *Perspectives—A Newsletter for Individuals with Alzheimer's Disease*, **2**: 7.

Vaihinger, H. (1925). *The Philosophy of 'as if'; a System of the Theoretical, Practical, and Religious Fictions of Mankind*. New York: Harcourt Brace.

WGN TV News, Chicago (2003). *The Buddy Program*.

Wittgenstein, L. (1958). *Philosophical Investigations*. Oxford: Blackwell.

Yale, R. (1995). *Developing Support Groups for Individuals with Early-Stage Alzheimer's Disease: Planning, Implementation, and Evaluation*. Baltimore: Health Professions Press.

Yeh, C., Truscott, T., Snyder, L. (2001). The benefits of a support group for persons with Alzheimer's disease. *Alzheimer's Care Quarterly*, **2**: 42–6.

17 From childhood to childhood? Autonomy and dependence through the ages of life

Harry Cayton

Alzheimer's; a second childhood

read the Headline on the BBC website (BBC 1999).

> People with Alzheimer's would be happier if treated as infants instead of adults researchers have said. Dr Barry Reisberg told the International Psychogeriatric Association that Alzheimer's patients lose physical and mental abilities in exactly the opposite order that children gain them. Eventually they return to an infant like state, he said.

When I read this report I reacted strongly; it seemed to patronize grown-up people. Nor did it match my own experience of people with dementia. But why was my resistance to seeing dementia as 'a second childhood' so strong? Suggesting that people with dementia are returning to childhood seemed to go against so much that progressive thinkers and researchers have been arguing for in dementia care; care that reinforces the autonomy, dignity, and agency of people with dementia—qualities we associate with adulthood. Nevertheless it is apparent that this metaphor for the frailties of age is universal. It appears in literature across cultures and epochs and it appears regularly in the way in which carers describe the person they care for. So I came to ask myself if the persistence of the metaphor of a second childhood had insights to give us into how to care for people with dementia and if a comparison of childhood and old age might help us to understand each better. This chapter is the result of that examination.

More than 2500 years ago, in the fifth century BC, the Greek playwright Aristophanes (1973) said, 'Men are children twice over', a sentiment echoed by Shakespeare (1951) in *Hamlet*, for instance, 'They say an old man is twice a child' (Act 2, Scene 2, 380–1). My title is taken from this quotation from a Native American Sioux, Black Elk:

> The seasons form a great circle in their changing and always come back again to where they were. The life of man is a circle from childhood to childhood.
> (Black Elk 1932)

We are accustomed in our age of progress to see life as linear, a line moving through time, developing and changing but constantly driving forward. If we are secular rationalists we may see the narrative of our lives as the onward march of the selfish gene, but for many with a religious view of the world the concept of the end stage of life being a restoration, a return to home, is a strong one. T. S. Eliot, the Christian poet wrote:

> We shall not cease from exploration
> And the end of all our exploring
> Will be to arrive where we started
> And know the place for the first time.   (Eliot 1942)

A sense of loss as well as of homecoming is fundamental to the Judeo-Christian view of the world and indeed to many religions. We have lost the innocence of Paradise and must journey through this vale of tears in the hope that through experience, or virtue, or faith, we shall ultimately regain it. In this cultural context the loss of self has particular resonance for us.

The sense of self has been a key concept in twentieth-century psychiatry and theories of child development. A secure and balanced sense of self, particularly in relation to the other, is understood to be necessary to mental health and social wellbeing. Alienation, disengagement, and loss of self have been powerful concepts in psychiatry, philosophy, and political theory.

The existentialist view, which developed out of the Second World War, inevitably values autonomy—self-governance—most highly as a human goal. Child development is seen, to a great extent, as a process for achieving this autonomy.

Indeed the life rituals, the *rites de passage* of many cultures, are symbolic of the achievement of autonomy and often legalize both the right to do 'adult' things (for instance, marrying without parental consent) and responsibility before the law for our actions. So becoming and being an adult are intimately linked to autonomy and responsibility.

This idea of the individual self as having a valid life separate from family and community is I think a late twentieth-century idea and particularly so in consumerist Western countries. In the UK, 31% of households contain a single person (Her Majesty's Stationery Office 2003). For many, though not of course for all, this is a desired choice. Yet it is a choice that would be as inexplicable as it is impossible for the peoples of many other societies.

Some people have suggested that the model of child development proposed by the French psychologist Jean Piaget (for example, Piaget (1962)) can be applied to people with dementia in reverse (Mahoney 2003). For example, Tessa Perrin suggests that,

> There has been considerable support over the years for the theory that the cognitive losses of dementia reflect (in an opposite direction) the cognitive gains of childhood.   (Perrin 1997)

I find this difficult. First, I am unable to find much serious literature that does give support to this theory though it has been discussed in a few journals.

Second, while it is true that some of the affective and functional behaviours of people with dementia and children are similar, the underlying neurological processes are totally different. We cannot deduce identical causes from phenomenological similarities.

For example, we know that in people with dementia, whether it be vascular dementia, Lewy body dementia, or Alzheimer's disease, brain cells are dying, chemical neurotransmitters are being disrupted, and brain volume is reducing. This is not the reverse of the process going on in children's brains. Children's brains change very little after birth in neurochemical or structural terms. Modern scanning techniques do show some neurological connections multiplying or changing in some specific areas of the brain, but these are not global changes as in dementia, nor are they the reverse of the route of damage. Brains in children are not growing in volume in the way that brains affected by Alzheimer's are shrinking. Babies' brains do develop, it seems, but one of the interesting things we know about babies' brains is how complete they are even at birth. They are already 'hard wired' (as it were) for crucial cognitive functions such as language, what Chomsky (1968) named deep structure. Plasticity—the capacity of the brain to change and create new neuronal connections—is most apparent in infants, but it is not lost entirely in older adults. Old brains can still make new neuronal connections. This is what enables people to recover, for example, from strokes or brain injury. So neurological decline in the brains of older people as a whole, or of people with dementia in particular, does not mirror the neurological development of babies.

Jean Piaget (Piaget 1962) described four phases of child development. Shakespeare of course had seven ages of man.[1] The psychologist Erik Erikson had eight (Erikson 1963), to which Naomi Feil (Feil 2002), creator of validation therapy, added a ninth to cover the old-old. It is common to talk of three stages of dementia. Dr Barry Reisberg (Reisberg *et al.* 2002) has described five. Tom Kitwood (Kitwood 1997) had no less than 17 aspects of malignant social psychology. There are four humours, twelve signs of the zodiac, and we have no idea how many angels might dance on the head of a pin.

I am not mocking these constructs but want, rather, to demonstrate that they are constructs: ways of codifying and describing human behaviour and the world we observe, of reducing complexity to enable us to see patterns and understand processes. These lists and tables are academic formulations, they are not facts and although they may represent part of the truth they are not the truth.

Piaget's four phases of child development are

(1) reflexive—responding to external stimuli (first month);

(2) sensory-motor—examining the world through sense and movement (until 2 years);

(3) representational—construction of mental symbols through parallel play (2–4 years);

(4) reflective—pattern, order, and rule enable social relationships through cooperative play (4–7 years).

Piaget validated these phases through experiment and observation and was careful to explain that they were complex. He showed that the driving force for child development is play.

Perrin (1997) asserts that people with dementia follow these stages in reverse. They can, therefore, be used with people with dementia to direct their care. For instance, using rule-based games, such as dominoes or quizzes, in the early stages of dementia; progressing, as cognitive powers decline, to sharing in fantasy worlds through conversation, music, and drama; and ultimately moving on to physical contact, as with small babies, through touching, rubbing, holding, and stroking.

I think this is sensible enough in relation to how we might modify our behaviour towards those with progressive dementia, but I find the underlying hypothesis difficult to believe. Piaget saw play as the behavioural building block of education. But according to Piaget, play is an instinctive and interactive response by a baby to its environment. If people with dementia were retracing their steps back into childhood, surely we would see spontaneous play behaviours. It is not that people with dementia cannot respond to playful behaviour by others; they sometimes do. It is that, unlike children, play in people with dementia does not seem to be spontaneous or regressive; we do not see them playing more as they get older. If people with dementia are 'playing backwards', because of changes in the brain, we would expect them to progress spontaneously from group to parallel and from parallel to solitary play. Observing the later stages of dementia it is possible to understand the rubbing or twitching of coloured threads or materials, which some, not all, people with dementia exhibit, not as childlike but as a common response to a restricted and deprived sensory environment as can be seen in any persons badly cared for in long-stay institutions whatever their age.

Reisberg (Reisberg *et al.* 1999, 2002) takes a functional approach to comparing child development with dementia. He has long been known for his descriptive tables of the 'stages' of dementia. In one he has produced in tabulated form a comparison of his 'stages of dementia' with some behaviours associated with child development. He calls this theory 'retrogenesis', which I take is 'growing backwards' in ancient Greek (Table 17.1).

There are four columns in each half of the table: reading up from the bottom in the case of child development and down from the top in the case of Reisberg's scales. If you look at the third column in each half of the table you will see a proposed progression of lost abilities. But are the behaviours of people with dementia really disease determined in this way? Reisberg's table seems to me to illustrate Kitwood's 'malignant social psychology'(Kitwood 1997). Such psychology, Kitwood argues, sees the symptoms of dementia as an inevitable, medically determined decline and reinforces that decline by our response to it. In fact, self-care, continence, mobility, and communication are all amenable to intervention, even to improvement with the right care and environment.

Table 17.1 Functional landmarks in normal human development and Alzheimer's disease*

Normal development approximate total duration: 20 years	Approximate age (approximate total duration: 20 years)	Approximate duration in development	Acquired abilities	Lost abilities	Alzheimer stage	Approximate duration (in Alzheimer's disease)	Develop mental age of patient
Adolescence	13–19 years	7 years	Hold a job	Hold a job	3 (incipient)	7 years	19–13 years (adolescence)
Late childhood	8–12 years	5 years	Handle simple finances	Handle simple finances	4 (mild)	2 years	12–8 years (late childhood)
Middle	5–7 years	2½ years	Select proper clothing	Select proper clothing	5 (moderate)	1½ years	7–5 years (middle childhood)
Early childhood	5 years	4 years	Put on clothes unaided	Put on clothes unaided	6a (moderately severe)	2½ years	5–2 years (early childhood)
	4 years		Shower unaided	Shower unaided	b		
	4 years		Toilet unaided	Toilet unaided	c		
	3–4½ years		Control urine	Control urine	d		
	2–3 years		Control bowels	Control bowels	e		
Infancy	15 months	1½ years	Speak 5–6 words	Speak 5–6 words	7a (severe)	7 years	15 months–birth (infancy)
	1 year		Speak 1 word	Speak 1 word	b		
	1 year		Walk	Walk	c		
	6–10 months		Sit up	Sit up	d		
	2–4 months		Smile	Smile	e		
	1–3 months		Hold up head	Hold up head	f		

I also wonder why the particular 'abilities' are selected for Reisberg's table. The idea of the 12-year-old stage of development progressing to the stage of 'holding a job' seems only there because it creates the illusion of a comparison with the person with mild dementia losing that capacity. It does not seem an appropriate descriptor for most of the 12 year olds I know.

The same applies to the comparison of language development with language decline. Although people with dementia do have progressive loss of language it seems far less systematic than this implies. Anyone involved in caring for a family member has, I am sure, observed moments of lucid communication in people in the last stage of dementia. Moreover, the pattern of language disorder varies considerably depending on the cause of the dementia. Vascular dementia and frontal lobe dementia may affect the language centres of the brain in very different ways.

To be precise, Reisberg's table refers only to 'Alzheimer's disease', but this raises the question as to why one particular cause of dementia should parallel normal child development while others do not. Indeed the comparison of Alzheimer's disease and normal human development in Reisberg's table does not really seem to me to be a comparison of like with like. Alzheimer's disease is not normal development. It is not an inevitable loss of function that comes with age in the way that acquiring new skills is an inevitable part of growing up. These losses may be associated with dementia, as they are with other chronic neurological conditions, but they are not normal aspects of ageing. One in five people over the age of 85 may have dementia but that means that four in five do not. Dementia is not inevitable in people in their 80s or 90s or even in those over 100 years of age.

Professor Tom Kirkwood (Kirkwood 1999) in his Reith lectures, *The End of Age*, argued that far from the frailties of old age being natural or inevitable they were the result of system failures. We are not genetically programmed to die, he says, our genes aim to live forever and could do so if disease were eliminated.

So there are a number of serious objections to the theory that dementia is a second childhood. We are not comparing like with like. We know that observed behaviours have complex links to underlying changes in the brain, they are also affected by the environment and by the way we interact with people, which can thus reinforce the expected behaviours. It is not clear either why we are comparing normal child development with loss of function in brains that are damaged rather than with normal ageing brains. Nor is it clear whether the exponents of the theory apply it to dementia as a syndrome or to Alzheimer's disease in particular.

Clearly I find both the observational and theoretical arguments for a second childhood seriously flawed. Might the concept help with appropriate care, as its supporters argue? I find accounts of the use of functional scales by caregivers dispiriting. As far as I can tell by reading carer's accounts on websites, seeing dementia as an ordered decline encourages a rigid, authoritarian, deficit-based approach to care. Caregivers anticipate and plan for the next failure, they concentrate on the loss of ability. They are indeed reinforced in all the ways of caring that Kitwood described as malignant: labelling, disempowerment, disparagement, and infantilization. Not surprisingly they describe their caring experience in negative terms as a constant battle against decline.

The most particular manifestation of the second childhood is in what is called 'doll therapy'. It is possible to buy life-sized dolls for people with dementia. To quote the sales pitch from a US website: 'When she looks at the doll the biggest smile you've seen comes across her face. The doll isn't a doll any more it is now a child. The proud owner has Alzheimer's and is 89 years old'. The Alzheimer's Association in the USA receives US$2.50 for every doll sold.

I can understand why some people like dolls. Lots of adults do and many of us cling onto a much-loved teddy bear or other soft toy long into adulthood. But I have to say, seeing the impact of my 2-year-old niece on a whole ward of people with severe dementia some years ago, that real children do the job better. But real children cannot always be pressed into service. So giving someone a doll if it makes them happy, less anxious, or more occupied seems like a creative way of caring, though a demeaning one.

What I have even more difficulty with is so-called 'doll therapy'. Ilse Boas (Boas 1998), a carer, suggested in the *Journal of Dementia Care* that a whole new range of 'therapies' are being invented to satisfy the needs of professionals rather than of people with dementia. It makes care workers feel important, she argued, to be providing 'therapy', but in fact the content is less important than 'the human interaction, the companionship of fellow human beings' (Boas 1998). Doll 'therapy' involves sessions in which dolls are 'introduced' to clients and used to stimulate memories of a rewarding life role, especially that of a parent and to act as a focus for reminiscence and conversation. But why only dolls? Why not toy therapy in general? Do men respond to dolls the way women do? Perhaps we could have some 'toy train therapy' for men.

I doubt that this 'doll therapy' is conscious play. I think it is deceit. The 'therapist' knows this is a doll. Do they share that fact with the client or do they pretend it is a baby? Are we colluding with a misunderstanding or are we asking people with dementia to collude with us? When children play make-believe, 'let's pretend' games they absolutely know it is pretend. That is why it is safe and liberating. It enables children to try out roles, take risks, and explore relationships. Real play is a conscious activity. Ask a child who is playing with a doll what they are doing and they may tell you matter-of-factly that they are going to the shops or that the doll is sick but they will also tell you that they are playing. A person with dementia does not do that I think.

One of the problems with the 'childhood' image is that it allows adults to take decisions on behalf of others and can be used to justify deceiving people 'for their own good'. In 2000, there was public debate in the UK about the ethics of giving people with dementia medicines without their knowledge or consent. Some of those who approved the practice said it was justified because people with dementia 'were like children' and we would not ask a child's permission to give them medicines.

In fact, good practice in childcare is moving increasingly towards reinforcing and supporting autonomy in children rather than making decisions on their behalf. So not only is the comparison with children inappropriate but the practice is not justified by that comparison.

I do think, however, acknowledging the childlike qualities that sometime seem apparent in people with dementia can help us to understand and respond to them effectively. I would like to make some different comparisons from those made by Reisberg.

Consider, for instance, the temper tantrums of a 3 year old. Could this be comparable with the catastrophic reaction that a person with dementia may experience? As an uncontrolled response to frustrated will and powerlessness in the face of an incomprehensible world they both seem explicable. Temper tantrums in children can be understood on a number of levels, but most simply as the painful response to discovering you are not the 'centre of the universe' and that you cannot always have your own way. As Christine Bryden (who has dementia) has said, 'a person with dementia responding abnormally to an abnormal situation can be regarded as normal' (personal communication). We can interpret such expressions as bursts of existential rage against a world you cannot control.

Consider, too, the role of food and eating. Children do not have to learn to eat—they do that from the moment they reach the breast—but an immense amount of time is spent by them and their parents in playing with food and accepting, rejecting, and giving food and thereby socializing the process of eating. Food and eating, or not eating, are also important in the lives of people with dementia: using inappropriate implements, eating with your hands, pushing food out of your mouth, tasting odd things, or eating strange combinations are all part of our relations to food in both childhood and dementia.

Eating behaviour in infants is primarily an expression of will and of control over the environment. I think we undervalue the importance of food and eating in dementia care. Having control over what you put into your mouth is an early autonomy we acquire and is almost the last we retain. Refusing to eat is a legitimate expression of self-determination. That is why feeding by tube is such an invasion of dignity and autonomy.

There is yet another sense in which accepting the childlike may help us care. The stress on choice and freedom, which rightly comes with person-centred care, may underestimate the need for safety and security. In a recent study of what quality meant to older people (Quereshi and Henwood 2000), feeling secure came high on their measures of well-being. In a thoughtful study from Sweden, Zingmark (2000) notes how many people with dementia in institutional care are preoccupied with talking about their parents and insist on going home. Leaving our childhood home is part of becoming an adult. Acknowledging the need for the feeling of home, of connectedness, of being safe, and of being cared for are all essential ingredients for the well-being of children and adults living in institutions.

Acknowledging the childlike in someone's behaviour does not require us to infantilize the whole person. Indeed the most harmful part of the second childhood metaphor is that it tricks us into responding to adults as though they were children, forcing them to respond in that way, generating powerlessness and dependency. A carer at a support meeting said about her husband, 'I knew when he was frightened as he came and stood next to me and held my hand like a child.' But then she concluded, 'People with dementia are not stupid, or children, or deaf, and shouldn't be treated as such.' Another carer describes her husband, a musician and music lecturer, as 'bouncing up and down like a baby' in time to the music. But his childlike pleasure does not lead her to conclude that he would prefer nursery rhymes to Mozart's Don Giovanni. These carers I think get the balance right.

If people with dementia are playful, respond to that playfulness. If they are fearful like a child, comfort them as you would a child. If they put themselves at risk, protect them. If they are lost, help them to find home. These things seem like empathy and good sense. They do not need to be dressed up as 'therapy' or justified by the construct of 'retrogenesis'.

So the objections to the idea of dementia as a second childhood are both scientific and moral. The science, unconvincingly in my view, tries to squeeze observed behaviours into an artificial construct, whether it is Piaget's theory of child development or Reisberg's retrogenesis. The consequence of such theories is to produce approaches to 'care' that reinforce dependence and decline, infantilizing and disabling people with dementia.

Childhood is indeed a compelling metaphor for some of the vulnerabilities and losses of old age. But it is just a metaphor. The sense of self and self-determination we have as adults is hard won through our childhood and adolescence. We should not take that away. We should aim to preserve it, not undermine it.

People with dementia are not going backwards; they are not going round in circles. They are going forwards, on a journey many of us will have to go on but none of us wants to make. They carry their childhood with them, as they do all the ages of their lives. We shall care best, and be cared for best, if we accept the child in all of us but never forget that, however disabled, we have grown into adults.

Endnote

1 See Bavidge, p. 46 in Chapter 2, this book.

References

Aristophanes (1973). [c.400 BC] *The Clouds* (trans. W. Arrowsmith). London: Penguin.

BBC (1999). *Health: Alzheimer's 'A Second Childhood'* (Available at http://newssearch.bbc.co.uk (accessed on 18 August 1999).)

Black Elk (1932). *Black Elk Speaks, Being the Life Story of A Holy Man of the Oglala Sioux* (ed. J. Neihardt, 1961) Lincoln: University of Nebraska Press.

Boas, I. (1998). Learning to be rather than do. *Journal of Dementia Care*, **6**: 13.

Chomsky, N. (1968). *Language and Mind*. New York: Harcourt Brace.

Eliot, T. S. (1942). *Little Gidding*. London: Faber and Faber.

Erikson, E. (1963). *Childhood and Society*. New York: Norton.

Feil, N. (2002). *V/F Validation; the Feil Method*. Cleveland: Edward Fiel.

Her Majesty's Stationery Office (2003). *Living in Britain 2001: Results of the 2001 General Household Survey*. London: Her Majesty's Stationery Office.

Kirkwood, T. (1999). *The Time of Our Lives: The Science of Human Ageing*. London: Weidenfield and Nicholson.

Kitwood, T. (1997). *Dementia Reconsidered; the Person Comes First*. Buckingham: Open University Press.

Mahoney, A. E. J. (2003). Age or stage appropriate? Recreation and the relevance of Piaget's theory in dementia care. *American Journal of Alzheimer's Disease*, **18**: 24–30.

Perrin, T. (1997). The puzzling, provocative question of play. *Journal of Dementia Care*, **3**: 15–17.

Piaget, J. (1962). *Play, Dreams and Imitation in Childhood*. London: Routledge.

Quereshi, H., Henwood, M. (2000). *Older People's Definitions of Quality Services*. York: Joseph Rowntree Foundation.

Reisberg, B., Kenowsky, S., Franssen, E. H., Auer, S. R., Souren, L. E. (1999). President's Report. Towards a science of Alzheimer's disease management: a model based upon current knowledge of retrogenesis. *International Psychogeriatrics*, **11**: 7–23.

Reisberg, B., Franssen, E. H., Souren, L. E., Auer, S. R., Akram, I., Kenowsky, S. (2002). Evidence and mechanisms of retrogenesis in Alzheimer's and other dementias; management and treatment import. *American Journal of Alzheimer's Disease and Other Disorders*, **17**: 202–12.

Shakespeare, W. (1951). *Hamlet*. In: *William Shakespeare: The Complete Works* (ed. P. Alexander), pp. 1028–72. London and Glasgow: Collins.

Zingmark, K. (2000). *Experiences Related to Home in People with Alzheimer's Disease*. Umea: Umea University.

18 Mind, meaning, and personhood in dementia: the effects of positioning

Steven R. Sabat

Introduction

The effects of dementia derive from a great deal more than the documented neuropathological changes in the brain of the person thus diagnosed and can be exacerbated or ameliorated to some degree by the way the person is positioned by others in the everyday social world. By analysing the nature of their social interactions with others we can readily come to appreciate that the ways in which the person with dementia is treated by others can have a profoundly positive or profoundly negative effect on (1) the subjective experience of the person with dementia; (2) the degree to which the person can display remaining intact cognitive abilities; (3) the ability of the person to meet the demands of everyday life; and (4) the quality of the person's social life and the meaning found in each day.

Umuntu ngumuntu ngabantu in Zulu conveys the idea that, 'a person is a person through others'. When we begin to think about the practical meaning of this Zulu idea as it applies to people with dementia, we are confronted with what might appear to be a disjunction in the way in which persons and their attributes are viewed socially and the way in which a person's attributes are understood in terms of biomedical approaches to disease. Likewise, we are also sensitized more deeply regarding the nature of the social interactions that occur between a person with dementia and healthcare professionals. In the biological model, the tendency is to attempt to understand the nature of a disease and its signs and symptoms by viewing the diagnosed person in isolation. Social interactions are limited to those with the examining clinicians. The effects of the disease are solely understood in terms of the physical and mental changes that have occurred in the person as a result of, in the case of dementia, neuropathology. Thus, by comparing the ways in which the person comported themselves in previous years to their present comportment, we note losses. Such losses are attributed to the neuropathology of the disease and these, taken together with the person's subjective complaints, are referred to as the signs and symptoms of the illness. Our biomedical conceptualization is further informed by the person's performance on neuropsychological tests and how that performance compares to that of age-matched, otherwise healthy, people. The ways in which family informants report the person's actions and discourse as being less coherent or efficient than previously are interpreted as being 'effects' caused by the illness alone. Thus, relatively little weight is given to the possibility that there might be psychosocial influences that also affect the person's actions. However, the medical literature has not always been antithetical to a broader approach.

It was Lipowski who noted that a disease is not to be understood as being separate from the afflicted person and that a person encompasses not only a biological organism but also the world of

> . . . feeling and symbolic activities in thought and language. Furthermore, he is a member of a social group with which he interacts. A concept of disease is incomplete unless it takes cognizance of these facts. How a person experiences the pathological process, what it means to him, and how this meaning influences his behaviour and interaction with others are all integral components of disease as viewed as a total human response.   (Lipowski 1969, p. 1198)

Taking this line of thinking further, Lipowski states rather pointedly,

> The response of the family caregiver and other meaningful people to the patient's illness or disability, to his communications of distress, and to his inability to perform the usual social roles may spell the difference between optimal recovery or psychological invalidism.   (Lipowski 1969, p. 1200)

Exactly what sorts of responses to the person with the diagnosis have the potential to promote recovery or 'psychological invalidism'? Before attempting to answer this question, it is important to recognize that in almost all types of dementia complete or near complete recovery is not currently possible. Still, even if we put aside the possibility of full recovery, optimal functioning, if attainable and sustainable for even a short time, could have profoundly positive effects not only on the person with dementia but also on their family and carers. That is to say, if it were possible to provide some interventions that might facilitate the ability of the person with dementia to communicate as effectively as possible, to interact with others as coherently as possible, and to sustain their sense of self-worth in the face of the effects of brain injury, it would be tremendously advantageous psychologically as well as financially to all concerned.

One purpose of the present chapter is to explore possible psychosocial interventions aimed at avoiding psychological invalidism. First, however, it is important to explore some subtle ways in which attitudes and actions of those deemed healthy may have untoward effects on the person with dementia.

Malignant positioning

Through the conversational exchanges that occur in the everyday social world, people often take for themselves, impose on others, and reject or accept positions that make their actions intelligible as social acts (van Langenhove and Harré 1999). Positions help to define, strengthen, or weaken a person's moral and personal attributes and help to create story-lines about persons. Through the process of positioning, people explain their own behaviour as well as that of others, so that to explain someone's actions in ways that emphasize the individual's negative attributes is to position that person in a potentially malignant way. Often in everyday life, when a person is negatively positioned by another, it is possible for that person to reject the positioning— social psychologists term this the fundamental attribution error (Ross 1977; Sabini *et al.* 2001). For example, Person A observes Person B trip and fall and comments to Person B that he or she is clumsy, thus positioning Person B as being ungainly. Person B might reject being positioned in this way and reply by saying, 'I'm not clumsy, I tripped and fell because I didn't see the crack in the pavement.' Hence, Person A has positioned Person B in a negative and potentially malignant way and attributed Person B's behaviour to something dispositional. Person B, however, rejects this initial positioning and, instead, attributes tripping and falling to the particular circumstances. Intimately related to the fundamental attribution error is the phenomenon known as the 'actor–observer bias'. Here, an observer attributes the behaviour (good or bad) to the disposition of the observed person; however, when we are the ones being observed (the 'actors'), we attribute our bad behaviour especially to situational factors (Jones and Nisbett 1972). The attribution of someone else's actions to their dispositions instead of to the situations they faced is not, however, universal among cultures—Miller has described a variety of different ways in which attributions are made (Miller 1984; Miller and Bersoff 1994).

Applying the notion of the fundamental attribution error to the case of a person with dementia, one can readily appreciate the predicament faced by the person thus diagnosed. The diagnosis itself sets the stage: actions taken by the person with dementia will usually be attributed to their disposition (in this case, the disease) rather than to the situation thay are facing. For example, the person with dementia is being given a battery of standard neuro-psychological tests and fails to answer questions that they know are relatively simple and that would have been easy to answer correctly in healthier times. They then begin to cry or perhaps becomes angry and adamantly refuse to go on with the testing, perhaps they even leave the room abruptly. Such a reaction is commonly labelled 'catastrophic' or an example of 'emotional lability', both of which are considered to be symptoms of dementia. Lost in this interpretation is the fact that the person reacting this way (1) is aware that there is a difference between what they can do now as compared to their previous abilities; (2) has evaluated the meaning of that difference correctly as being frightfully negative; (3) is reacting appropriately for the most part to the loss that is thereby evidenced; and (4) is therefore a person whose behaviour is driven by the meaning of the situation and is thus a 'semiotic subject' (Shweder and Sullivan 1990).

Often in everyday social interaction, it is quite simple for a person to reject being positioned in a negative or undesirable way, but if the person being positioned negatively happens to have dementia, the ability to reject such positioning and reposition themselves in a positive way may be compromised owing to word-finding problems, syntactical problems, and the like. Thus, what is initially negative positioning can become malignant, or dangerous, because (1) the behaviour of the person with dementia is increasingly inter-preted in defective terms; (2) the person thus positioned is then treated as being defective so that 'malignant social psychology' ensues (Kitwood 1998; Kitwood and Bredin 1992); (3) the person can then come to see themselves in progressively more defective terms and lose a sense of self-worth; (4) if their behaviour is negatively affected by the ways in which they are treated by others, this possibility may go unnoticed and will continue; and (5) the dysfunctional relationship will continue to have a negative impact on the person with dementia and the results of that impact will be attributed to the disease and may generate a vicious cycle whereby the effects of the dysfunc-tional relationship are perceived as evidence validating the original negative positioning.

To illustrate the process, let us examine the following (sadly all too common) scenario. The person with dementia and the primary carer are meeting with a healthcare professional and the carer and professional discuss the person with dementia as if they were not present, illustrating a form of malignant social psychology called 'ignoring'. Suppose further that the topic being discussed is one or another deficit displayed by the person with dementia and the carer's negative reaction to the deficit. Sometime after the meeting is over, the person with dementia expresses anger towards the carer. If the carer then describes the displayed anger as 'irrational hostility', another form of malignant social psychology is occurring, namely 'labelling'. What is prob-lematic in this situation is that the two individuals deemed as being healthy would rarely, if ever, talk about another otherwise healthy person in that way if the person being discussed were present, for it would be understood that to do so would be potentially humiliating.

Why, then, are the carer and professional behaving disrespectfully towards the person with dementia? Surely it is unlikely to be intentional. What I propose here as an explanation entails the following train of interpretive thinking: The person with dementia is initially positioned malignantly due to defects that result directly from neuropathology, such as damage to the hippocampus, which makes the recall of recent events problematic. Also at play are cultural stereotypes about people with dementia that emphasize aberrant behaviour and defective cognitive function, such that persons with the diagnosis are viewed and defined primarily in defective terms. Now, in the interview situation described above, it is tacitly assumed to one or another degree by the healthy interlocutors that it is not problematic to talk about the person with dementia in negative ways as if the person were absent because the person with dementia is (1) unaware of what is transpiring; and (2) if not unaware, will soon forget what was said; and so (3) the person will not be affected negatively by unacceptable and insensitive comments. Under these conditions, when the person with dementia displays anger toward the carer, the carer can see no logical reason for the anger and thus concludes that the anger is due to dementia, for 'irrational hostility' is considered to be a symptom of dementia. That the anger is labelled 'irrational' as opposed to 'righteous indignation' follows directly from the initial malignant positioning and the dysfunctional treatment accorded the person with dementia on the basis of that positioning.

Let us now explore and analyse some instances of malignant positioning as they occur in the professional literature as well as in the lay public press.

> Patients with Alzheimer's disease experience fear throughout their disease course. As they decline and lose capacities, part of what is also lost is the ability to articulate their fears and cope with them. Essentially, what is lost is the person's ability to self-soothe if fears become overwhelming. This is akin to the behaviour seen in infants who do not have the neurological and cognitive capacities to overcome their unrealistic fears.   (Raia 1999, p. 33)

Although it is quite doubtful that the author intended to do so, it is the case that the person with dementia is being positioned herein as being akin to an infant and burdened by unrealistic fears. The fact that a healthy person, for one or another reason, does not understand the basis of fears as experienced by a person with dementia does not mean those fears are 'unrealistic' to the person with dementia. An individual's private experience is quite real to them (Laing 1965) and to deny that reality is unhelpful in any therapeutic or supportive sense. Furthermore if, as the author states above, the person with dementia has lost the ability to articulate their fears, it is more than difficult for another person to assess those unarticulated fears as being unrealistic. It is also not necessarily the case that the person with dementia has lost the ability to articulate their fears. There is evidence that with the aid of conversational facilitation, such as indirect repair, people with dementia who are thought to be unable to communicate can indeed convey their thoughts and feelings (Sabat 1991).

Malignant positioning can lead to the creation of story lines that confirm the initial positioning of the person in question. The following example is illustrative:

> . . . nurses reported that patients receiving validation therapy were less physically and verbally aggressive, less depressed, but more nonphysically aggressive in terms of increased wandering, pacing, and repetitive movement. (Benjamin 1999 p.124)

Exactly what makes the actions described above examples of aggressive behaviour, even if 'non-physically aggressive', is not at all clear. People might walk about or pace or engage in repetitive movement for many different reasons, including having nothing else to do or feeling anxious and unable to sit still. Neither of these reasons necessarily involves aggression toward anyone else. Perhaps when people with diagnoses of dementia engage in such actions, staff members find it more difficult or frustrating to deal with the situations, or are possibly annoyed by them, but that does not mean that the people with dementia are being 'non-physically aggressive' toward anyone. Still, it remains true that such behaviour is interpreted this way because, at least to some degree, the staff have positioned the people thus on the basis of their being 'dementia patients' who live in a nursing home. Hence, any actions of such people are quite easily construed as being pathological.

Another example of malignant positioning may be found in the commentary regarding a situation in which staff members kept track of the moods of military veterans who had dementia and who were participating in a programme developed for them.

> Staff members are amazed at the relaxed manner and sometimes candor with which the men talk to each other about their forgetfulness and difficulty with their everyday problems. (Maddox and Burns 1999, p. 69)

The type of malignant positioning occurring here may be called 'implicit malignant positioning' in that it is in the amazement of the staff members that we discover the way in which they had positioned the veterans with dementia in the first place. That is, the staff members expected in advance that these veterans would not share their concerns with one another. Their expectations were not met, but were disconfirmed soundly. It may be that such expectations were developed on the basis of the staff members' previous experiences with people with dementia, but it remains an open question as to whether or not such previous experiences were themselves affected by the way in which people with dementia were then implicitly positioned! In other words, if the staff members had not experienced the disconfirmation of the way in which they had implicitly positioned the men with dementia, would the same staff members interact with these men with dementia in such a way as to encourage discussion of such problems and sympathize with such expressions? In this way, the expectations of others, based on the way they position people with dementia, can and do have an effect on the behaviour of the latter. (An alternative explanation is likewise possible in that perhaps the staff members' amazement occurred because they had positioned men in general as not being willing or able to discuss their problems in a relaxed manner. But here, too, we see the application of yet another erroneous stereotype—men do not discuss their feelings openly—and the positioning that is involved.)

What I should like to propose is that when carers position people with dementia in malignant ways, what can often follow is behaviour referred to earlier as 'malignant social psychology'. The forms of behaviour engaged in by healthy carers fall into the category of malignant social psychology if the behaviour in question (1) constitutes an assault on the personhood of individuals with dementia and (2) produces negative reactions such as anger and depression in response to what can be seen as instances of humiliation and embarrassment. One would not intentionally or maliciously act in a way that would humiliate another person, so why would healthy others engage in such behaviour toward people with dementia? One possible reason is that the persons with dementia have been positioned in advance so as to create story lines about them in which they are deemed incapable of a level of understanding that would be required to know that they are being treated in a humiliating or embarrassing way. Another possible reason is that persons with dementia are deemed incapable of remembering that they had, in fact, been treated in a humiliating or embarrassing way. That these possibilities are not merely remote hypotheses can be seen in the following example taken from the popular press.

In an article called 'My father's brain: what Alzheimer's takes away', author Jonathan Franzen describes an episode in which he, his wife, and his mother took his father (who had dementia) home for Thanksgiving dinner and then brought his father back to the nursing home where the father lived. Franzen claimed in advance of his discussion of this episode that '. . . a change in venue no more impressed my father than it does a one-year-old' (Franzen 2001, p. 89) and

> . . . the patient himself has lost the cerebral equipment to experience anything as a repetition . . . if your short-term memory is shot, you don't remember, as you stoop to smell a rose, that you've been stooping to smell the same rose all morning . . . Hence, the ghost-like apparition of the middle-stage patient who continues to walk and feed herself even as she remembers nothing from hour to hour . . . Neurologically speaking, we're looking at a one-year old. (Franzen 2001, p. 86)

What follows in the story is quite remarkable, for when about to re-enter the nursing home following the dinner at home with his loved ones, the father is said to have remarked, 'Better not to leave, than to have to come back.'

Here we appreciate that the father's statement is a striking contradiction to the author's previous assessment that his father would be unable to appreciate a change of venue any more than would a 1-year-old child. Indeed, the father not only appreciated the change of venue, but also made an extraordinary evaluative statement.

How Franzen attempts to make sense of this apparent contradiction is an excellent example of how a carer, having already positioned the person with dementia in a malignant way, will weave together a story line that will attempt to preserve the accuracy of the original malignant positioning. This is achieved by providing an account or explanation for the apparent contradiction between the statement made by his father and the original malignant positioning, which is deemed to highlight his father's pathology. The author goes on to discuss his father's 'self' and comments that it is mostly correct that the person with dementia loses their 'self' long before the death of the body. In light of this belief, the author asserts that there was in his father a 'bodily remnant of his self discipline . . . when he pulled himself together for the statement he made . . . outside the nursing home' (Franzen 2001, p. 89). The idea that it was a 'bodily remnant of his [father's] self-discipline' that allowed the father to make the insightful statement ignores or, at the very least, diminishes the possibility that his father had retained the mental/cognitive ability to make such an evaluative statement. To the author, it was not a deliberately provided opinion or a report of a subjective experience that his father offered, but rather something that emerged from a 'bodily remnant', or some reflexive, knee-jerk reaction stemming from what was a 'remnant' of his father's self-discipline (whatever that means). By diminishing the significance of his father's statement, the author is able to maintain his original malignant positioning of his father, even though his father's most 'consistently near-coherent theme [of conversation that night] was his wish to be removed from "this hotel" [the nursing home] and his inability to understand why he couldn't live in a little apartment and let my mother take care of him' (Franzen 2001, p. 89).

To acknowledge that his father's rather astute, even poignant, observation required quite a significant level of mental functioning, would mean that Franzen would have to recognize that his malignant positioning of his father was itself incorrect in the first place: his father was, in fact, powerfully impressed by a change of venue. The degree of contradiction in Franzen's account is shown by the unlikelihood of there ever being a 1 year old who could possibly make such a statement.[1]

In a final example of malignant positioning, the author describes sorting through his father's papers and other belongings after his father went to live in a nursing home:

> I helped my mother sort through his desk (it's the kind of liberty you take with the desk of a child or a dead person). (Franzen 2001, p. 89).

Now, in addition to positioning his father as 'neurologically' a 1 year old and 'a child', he has positioned his father as, in essence, a dead person. Once again, this sort of positioning is malignant because it sets the stage for treatment that might be described accurately as 'malignant social psychology', for such treatment depersonalizes the individual with dementia, leads to a diminished sense of self-worth, and essentially pours salt on an already open wound. Ironically, the second part of the title of Franzen's article, 'What Alzheimer's takes away', is an example of how a carer fails to see that, to a significant degree, it is not what Alzheimer's alone takes away, but what is taken away by carers too when they malignantly position the person with dementia. There is some preliminary evidence that this sort of malignant positioning begins even in the mild to moderate stages of the disease (Sabat *et al.* 2004), so by the time a person is in the moderate to severe stages, malignant positioning and its effects already may have become a way of life. It must be reiterated, though, in the words of Kitwood,

The strong word malignant signifies something very harmful, symptomatic of a care environment that is deeply damaging to personhood . . . The term malignant does not, however, imply evil intent on the part of caregivers; most of their work is done with kindness and good intent. The malignancy is part of our cultural inheritance. (Kitwood 1997, p. 46)

An alternative to malignant positioning

In the foregoing examples of malignant positioning I have pointed out the faulty reasoning that they entail and would suggest that such errors of positioning persons with dementia are commonplace. I have attempted to show that such positioning is the foundation of malignant social psychology, which can have profoundly negative effects. I shall now turn to an alternative, more constructive way of approaching and interacting with people with dementia.

One might begin by recognizing that many aspects of the cognitive life of people with dementia survive into the moderate to severe stages of the disease. These cognitive abilities include (amongst others) the ability to behave on the basis of the meaning of situations, to experience a range of emotions, to experience and seek to avoid embarrassment, to feel pride and seek to maintain self-respect, to feel concern for others, to communicate effectively with facilitation by others (for a more detailed account, see Sabat 2001), and to display at least implicit short-term and long-term memory (Grosse *et al.* 1990; Heindel *et al.* 1989; Knopman and Nissen 1987). All these aspects of cognitive function are, of course, exhibited by people without dementia and are considered to be important in everyday life. In these ways, people with dementia and people without dementia have much in common, to be sure; they also share a common humanity.

On the basis of all these instances of commonality, it follows that the way in which we relate to people with dementia should be, in the most important respects, no different from the considerate, caring, and honourable ways in which we relate to other people. That is to say, we would do well to avoid being so quick to interpret behaviour as being pathological simply because it is being displayed by someone with a diagnosis of one or another form of dementia. Thus, if a person objects to being ignored, patronized, embarrassed, or humiliated, we should recognize the reaction as 'righteous indignation' instead of 'irrational hostility' or 'emotional lability', because the person with dementia has the ability to experience embarrassment, humiliation, and the pain of being ignored. If a person did not react negatively to being treated in these ways, we would be rather quick to be concerned that the person was lacking in self-respect or self-worth or was without the necessary cognitive abilities to understand what was transpiring. The man with dementia who cannot find a particular possession and accuses others of having stolen it is not necessarily paranoid, but most certainly has a problem with recall. The woman with dementia who cries inconsolably may not be exhibiting a 'catastrophic reaction' but may be reacting quite appropriately to the losses that she has sustained and the correctly understood meaning of those losses in light of the goals, desires, and dispositions that formed much of the fabric of previous decades of adult life. The person who walks back and forth over and over again through the halls of a day centre or residential home may not be engaged in 'irrational wandering', but may have nothing else to do and would prefer not to sit still ('aimlessly') in one place for long periods of time. Then, too, the person might be anxious and need to move around, even pace back and forth—much the way many people without dementia do when they are upset about something and cannot sit still.

It would appear logical, therefore, that carers of all types, formal as well as informal, should refrain from positioning people with dementia in malignant ways. For this is precisely how we, who are deemed healthy, expect to be treated, as befits our shared humanity. One possible way to avoid engaging in malignant positioning and malignant social psychology is to consider the meaning of a simple, yet profound, statement uttered by the late actor Christopher Reeve. Following the accident that left him paralysed from the neck down, Reeve considered suicide, but changed his mind and instead devoted the rest of his life not just to trying to recover, but to supporting research aimed at ameliorating the effects of spinal cord injuries. When asked what led to this rather striking change of mind, he said, 'I had to stop being a patient and start being a person.' Clearly, being a person led him to live his remaining years meaningfully, inspiring many to join his cause as well as inspiring the deep admiration and respect of countless others. In Reeve's mind, being a 'patient' would not have allowed him to live his remaining years in ways that were even remotely as meaningful. Reeve was paralysed but was not otherwise prevented from articulating his thoughts as well as, or perhaps better than, he had in the years prior to his accident. Perhaps that fact allowed him to reject being positioned by others and by himself as being a 'patient' and instead allowed him to reposition himself as a person.

For the person with one or another form of dementia, the situation is often quite different. Word-finding problems, syntactical problems, and losses in the ability to retrieve information from memory via recall, along with the frustration and possible anger and sadness in response to such problems, may all prevent the person from articulating their thoughts fluently. Thus the person with dementia may lose the ability to reject malignant positioning and then to reposition themselves in a more favourable way. By observing and understanding this complex predicament, we come to appreciate the vulnerability of the person with dementia and the striking importance of others in their social milieu. We appreciate that many people with dementia are semiotic subjects, given that the meaning of the situations they confront drives their behaviour. All this redounds to the fact that to be positioned malignantly can and does mean something to people with dementia and often prevents them from living a life that is as positive and meaningful as it otherwise might be.

Generalizing the 'patient' label

All too often, people who are not physicians or other medical personnel refer to people with dementia as 'patients'—as if 'patient' denoted their social identity in every social situation. It is clear that in relation to one's physician or nurse or dentist, one is a 'patient'. It should be just as clear that, in relation to everyone else in the world, a person with dementia is a person who can have a variety of valued social identities, as is the case with people who have heart conditions or paralysis or some other ailment. Yet, in the case of people with dementia, we find, as Hockey and James (1993) point out, that the metaphors used to describe them most often are those that emphasize their helplessness and dependency in such a way as to imply that these attributes are the direct results of physical illness and not linked at all to the ways in which they are treated or to the expectations of those who provide care. To restrict a person's social identity to 'the patient' or 'the burdensome patient' is to put them at risk of malignant positioning and the ensuing treatment, malignant social psychology, that leads to depersonalization and a loss of self-worth, whilst simultaneously obscuring the person's remaining intact cognitive and social abilities. Viewing a person with dementia primarily, if not solely, as 'the patient' stems directly from the dominance of neuropathological explanations of dementia and the tendency of those who proffer such explanations to pay scant attention to the social contexts in which people with dementia live (Bender and Cheston 1997). It has been noted, for example, that among the situations confronted by people with dementia is that of relocation and the related emotional and cognitive effects thereof (Anthony *et al.* 1987). And still, we find a relative absence of attention to the effects of relocation to institutions on the cognitive and linguistic abilities of people who have experienced this significant change in their lives (Bender and Cheston 1997), as if such momentous social changes are of little consequence. It is the case, however, as has been noted with more and more frequency in the past decade, that the individual with dementia and the kind of meaning to be experienced in the day-to-day life of that person, is affected as much by their social world as by the neuropathological changes in the brain (Kitwood 1997; Snyder 1999; Killick and Allan 2001; Sabat 2001; Harris 2002; Hubbard, *et al.* 2003). One way to begin to improve the lives of people with dementia (and those of their carers as well) is to recognize that such persons are, if given the proper kinds of support, able to enjoy positive, valued social identities far beyond the restrictions imposed by that of 'patient'.

Conclusion

From the outset of this book, we began to understand that,

> There are biological structures within which we think and act and there are
> social structures which determine the options we take ourselves to have.
> (Chapter 2, by Bavidge, p. 42)

Thus, the neuropathology involved with dementia sets one kind of limit on
what a person can experience and the social situations that the person faces can
set still other limits. Bavidge suggests that,

> We should think of old age as offering alternative rather than impaired ways
> of experiencing life. (Chapter 2, by Bavidge, p. 49)

Surely, the limits set by the neuropathological and social constraints of
dementia provide the foundation for either an alternative or an impaired way
of life. Perhaps, it is more accurate to say that dementia can lead to both kinds
of life, each in its own way. Yet it is primarily, but not solely, in the social
domain that a large number of possibilities exist for minimizing impairment at
the present time.

In order to realize those possibilities for minimizing impairment, it would
seem fruitful to examine the social interactions that occur between people with
dementia and their carers, so as to minimize or eliminate the instances of
malignant social psychology that lead to the depersonalization of the
individual with dementia. In order to do so it would seem fruitful, likewise, to
explore the thought processes that carers bring to those interactions.
Specifically, an examination of the ways that carers position people with
dementia would seem in order, for to reduce or eliminate malignant positioning can lead, in principle, to a reduction or elimination of the ways in which
the person with dementia is subsequently depersonalized. As Kitwood notes,
among the qualities that the carer must bring to the interaction are 'recognition', which is 'an open and unprejudiced attitude, free from tendencies to
stereotype or pathologize' (Kitwood 1997, p. 119) and 'validation', which
occurs when the carer

> goes beyond his or her own frame of reference, with its many concerns and
> preoccupations, in order to have an empathic understanding of the other . . .
> (Kitwood 1997, p.120)

It is in the social dynamics of everyday life beyond the neuropathological
processes in their brains that people with dementia can be supported in, or
experience assaults on, their personhood. In order to experience depersonalization in the ways that stem from malignant positioning and malignant social
psychology, there must be in existence a person who has that experience. The
person in question may not be able to recall the date, day of the week, year,
season, or month, to perform rudimentary mathematical operations, or to
speak without mispronouncing some words or failing to recall others. The
person might not be able to speak in syntactically correct sentences or spell
rather simple words correctly, to get dressed efficiently (or at all), or use eating
utensils properly. Indeed, the person in question might, in an attempt to

maintain their dignity or to avoid humiliation (as opposed to being apathetic), withdraw from social situations by not speaking or not attempting to do things that used to be easy to do, but that are now very difficult. They may, on the other hand, try to do something around the home to be of help to the primary carer and, as one carer reported about his wife, 'she purposefully puts things away in random places' and the person may, when confronted with failure, become sullen, angry, or tearful for what is often described as 'no apparent reason' or have a 'catastrophic reaction'. They may seem on edge and agitated and when asked why, might reply by saying, 'I don't know'.

On the other hand, the person in question might attend a day centre where they might be observed to engage in conversation with another person with dementia, but closer examination of what is being said by each of the interlocutors reveals that there is little to nothing of coherence regarding the comments that are being uttered. Yet, each of the partners in conversation seems animated, seems to be enjoying the other's company, and seems to be relating in very warm and solicitous ways to the other. They are clearly communicating something of value to one another even if a staff member who is eavesdropping on the conversation does not understand what is being communicated by the words being exchanged. One of the interlocutors might suddenly see someone in a wheelchair trying with apparent difficulty to exit the room, get up to help the person through the doorway, and then return to where they were previously sitting and continue the conversation.

In each of the above situations, there is a person with dementia engaging the social world in one or another way, which indicates the ability to evaluate, interpret, and derive meaning from the situations at hand. In other words, there is a person with dementia who is also acting in ways that indicate a semiotic ability, such that the actions taken by the person are driven by meaning. It is when the carers fail to see or to look for the meaningful nature of the actions taken by persons with dementia that we find the beginnings of depersonalization in malignant positioning. Indeed, it is when carers assume in advance that there *can be* no meaningful action authored by a person with dementia that we find that the process of depersonalization has already begun. In a sense, then, despite all sorts of losses in this or that cognitive function, the person with dementia is just that: a person who shares a significant degree of common ground with others who may or may not have a diagnosis of dementia. And, as a person, the individual with dementia must be treated in the same dignified way that would be appropriate if they did not have the diagnosis and did not experience all of the losses that result directly from neuropathology.

We who are deemed healthy and those of us who are diagnosed with dementia are part of the same human family. In this chapter I have attempted to show that from the philosophical, psychological, and interpersonal viewpoints, people with dementia still possess meaning-making abilities and personhood and can experience a variety of important psychological dimensions of life and that this experience may be enhanced as a result of the quality of their interactions with others. It is the case, however, that the degree to which persons with dementia can be recognized as having those abilities and qualities depends a great deal on the ways in which they are positioned, understood, and subsequently treated by others. Indeed, in the words of Snyder, 'we must listen to them as if the well-being of humanity depended on our understanding' (Chapter 16, by Snyder, p. 274) for our own quality of life is intimately connected to that of the people with dementia with whom we are connected in formal as well as in informal relationships. To the extent that our understanding of and respect for the personhood and experience of people with dementia are deepened, we likewise find greater depth and fulfillment in our own lives. So, in a very real sense, the notion of *umuntu ngumuntu ngabantu*, a person is a person through others, applies not only to the person with dementia, but also to those who interact with and care for them. For, in the words of McCurdy (1998), '. . . the awareness of a deeply shared humanity . . . might permit caregiver and (nursing home) resident to become means of grace (Niebuhr 1963) to each other.'

Endnote

1 For further discussion of this theme see Chapter 17 of this book, by Cayton.

References

Anthony, K., Proctor, A. W., Silverman, A. M., Murphy, E. (1987). Mood and behaviour problems following the relocation of elderly patients with mental illness. *Age and Ageing*, **16**: 355–65.

Bender, M. P., Cheston, R. (1997). Inhabitants of a lost kingdom: A model of the subjective experiences of dementia. *Ageing and Society*, **17**: 513–32.

Benjamin, B. (1999). Validation: A communication alternative. In: *Enhancing Quality of Life in Advanced Dementia* (ed. L. Volicer and L. Bloom Charette), pp. 107–25. Philadelphia, Pennsylvania: Brunner/Mazel.

Franzen, J. (2001). My father's brain: What Alzheimer's takes away. *The New Yorker*, **September 10**: 81–91.

Grosse, D. A., Wilson, R. S., Fox, J. H. (1990). Preserved word-stem completion priming of semantically encoded information in Alzheimer's disease. *Psychology and Aging*, **5**: 304–6.

Harris, P. B. (2002). *The Person with Alzheimer's Disease: Pathways to Understanding the Experience*. Baltimore: Johns Hopkins University Press.

Heindel, W. C., Salmon, D. P., Shults, C. W., Walicke, P. A., Butters, N. (1989). Neuropsychological evidence for multiple implicit memory systems: A comparison of Alzheimer's, Huntington's, and Parkinson's disease patients. *Journal of Neuroscience*, **9**: 582–7.

Hockey, J., James, A. (1993). *Growing Up and Growing Old: Ageing and Dependency in the Life Course*. London: Sage.

Hubbard, G., Tester, S., Downs, M. (2003). Meaningful social interactions between older people in institutional care settings. *Ageing and Society*, **23**, 99–114.

Jones, E. E., Nisbett, R. E. (1972). The actor and the observer: divergent perceptions of the cause of behaviour. In: *Attribution Perceiving the Causes of Behaviour* (eds. E. E. Jones, D. E. Karouse, H. H. Kelley, R. E. Nisbett, S. Valins, and B. Weiner), pp. 79–94. Morristown, New Jersey: General Learning Press.

Killick, J., Allan, K. (2001). *Communication and the Care of People with Dementia*. Buckingham: Open University Press.

Kitwood, T. (1997). *Dementia Reconsidered: the Person Comes First*. Buckingham: Open University Press.

Kitwood, T. (1998). Toward a theory of dementia care: ethics and interaction. *Journal of Clinical Ethics*, **9**: 23–34.

Kitwood, T., Bredin, K. (1992). Towards a theory of dementia care: Personhood and well-being. *Ageing and Society*, **12**: 269–87.

Knopman, D. S., Nissen, M. J. (1987). Implicit learning in patients with probable Alzheimer's disease. *Neurology*, **37**: 784–8.

Laing, R. D. (1965). *The Divided Self*. Baltimore, Maryland: Penguin Books.

Lipowski, Z. J. (1969). Psychosocial aspects of disease. *Annals of Internal Medicine*, **71**: 1197–206.

Maddox, M. K., Burns, T. (1999). Adapted work program: A sheltered workshop for patients with dementia. In: *Enhancing Quality of Life in Advanced Dementia* (ed. L. Volicer and L. Bloom-Charette), pp. 56–79. Philadelphia, Pennsylvania: Brunner/Mazel.

McCurdy, D. B. (1998). Personhood, spirituality, and hope in the care of human beings with dementia. *Journal of Clinical Ethics*, **9**: 81–91.

Miller, J. G. (1984). Culture and the development of everyday social explanation. *Journal of Personality and Social Psychology*, **46**: 961–78.

Miller, J. G., Bersoff, D. M. (1994). Cultural influences on the moral status of reciprocity and the discounting of endogenous motivation. *Personality and Social Psychology Bulletin*, **20**: 592–602.

Niebuhr, H. R. (1963). *The Responsible Self: An Essay in Christian Moral Philosophy*. New York: Harper and Row.

Raia, P. (1999). Habilitation therapy: A new starscape. In: *Enhancing Quality of Life in Advanced Dementia* (ed. L. Volicer and L. Bloom-Charette), pp. 21–37. Philadelphia, Pennsylvania: Brunner/Mazel.

Ross, L. (1977). The intuitive psychologist and his shortcomings: distortions in the attribution process. In: *Advances in Experimental Social Psychology: Volume 10* (ed. L. Berkowitz), pp. 172–214. New York: Academic Press.

Sabat, S. R. (1991). Facilitating conversation via indirect repair: A case study of Alzheimer's disease. *Georgetown Journal of Languages and Linguistics*, **2**: 284–96.

Sabat, S. R. (2001). *The Experience of Alzheimer's Disease: Life through a Tangled Veil*. Oxford: Blackwell.

Sabat, S. R., Napolitano, L., Fath, H. (2004). Barriers to the construction of a valued social identity: A case study of Alzheimer's disease. *American Journal of Alzheimer's Disease and Other Dementias*, **19**: 177–85.

Sabini, J., Sietman, M., Stein, J. (2001). The really fundamental attribution error in social psychological research. *Psychological Inquiry*, **12**: 1–15.

Shweder, R. A., Sullivan, M. (1990). The semiotic subject of cultural psychology. In: *Handbook of Personality Theory and Research* (ed. L. Previn), pp. 399–416. New York: Guilford.

Snyder, L. (1999). *Speaking our Minds: Personal Reflections from Individuals with Alzheimer's Disease*. New York: W. H. Freeman.

van Langenhove, L., Harré, R. (1999). Introducing positioning theory. In: *Positioning Theory* (ed. R. Harré and L. van Langenhove), pp. 14–31. Oxford: Blackwell.

Index